Contemporary Cardiology

Series Editor

Peter P. Toth
Ciccarone Center for the Prevention of Cardiovascular Disease
Johns Hopkins University School of Medicine
Baltimore, MD
USA

For more than a decade, cardiologists have relied on the Contemporary Cardiology series to provide them with forefront medical references on all aspects of cardiology. Each title is carefully crafted by world-renown cardiologists who comprehensively cover the most important topics in this rapidly advancing field. With more than 75 titles in print covering everything from diabetes and cardiovascular disease to the management of acute coronary syndromes, the Contemporary Cardiology series has become the leading reference source for the practice of cardiac care.

More information about this series at http://www.springer.com/series/7677

Keith C. Ferdinand
Herman A. Taylor, Jr.
Carlos J. Rodriguez
Editors

Cardiovascular Disease in Racial and Ethnic Minority Populations

Second Edition

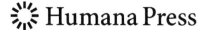 Humana Press

Editors
Keith C. Ferdinand
Tulane University School of Medicine
New Orleans, LA
USA

Herman A. Taylor, Jr.
Cardiovascular Research Institute
Morehouse School of Medicine
Atlanta, GA
USA

Carlos J. Rodriguez
School of Medicine
Albert Einstein College of Medicine
Bronx, NY
USA

ISSN 2196-8969   ISSN 2196-8977   (electronic)
Contemporary Cardiology
ISBN 978-3-030-81036-8   ISBN 978-3-030-81034-4   (eBook)
https://doi.org/10.1007/978-3-030-81034-4

This Humana imprint is published by the registered company Springer Nature Switzerland AG
The registered company address is: Gewerbestrasse 11, 6330 Cham, Switzerland

Preface

Social Justice and Health Equity: Identification and Elimination of Cardiovascular Disparities by Race/Ethnicity and Socioeconomic Status

The worst part of the storm is going back to clean up. Everything is a total loss. The furniture broke up into splinters. We have not found the chest of drawers which we used to step into the attic. What is not destroyed is so filled with stench & slime that you'll throw it away. ...We learned: that communication and cooperation are necessary factors for survival in a disaster; that water is the most destructive force in the world; that ice, electricity, and telephone are precious possessions; that people are great.

Yours, Inola

Excerpts from a letter by my late mother, Inola Copelin Ferdinand, to her sister, Narvalee, after our family's dreadful days outside on the roof, subsequent to the drowning death of my paternal grandfather and many neighbors, and the wide-spread devastation of Hurricane Betsy, Lower Ninth Ward, New Orleans, Louisiana USA, September 9, 1965.

Keith C. Ferdinand

This written note from my mother in 1965 reflects the terrible intersection of social injustice and adverse outcomes, while holding out the hopes and dreams of a better tomorrow. This personal life-changing experience of my childhood was not only reflected in the immediate aftermath of Hurricane Betsy but was unfortunately repeated by thousands in New Orleans post-Katrina and many more nationally during the COVID-19 pandemic. These were terrible storms (Hurricanes Betsy and Katrina, along with disparate minority morbidity and mortality in the COVID-19 pandemic). The United States and, indeed, the world have been deeply affected by the devastating effects of the COVID-19 pandemic. The root causes that fueled the disparate outcomes during Hurricanes Betsy and Katrina harken the need for deeper understanding and action. The social determinants of health (SDOH)—poverty, higher housing density, high-crime neighborhoods, substandard education, and poor access to healthy food—left African Americans, Hispanic/Latinx, and other disadvantaged populations ill-equipped to deal with the ravages of the pandemic [1].

Forward-thinking organizations, such as the Association of Black Cardiologists (ABC), recognize that the COVID-19 pandemic represents an opportunity to decisively address race and ethnic inequalities in cardiovascular (CV) health that fueled and compounded the effects of the coronavirus [2]. One aspect of this once-in-a-century public health crisis has been to reveal the persistent, distressing, and unacceptable disparities in health among special populations in the United States, including African Americans, Hispanics/Latinx, Native Americans, and other disadvantaged populations. Health life expectancy and care have improved dramatically for all Americans over the last 100 years; nevertheless, the distribution of these benefits has not occurred equitably. Most distressing, there has been a persistent mortality gap between Whites and Blacks since the 1960s, and African Americans have a higher risk for conditions including hypertension, type 2 diabetes, obesity (especially in Black females), stroke, chronic kidney disease, end stage renal disease, myocardial infarction, and overall CV mortality, especially premature cardiac death [3].

Life expectancy in 2017 for non-Hispanic Black males was 71.5 years and 76.1 years for non-Hispanic White males. Among females, non-Hispanic Black's life expectancy was 78.1 years and 81.0 years among non-Hispanic Whites. It is a conundrum that the US life expectancy of Hispanic males (79.1 years) and females (84.3 years) has not been shown to be shorter than that of non-Hispanic Whites. Given the high rates of diabetes and cardiometabolic conditions in Hispanics/Latinx communities, our understanding of the reasons for so-called "Hispanic paradox" remains unclear and may change with disaggregation of Hispanics, more granular data, and the aging of a growing population [4]. On the other hand, the persistent, adverse outcomes in African Americans are not only seen for various forms of cardiovascular diseases (CVD), but also many cancers [5]. Recent analysis on the Black–White differences in CVD mortality, especially in the Southern United States, suggests that socio-economic status (SES) and poor control of CVD risk factors are a substantial proportion of the mortality difference [6]. The data therefore demand implementing national policies addressing SDOH and controlling modifiable risk factors.

On the other hand, understanding the complexity of heart failure risk in African American patients demands not only addressing traditional risk factors, while recognizing the adverse environmental contributions, but also possible genetic aspects. The V122I variant, carried by approximately 3–5% of African Americans, is an increased risk for the most prevalent transthyretin cardiomyopathy (ATTR-CM) [7]. However, regardless of any postulated genetic factors or even traditional risk factors, healthcare system and policy factors predominate as causal factors for much of the death and disability among minorities, including less insurance access, CV and primary care, implicit bias, imbalance in the application of guideline-directed medical therapy, and suboptimal workforce diversity [7].

As with the imbalances in COVID-19 outcomes, CVD disparities reflect a mixture of difficulties faced by minorities such as discrimination, barriers to quality education, lower income, inferior or insecure housing, poor healthcare access, and wealth gaps. This textbook specifically details unique aspects of CVD and associated risk factors in African Americans and Hispanics/Latinx, which will inform targeted programs to address inequities including obtaining reliable information on prevention, providing the medical communities with best practices for treating underlying medical conditions, and ensuring availability and ease of access for preventive and therapeutic healthcare for all communities. Therefore, recognizing the confluence of race/ethnicity and associated SDOH in persistent imbalances in CVD risks and outcomes, this textbook focuses on two of the largest racial/ethnic groups in the United States, African Americans (14.1% of the population) and Hispanics/Latinx (18.3% of the population).

The editors are a trio of clinicians and researchers: Herman A Taylor, Jr., MD, MPH, FACC, FAHA, endowed professor and director of the Cardiovascular Research Institute at Morehouse School of Medicine, Atlanta, GA; Carlos J Rodriguez, MD, MPH, FACC, FAHA, the director of clinical cardiology and cardiovascular epidemiology at Albert Einstein College of Medicine, NY; and the lead editor Keith C. Ferdinand, MD, FACC, FAHA, FNLA, FASPC, FNLA, the Gerald S. Berenson Endowed Chair in Preventive Cardiology and professor of medicine at Tulane University, School of Medicine, New Orleans. The editors thank all the esteemed authors for their contributions addressing these inequities and the tolls they have indeed taken (and continue to take).

Dr. Taylor has recently highlighted the importance of recognizing in Blacks the wide heterogeneity in outcomes, suggesting the existence of substantial individual and collective resilience among African Americans. Perhaps, this text will also stimulate discussion and research that explores resilience in a population in which "overcoming" and "bouncing back" from adversities (ranging from minor incidents to legally ordained, chronic and horrific oppression) has been a requirement for survival. Black resilience, as detailed by Dr. Taylor and others, may yield important insights into the phenomenon of human resilience that transcends race [8]. In addition, Dr. Rodriquez has cautioned researchers and public health officials against "lumping" Hispanic/Latinx populations when defining risks and CVD outcomes. Therefore, he is pleased with the detailed efforts of several authors in this text to address the under-recognized need for disaggregation in data from Hispanic/Latinx communities [9].

Hopefully, new legislative initiatives and recent social activism will be able to successfully confront and overcome these unacceptable racial/ethnic disparities in healthcare. The COVID-19 pandemic, while a source of terrible economic and adverse health outcomes, may also be an opportunity to finally and successfully address issues of health equity for all populations regardless of race/ethnicity, sex/gender, social economic status, or geography. We live in a very special country. The United States is one of the wealthiest countries in the world and has demonstrated exceptional leadership in science, medicine, finances, and law, but we overcome these persistent inequities.

Of all the forms of inequality, injustice in health care is the most inhumane.
Martin Luther King, Jr,
Medical Committee for human rights Chicago, IL 1966

New Orleans, LA, USA   Keith C. Ferdinand
Atlanta, GA, USA   Herman A. Taylor, Jr.
Bronx, NY, USA   Carlos J. Rodriguez

References

1. Van Spall HGC, Yancy CW, Ferdinand KC. COVID-19 and Katrina: recalcitrant racial disparities [published online ahead of print, 2020 Jun 13]. Eur Heart J. 2020;ehaa488. https://doi.org/10.1093/eurheartj/ehaa488.
2. Chin-Hong P, Alexander KM, Haynes N, Albert MA; Association of Black Cardiologists. Pulling at the heart: COVID-19, race/ethnicity and ongoing disparities. Nat Rev Cardiol. 2020;17(9):533–5. https://doi.org/10.1038/s41569-020-0416-6.
3. Institute of Medicine (US) Committee on Understanding and Eliminating Racial and Ethnic Disparities in Health Care, Smedley BD, Stith AY, Nelson AR, editors. Unequal treatment: confronting racial and ethnic disparities in health care. Washington, DC: National Academies Press (US); 2003.
4. Ferdinand KC, Nasser SA. African-American COVID-19 Mortality: a sentinel event. J Am Coll Cardiol. 2020;75(21):2746–8. https://doi.org/10.1016/j.jacc.2020.04.040.
5. Sidney S, Quesenberry CP Jr, Jaffe MG, et al. Recent trends in cardiovascular mortality in the United States and Public Health Goals. JAMA Cardiol. 2016;1(5):594–9. https://doi.org/10.1001/jamacardio.2016.1326.
6. Tajeu GS, Safford MM, Howard G, et al. Black-White differences in cardiovascular disease mortality: a prospective US Study, 2003–2017. Am J Public Health. 2020;110(5):696–703. https://doi.org/10.2105/AJPH.2019.305543.
7. Nayak A, Hicks AJ, Morris AA. Understanding the complexity of heart failure risk and treatment in black patients. Circ Heart Fail. 2020;13(8):e007264. https://doi.org/10.1161/CIRCHEARTFAILURE.120.007264.
8. Taylor HA Jr, Washington-Plaskett T, Quyyumi AA. Black Resilience - Broadening the Narrative and the Science on Cardiovascular Health and Disease Disparities. Ethn Dis. 2020;30(2):365–8. Published 2020 Apr 23. https://doi.org/10.18865/ed.30.2.365.
9. Rodriguez CJ, Allison M, Daviglus ML, et al. Status of cardiovascular disease and stroke in Hispanics/Latinos in the United States: a science advisory from the American Heart Association. Circulation. 2014;130(7):593–625. https://doi.org/10.1161/CIR.0000000000000071.

Contents

Contributors

Kevin M. Alexander, MD Stanford University School of Medicine, Stanford, CA, USA

Jamy D. Ard, MD Department of Epidemiology and Prevention, Wake Forest School of Medicine, Winston-Salem, NC, USA

Ivor J. Benjamin, MD, FAHA, FACC Cardiovascular Center, Department of Physiology, Medical College of Wisconsin, Milwaukee, WI, USA
Cardiovascular Center, Division of Cardiovascular Medicine, Department of Medicine, Medical College of Wisconsin, Milwaukee, WI, USA

Vanessa Blumer, MD Division of Cardiology, Duke University Medical Center, Durham, NC, USA

Matthew Budoff, MD David Geffen School of Medicine at UCLA, Division of Cardiology, Harbor-UCLA Medical Center, Torrance, CA, USA

Adolfo Correa, MD, MPH Jackson Heart Study, Jackson, MS, USA
Department of Medicine, University of Mississippi Medical Center, Jackson, MS, USA

Leonor Corsino, MD, MHS Duke University School of Medicine, Division of Endocrinology, Metabolism, and Nutrition, Durham, NC, USA

Bradley Deere, MD Tulane University School of Medicine, New Orleans, LA, USA

Keith C. Ferdinand, MD, FACC, FAHA, FASPC, FNLA Tulane University School of Medicine, New Orleans, LA, USA

Icilma V. Fergus, MD Icahn School of Medicine at Mount Sinai, New York, NY, USA

Ervin R. Fox, MD, MPH Division of Cardiovascular Diseases, Department of Medicine, University of Mississippi Medical Center, Jackson, MS, USA

Robert Gillespie, MD, FACC Sharp Rees-Stealy Medical Group, San Diego, CA, USA

Carola Maraboto Gonzalez, MD Tulane University School of Medicine, New Orleans, LA, USA

Manuel Hache-Marliere, MD Internal Medicine, Jacobi Medical Center, New York City, NY, USA

Robert C. Hendel, MD Tulane University School of Medicine, New Orleans, LA, USA

Frances C. Henderson, EdD Jackson Heart Study, Jackson, MS, USA

César J. Herrera, MD, FACC Montefiore Center for Heart and Vascular Care, New York City, NY, USA

CEDIMAT Cardiovascular Center, Santo Domingo, Dominican Republic

Virginia J. Howard, PhD, MSPH Department of Epidemiology, School of Public Health, University of Alabama at Birmingham, Birmingham, AL, USA

Kenneth A. Jamerson, MD University of Michigan Health System, Division of Cardiovascular Medicine, Ann Arbor, MI, USA

Adedoyin Johnson, PhD Tulane University School of Medicine, New Orleans, LA, USA

Muin J. Khoury, MD, PhD Office of Genomics and Precision Public Health, Centers for Disease Control and Prevention, Atlanta, GA, USA

Latrice Landry, MS, PhD, MMSc Harvard Medical School/Harvard School of Public Health, Brigham and Women's Hospital and Dana Farber Cancer Institute, Boston, MA, USA

Matthew S. Maurer, MD Columbia University Irving Medical Center, New York Presbyterian Hospital, New York, NY, USA

George A. Mensah, MD Center for Translation Research and Implementation Science (CTRIS), National Heart, Lung, and Blood Institute, National Institutes of Health, Bethesda, MD, USA

Nia S. Mitchell, MD, MPH Division of General Internal Medicine, Department of Medicine, Duke University School of Medicine, Durham, NC, USA

Solomon K. Musani, PhD University of Mississippi Medical Center, Statistical Geneticist, Jackson Heart Study, Jackson, MS, USA

Samar A. Nasser, PhD, MPH, PA-C School of Medicine and Health Sciences, The George Washington University, Washington, DC, USA

Ronald R. Nelson Jr, BS Columbia University Medical Center-College of Physicians and Surgeons, New York City, NY, USA

Ike S. Okwuosa, MD Division of Cardiology, Department of Medicine, Northwestern University, Feinberg School of Medicine, Chicago, IL, USA

Gissette Reyes-Soffer, MD Columbia University Medical Center-College of Physicians and Surgeons, New York City, NY, USA

Carlos J. Rodriguez, MD, MPH, FACC, FAHA Montefiore Center for Heart and Vascular Care, New York City, NY, USA

Division of Cardiovascular Medicine, Albert Einstein College of Medicine, New York City, NY, USA

Fatima Rodriguez, MD, MPH Division of Cardiovascular Medicine, Stanford University, Stanford, CA, USA

Herman A. Taylor, Jr., MD, MPH Cardiovascular Research Institute, Morehouse School of Medicine, Atlanta, GA, USA

Nnamdi Uche Cardiovascular Center, Department of Physiology, Medical College of Wisconsin, Milwaukee, WI, USA

Jonathan D. Velez-Rivera, MD Duke University School of Medicine, Division of Endocrinology, Metabolism, and Nutrition, Durham, NC, USA

Karol Watson, MD, PhD David Geffen School of Medicine at UCLA, Los Angeles, CA, USA

Peter W. F. Wilson, MD Atlanta VAMC and Emory Clinical Cardiovascular Research Institute, Atlanta, GA, USA

Clyde W. Yancy, MD, MSc Division of Cardiology, Department of Medicine, Northwestern University, Feinberg School of Medicine, Chicago, IL, USA

Quentin R. Youmans, MD Division of Cardiology, Department of Medicine, Northwestern University, Feinberg School of Medicine, Chicago, IL, USA

Overview and Perspectives: Cardiovascular Disease in Racial/Ethnic Minorities in the Era of COVID-19

Adedoyin Johnson, Bradley Deere, and Keith C. Ferdinand

Introduction

This textbook is urgently needed, as demonstrated by the recent higher adverse outcomes in the COVID-19 pandemic, which can be catastrophic in racial/ethnic minorities and disadvantaged populations. The disparate mortality rate seen in African Americans, Hispanic/Latino Americans, and other racial/ethnic minorities confirms the inadequate societal efforts to eradicate imbalances in cardiovascular disease (CVD) and cardiometabolic risk. African Americans, Hispanic/Latino groups, and other minorities are not genetically predisposed to coronavirus infection but may have a higher incidence of co-morbid conditions such as CVD, HTN, diabetes, chronic kidney disease (CKD), and obesity that contribute to higher COVID-19 mortality [39]. This publication is an update to the previous textbook, *Cardiovascular Disease in Racial and Ethnic Minorities* published in 2010 [4]. The various contributors, all leaders in their respective fields, build on many of the concepts and data presented previously with updated information that includes recently developed national guidelines and relevant peer-reviewed literature. Specifically, this textbook focuses on CVD risk factors, morbidity, and mortality in non-Hispanic Black and Hispanic/Latino Americans, the two largest minority populations in the United States.

Hypertension is the most prevalent and potent risk factor for CVD, especially in African Americans. The 2017 American College of Cardiology/American Heart Association (ACC/AHA) and Multi-Society Guideline for the Prevention, Detection, Evaluation, and Management of High Blood Pressure in Adults [1] recommends antihypertensive medications for most adults with systolic blood pressure (BP) ≥130 mm Hg or diastolic blood pressure (BP) ≥80 mm Hg to help combat the associated morbidity and mortality. Similarly, the 2018 ACC/AHA Guideline on the Management of Blood Cholesterol [2] and the 2019 ACC/AHA Guideline on the Primary Prevention of Cardiovascular Disease [3] outline impactful information and provide optimal identification, prevention and management of hypercholesterolemia and associated conditions.

The goal of this collection of evidence-based chapters, including contributions by leading researchers, clinicians, and experts in various fields of study, is to find the best pathways to better understand, decrease, and potentially eliminate persistent and unacceptable disparities in CVD morbidity and mortality. The authors have all provided a comprehensive depiction of current and evolving research in their respective areas, constructing a compilation of current

A. Johnson · B. Deere · K. C. Ferdinand (✉)
Tulane University School of Medicine,
New Orleans, LA, USA
e-mail: ajohns34@tulane.edu; bdeere@tulane.edu;
kferdina@tulane.edu

© Springer Nature Switzerland AG 2021
K. C. Ferdinand et al. (eds.), *Cardiovascular Disease in Racial and Ethnic Minority Populations*,
Contemporary Cardiology, https://doi.org/10.1007/978-3-030-81034-4_1

considerations and perspectives. This state-of-the-art review of research and clinical practice will hopefully add important information to successfully address ongoing disparities.

The burden of CVD remains costly and deadly despite unprecedented advancements in the diagnosis and treatment of CVD. Despite the decline in US cardiovascular mortality over the last several decades, CVD remains the foremost cause of death. Furthermore, there has been a disturbing trend towards an actual increase in CVD mortality with persistent racial/ethnic disparities. African Americans continue to have the highest rate of stroke, heart failure (HF), coronary heart disease (CHD), T2D, HTN, and obesity (in females), compared to other groups [5, 6]. Since the 2010 edition, the several ACC/AHA and Multi-Society Guidelines remain essential to assist clinicians in determining optimal clinical care. The various authors have used these recommendations, along with best recent evidence, to make impactful commentary.

Introduction to Precision Medicine: Minority Populations and Cardiovascular Health

Latrice Landry, PhD, MS, builds on her previous work demonstrating the lack of diversity in genomic databases and how this creates a barrier for precision medicine to be translated into clinical care. Landry elucidates that biomarkers are the mainstay for translational medicine. However, non-European populations are not properly represented. Reviewing the National Institutes of Health (NIH) genome-wide association study catalog, of the 52 hematologic/lymphatic cancer studies and 47 digestive tract cancer studies, none of the studies focused on underrepresented minorities [16]. Since 2015 and beyond, federal efforts have included the precision medicine initiative, with a goal to personalize approaches to health and treating disease. Subsequent programs to maintain and further develop data, such as the All of Us Research Program, seek to carry out this vision. This novel prospective cohort initiative takes into consideration population biases that exist in prior research and leverages the diversity of the United States to account for individual variation [31]. The foundation of the All of Us Research Program takes into consideration structural issues that affect biomedical research and can account for factors related to health disparities. This data repository has promise to usher in personalized and precision medicine. By accounting for individual variation, there is hope for reducing the disparities that exist in CVD prevention, diagnosis, and management.

Lipoprotein(a): A Cardiovascular Risk Factor Affecting Ethnic Minorities

Low-density lipoprotein cholesterol (LDL-C) is an established major risk factor for atherosclerotic development, progression, and increased atherosclerotic cardiovascular disease (ASCVD) [21]. In this chapter, Gissette Reyes-Soffer, MD, Ronald R. Nelson Jr., MD, and Karol Watson MD, PhD, build on their previous work on dyslipidemia and CVD. A prior study demonstrates racial/ethnic disparities in patients with familial hypercholesterolemia, an underdiagnosed, but high-risk group for ASCVD. African Americans were diagnosed at older ages and were 50% less likely to achieve LDL-C <100 mg/dl, which shows significant under-treatment [22]. Research in the future should better elucidate how emerging and known risk factors for CVD affect minority populations. Studies utilizing Mendelian randomization may prove to be a powerful tool to determine mechanisms and potential effects of modifiable exposures and health outcomes. A recent analysis involving 438,952 participants of European ancestry demonstrated that life-long genetic exposure to lower levels of LDL and lower SBP was associated with a significantly lower cardiovascular risk [23]. While Mendelian randomization studies have been successful within CVD research (i.e., providing evidence for causality for biomarkers and drug targets such as Lp(a) and PCSK9, respectively), more work is needed to determine the benefit of this tool for among racial/ethnic minority populations.

Emerging Precision Medicine Concepts and Cardiovascular Health in African Americans and Hispanics

This chapter by George A. Mensah, MD, delves into the current concepts and approaches to tackling medical issues related to precision medicine. Mensah details the importance of rapidly evolving advances within precision medicine and its contributions to CVD. Differences in minority representation in genomic research are noted and the future implications are discussed [17]. Improvements are currently being sought in the African American community to bridge the gap in the delivery of personalized medicine, such as the African American Cardiovascular Pharmacogenetic Consortium (ACCOuNT) group. Their goal is to discover new genetic variants in African Americans associated with cardiovascular phenotypes and to integrate African American-specific sequence variations into clinical guidelines [18]. As a leader in public health, Mensah's work has helped determine best pathways forward to reveal and eliminate disparities in the United States.

The Implementation Frontier: Impact on Cardiovascular Health in Racial and Ethnic Minority Populations

In addition to his work in the emerging field of precision medicine, Mensah introduces the importance of implementation science and its unique potential within the realm of CVD and minority populations. He expertly demonstrates how minority populations are at greatest risk to suffer from the underuse of high-value interventions and overuse of ineffective or low-value interventions. Implementation science is poised to address these disparities and improve the delivery of health care to all racial/ethnic and socioeconomic groups. Using HTN as an example, Black individuals are less likely than White individuals to achieve blood pressure control despite receiving drug treatment. Even when pro-

viding equal access to antihypertensive regimens (i.e., in clinical trials), an individual's socioeconomic context is independently associated with worse cardiovascular outcomes and blood pressure control. For instance, participants in the ALLHAT study (Antihypertensive and Lipid-Lowering Treatment to Prevent Heart Attack Trial) with lower household income had poorer blood pressure control and worse CVD outcomes such as all-cause mortality, heart failure hospitalizations, and end-stage renal disease [32].

A comprehensive, evidence-based approach to implementing interventions is needed to reduce the burden of CVD risk factors and disparities in a cost-effective manner. For instance, the Heart Outcomes Prevention and Evaluation 4 (HOPE 4) program, a cluster-randomized controlled trial, implemented community-based interventions that addressed barriers to effective disease management. The intervention group had a significant reduction in the Framingham Risk Score for 10-year risk (−11.2%) in addition to greater absolute reduction in systolic blood pressure, total cholesterol, and LDL-cholesterol levels when compared to standard-care group [33]. It will be critical for future implementation research to consider barriers to care and account for potential harms or lack of benefit of interventions to improve CVD disparities in high-burden populations.

Genomic Approaches to Hypertension

Genetic variants associated with susceptibility for various CVD conditions are delineated by Ivor J. Benjamin, MD, FAHA FACC, and other authors. Benjamin initiates a detailed understanding of genetics, genomics, and human disease. Recent data have shown that African Americans and Hispanic/Latino Americans represented 14% and 3%, respectively, of NIH-funded genome-wide association studies (GWAS) using the Research Portfolio Online Reporting Tools (RePORT) [15]. One of the key themes underlying the work of Benjamin and others is the need for diversity in large-scale genome-wide association studies (GWAS). There is a large over-representation of participants of European ancestry in genetic research. As of 2019, only 3.8% of polygenic studies involved African, Hispanic/Latino, or Indigenous peoples [29]. When analyzing datasets over decades, most studies included exclusively European ancestry participants 67% and another 19% included only East Asian ancestry participants [30]. Additionally, research has found that the predictive performance of European ancestry-derived PRS was lower among those in non-European ancestry samples [29]. Given the over-representation of participants of European ancestry in genetic datasets, more studies will be needed before genetic research can be translated into clinical practice. Elucidating the causes of differences in genetic risk score distributions across populations and risk score relationships to phenotypes may help address current gaps. Until well-powered GWAS in diverse populations are available, the benefit of PRS as a precision medicine tool remains unclear.

Heart Failure in African Americans and Hispanic Americans: A Persistent and Disproportionate Burden in Underrepresented Minorities

The care available for HF patients is influenced by different variables, such as access to ambulatory care, presence of comorbid conditions, and racial/ethnic disparities. Clyde W. Yancy, MD, MSc, MACC, FAHA, MACP, Quentin R. Youmans, MD, and Ike S. Okwuosa, MD, discuss the various factors in this chapter. A study documented differences in readmission rates of racial/ethnic groups after HF hospitalization in a large hospital system in New York City. Readmission was substantially higher among Hispanic/Latino patients at 30 and 90 days and 90 days for Black patients when compared to White patients [13]. A key priority moving forward will include strategies that improve tools and concepts within the realm of risk prediction. A better understanding of the unique aspects of

HF risk factors among racial/ethnic minorities may offer opportunities for implementing primordial or primary prevention. Cumulative exposure to modifiable risk factors is largely responsible for HF. Data continue to indicate that racial/ethnic minorities, particularly young and middle-aged African Americans, experience a higher burden of HF-related CVD mortality. When compared to White men and women, the age-adjusted HF-related CVD death rates were 2.6- and 2.97-fold higher for young Black men and women, respectively [34]. Age-adjusted rates for heart failure-related CVD death are increasing. Given that the HF rates in African Americans are more pronounced among younger adults and significant disparities exist, identifying those at higher risk and preventing heart failure development is paramount.

Heterogeneity, Nativity, and Disaggregation of Cardiovascular Risk and Outcomes in Hispanic Americans

As previously documented from the Hispanic Community Health Study/Study of Latinos (HCHS/SOL) [8], Fatima Rodriguez, MD, MPH, FACC, and Vanessa Blumer, MD, add to our understanding of the importance of nativity and disaggregation in the disease burden of a heterogeneous Hispanic/Latino population. Disaggregation of Hispanic/Latino subgroups has revealed marked heterogeneity in CVD mortality. Data show significant differences in premature CVD mortality among Hispanic/Latino subgroups with years of potential life loss that persists over a decade [11]. These findings emphasize the importance of a comprehensive evaluation of demographics and ancestry when implementing measures to improve cardiovascular health of diverse, minority populations. Additionally, NIH funding for clinical research involving racial and ethnic minorities will need to match the proportion and significance of disease burden [31]. Appropriate funding that addresses health disparities is critical for future research funding and prioritization.

Cardiovascular Epidemiology in Hispanics/Latinos: Lessons Learned from HCHS/SOL

In this chapter, Cesar J Herrera, MD, Manuel Haché, MD, and Carlos J. Rodriguez, MD, MPH, continue to build on previous studies, especially newer data from Prevalence of Hypertension, Awareness, Treatment, and Control in the HCHS/SOL [8]. Hispanic/Latino Americans are heterogeneous and there is difficulty making accurate statements regarding CVD risk and disease across such diverse and large subpopulations. Nevertheless, understanding the epidemiology of CVD burden in Hispanic/Latino Americans is paramount. As highlighted in this chapter, health risks differ greatly among Hispanic/Latino individuals, who may be of any self-identified race or admixture based on the presence of DNA. This complexity of genetic origin makes general comments regarding CVD burden in Hispanic/Latino populations difficult and at times inexact when compared to non-Hispanic/White populations. There is a differential burden of CVD risk including T2D and HTN among Hispanic/Latino groups. Hispanic/Latino individuals have been noted to have increased triglycerides levels which appears to be inversely associated with data seen among various nationals within the subpopulations studied [9]. Furthermore, Central Americans were shown to have higher prevalence of valvular heart disease [10]. Finally, given that Hispanic/Latino Americans are the largest racial/ethnic minority population in the United States and are on average 15 years younger than White Americans, preventive efforts to reduce CVD risk factors such as T2D and obesity must be ongoing research priority [11].

Lessons Learned from the Jackson Heart Study (JHS)

As highlighted in this chapter by Ervin R. Fox, MD, MPH, Solomon K. Musani, PhD, Frances C. Henderson, EdD, Adolfo Correa, MD, MPH, and Herman A. Taylor, MD, MPH, the Jackson Heart Study continues to make important contri-butions to the field of CVD epidemiology in African Americans. The longitudinal investigation of genetic and environmental risk factors associated with CVD has paved the way for effective interventions to reduce risk burden. Yet, the epidemiology of CVD is shifting with the ongoing obesity and diabetes epidemic and understanding risk factor trends is an active research priority, particularly among young adults. Prospective cohort studies such as the Jackson Heart Study (JHS) will continue to enrich our understanding of CVD epidemiology and play a critical role in the advancement of cardiovascular health disparities research [36, 37]. Racial/ethnic disparities in HF incidence and outcomes are markedly prevalent and identifying vulnerable individuals with pre-clinical HF phenotypes may offer opportunities for prevention. In turn, a recent JHS study identified a malignant preclinical, high-risk phenotype that was independently predictive of incident HF in this African American population [38]. Another study including JHS participants found that the population-attributable risk of CVD associated with HTN was 32.5% [26]. These data highlight the importance of the JHS contribution to our understanding of CVD in vulnerable populations and pave the way for those who may benefit from targeted preventive efforts.

Cardiovascular Disease Risk Factors in the Hispanic/Latino Population

Overall diabetes prevalence is increased among racial/ethnic groups. Obesity and metabolic syndrome and diabetes in African and Hispanic/Latino Americans are discussed by Jonathan Velez-Rivera, MD, and Leonor Corsino, MD, MHS, FACE. Some of the topics explored include bariatric surgery of which racial disparities in long- and short-term weight loss outcomes are being documented [24, 25]. Recent data have shown that African Americans have higher risks for postoperative complications, readmission, and re-intervention within 30-days post-operation for Roux-en-Y gastric bypass (LRYGB) or laparoscopic sleeve gastrectomy (LSG) bariatric surgery [25]. Metabolic issues vary by race/ethnicity. Our understanding is informed by a growing body of research that demonstrates the impact of metabolic syndrome on racial/ethnic populations. For instance, T2D is disproportionately prevalent among Hispanic/Latino Americans when compared to White or Black Americans. Within this subgroup, the burden of metabolic syndrome and diabetes is greater in Mexican Americans compared to White individuals or Puerto Rican individuals, whereas African Americans have increased diabetes and HTN. Finally, features of metabolic syndrome vary by group and within groups and abdominal adiposity is a factor that may portend an increased risk [2].

Progress in ASCVD Risk Assessment in African American and Hispanics

Peter W F Wilson, MD, expands on identifying the risk of ASCVD and its profound implications on the natural history of CVD. ASCVD risk assessment continues to evolve. There is marked heterogeneity across sex, race/ethnicity, family history, and socioeconomic status which may result in under- or overtreatment of individuals. To estimate an individual's 10-year risk for hard CVD events, the 2018 Multi-Society Guideline on the Management of Blood Cholesterol and 2017 Multi-Society Guideline for High Blood Pressure in Adults [1, 2] recommend the use of the US-derived pooled cohort equations (PCE). However, factors such as socioeconomic status, acculturation level, and ancestry or country of origin (i.e., Mexican vs Puerto Rican) pattern risk burden in Hispanic/Latino Americans. Black women consistently demonstrate greater ASCVD risk when compared to White women. And while the PCE appears to be accurate in Black subjects, there is no separate PCE available for Hispanic/Latino subjects [2]. Inclusion of ancestry or country-specific race/ethnicity along with consideration of socioeconomic status may improve risk estimation in racial/ethnic minority populations. Given the recent increase in CVD mortality rates in certain groups, particularly among young adults and racial/ethnic minorities [13], progress is needed to better identify those at increased risk of ASCVD in order to guide prevention efforts. Technological advances such as artificial intelligence may improve CVD risk prediction. For instance, a Machine Learning-based risk calculator outperformed the ACC/AHA Risk Calculator by recommending less drug therapy while missing fewer cardiovascular disease CVD events [14]. However, the potential for these tools to improve risk prediction and assist with clinical decision-making among racial/ethnic minority groups is yet to be determined.

Cardiovascular Disease in Minorities: Unique Considerations Hypertension in African and Hispanic Americans

Kenneth A. Jamerson, MD, and Samar Nassar, PhD, MPH, offer a comprehensive and relevant review of this important topic and provide additional insight regarding the impact of the leading risk factor for mortality and disability in the United States [21]. The impact of HTN among African Americans is especially profound with an estimated CVD population-attributable risk of 33%; meaning that up to 1 in 3 cases of CVD in Black adults is attributed to HTN [26]. While there is promise for effective novel HTN pharmacologic therapies such as SGLT2 inhibitors, brain aminopeptidase A inhibitors, and neprilysin inhibitors, primordial prevention may offer the greatest impact to reduce the burden of HTN-related CVD. Preventing CVD risk factors and maintaining ideal cardiovascular health over the life course will likely prove to be the most impactful intervention to reduce the burden of metabolic disorders among African and Hispanic/Latino Americans. By harnessing the ability of machine learning to analyze and integrate vast amounts of data from multiple sources ("-omics" data, health records, imaging, environmental and lifestyle data such as heart rate, blood pressure, physical activity, dietary habits, and sleep quality), there is the possibility to glean valuable insights into the epidemiology of HTN and CVD risk.

Weight Loss, Lifestyle, and Dietary Factors in CVD in African Americans and Hispanics

In this chapter, the relationship between weight loss, diet, and CVD is explored by Jamy Ard, MD, Nia Schwann Mitchell, MD, Tiffany Carson, Stephanie L. Fitzpatrick, and Chiadi Ndumele, MD, PhD, FAHA. Current evidence shows that African and Hispanic/Latino American women are inclined to lose less weight than other racial/ethnic groups due to numerous factors [19]. Among overweight patients with increased ASCVD, African and Hispanic/Latino American women were less likely to report a healthy diet and physical activity when compared to White Americans [20]. Additional consideration should be given to how weight loss is tracked (i.e., body mass index (BMI), weight, visceral adiposity) and the social environment contribution to cardiometabolic health. CVD mortality rates have plateaued and are likely increasing largely due to the obesity and diabetes epidemic. Thus, understanding the primary drivers of these epidemics will be critical to optimize early preventive care strategies. Dr. Ard and co-authors expertly navigate the nuances of this broad, important topic and relevant research.

Coronary Calcium Scoring in African American and Hispanic Patients

Robert Gillespie, MD, and Matthew Budoff, MD, offer an invaluable perspective on coronary artery calcification (CAC) and ASCVD in racial/ethnic minorities. Providing an excellent historical perspective and highlighting future directions, the authors establish the powerful predictive value of CAC in asymptomatic patients. The use of CAC scan scoring via computed tomography (CT) is increasingly recognized as a valuable tool to further risk estimation either upward or downward among patients at intermediate risk of ASCVD [3]. Given a large proportion of patients who fall at intermediate risk based on pooled cohort equations, measuring CAC has definite value. Importantly, this tool refines risk and may offer potential life-saving therapies or avoid unnecessary therapeutic interventions. The potential utility of this approach for improving CVD risk assessment is evident and will continue to be important in the era of personalized and precision cardiovascular health. The possibility of integrating patient data with artificial intelligence technology such as machine learning may improve CV imaging diagnostic efficacy ushering in a new era of CVD diagnosis and management.

Epidemiology CVD in African Americans

To address disparate CVD morbidity and mortality, it is important to document the extent of various conditions with specific data related to health disparities. Virginia J Howard, PhD, FAHA, FSCT, sets the table for understanding the unique aspects of CVD epidemiology in African American populations. By 2030, CVD prevalence in the United States is projected to be 40.5% and CVD total direct medical costs are projected to triple [12]. Progress in CVD epidemiology is critical to assess disease burden and risk factors for health in African American populations. The burden of CVD continues to shift and evolve while health disparities persist. Howard has detailed our best understanding of the extent and nature of CVD morbidity/mortality and provides a road map by which clinical research and interventions can better address areas of concern. In addition to her landmark REGARDS study (Reasons for Geographic and Racial Differences in Stroke) [7], Howard's writing provokes needed insights. Dr. Howard and colleagues explore basic epidemiology of prevalence, incidence, and mortality and set the stage for others to further detail unique aspects of risk factors, specifically as related to non-Hispanic Black or African Americans in comparison to other race/ethnic groups.

Cardiac Amyloid Heart Disease in Racial/Ethnic Minorities: Focus on Transthyretin Amyloid Cardiomyopathy

In this chapter, amyloid cardiomyopathy, Icilma V. Fergus, MD, FACC, Matthew Maurer, MD, and Kevin Alexander, MD, FACC, build on previous work regarding transthyretin cardiac amyloidosis (TTR CA) in US Black individuals. The authors noted that the valine-to-isoleucine substitution at codon 122 on the transthyretin (TTR) gene was more common in Black subjects compared to the wild type mutation that was predominantly White subjects. US Black individuals with the Val122Ile mutation were misdiagnosed and underdiagnosed because it mimics hypertrophic hypertensive heart disease and other common pathologies such as diabetes, obesity, and HTN are considered as the main reasons without adequately considering all options. Hence compared to White Americans, Black Americans presented with more advanced disease despite genetic testing and non-invasive methods such as nuclear imaging that can aid diagnosis [27]. Additional evidence of cardiac amyloid (CA) underdiagnoses in African Americans is suggested by geographic disparities which found that temporal and regional trends in age-adjusted mortality rates of CA were greater by proximity to amyloidosis centers rather than regions with greater proportion of Black residents in the United States [35]. This regional variability suggests an underdiagnoses of CA among African Americans and highlights the prevalent racial disparities in diagnosing and reporting amyloid mortality. With non-invasive nuclear medicine techniques for identifying TTR CA and the advent of disease modifying therapies (TTR stabilizers and TTR silencers) [28], there is an opportunity to improve early diagnosis and

change the natural history of this relentless form of HF.

Imaging for the Assessment and Management of Cardiovascular Disease in Women and Minority Populations

Carola Maraboto Gonzalez, MD, Vanessa Blumer, MD, and Robert C. Hendel, MD, summarize the expansive and evolving field of CV imaging. They highlight the value of CV imaging with CVD risk assessment while optimizing diagnoses and management. From facilitating catheter-based treatment of atrial fibrillation or improving identification of individuals with ATTR cardiomyopathy, imaging continues to drastically improve the diagnosis and management of CVD. In this multimodality imaging era, the appropriate use of emerging and novel technology is critical for improving outcomes in diverse populations. Citing work from population-based studies, they report key racial/ethnic differences across multiple imaging modalities and CVD and emphasize the importance of diagnostic accuracy and reference values by race and gender. The authors insightfully address current multimodality imaging techniques and clinical implications for racial/ethnic minorities while developing a strong case for their application in CV risk assessment in underrepresented, underserved populations. The early diagnosis of CVD is necessary to appropriately address specific interventions that are needed to decrease morbidity and mortality. While advanced imaging is often less utilized in racial/ethnic minorities, barriers based on insurance status or access must be overcome so unique findings can be revealed that may better help target appropriate interventions.

In the final analysis, unique aspects of cardiovascular disease and associated risks remain complex and at times difficult to fully understand, nevertheless as identified by the unacceptable disparities in COVID-19 hospitalizations and death, adverse outcomes in African Americans and Hispanic/Latino Americans must be identified, addressed, and eventually eliminated. It is therefore important to continue to accumulate data and develop concepts that lead to not only better understanding of unique aspects of CVD and cardiometabolic risks in minorities but most importantly appropriate intervention.

References

1. Whelton PK, Carey RM, Aronow WS, Casey DE Jr, Collins KJ, Dennison Himmelfarb C, DePalma SM, Gidding S, Jamerson KA, Jones DW, MacLaughlin EJ, Muntner P, Ovbiagele B, Smith SC Jr, Spencer CC, Stafford RS, Taler SJ, Thomas RJ, Williams KA Sr, Williamson JD, Wright JT Jr. 2017 ACC/AHA/AAPA/ABC/ACPM/AGS/APhA/ASH/ASPC/NMA/PCNA guideline for the prevention, detection, evaluation, and management of high blood pressure in adults: a report of the American College of Cardiology/American Heart Association Task Force on Clinical Practice Guidelines. Hypertension. 2018;71:e13–e115.
2. Grundy SM, Stone NJ, Bailey AL, Beam C, Birtcher KK, Blumenthal RS, Braun LT, de Ferranti S, Faiella-Tommasino J, Forman DE, Goldberg R, Heidenreich PA, Hlatky MA, Jones DW, Lloyd-Jones D, Lopez-Pajares N, Ndumele CE, Orringer CE, Peralta CA, Saseen JJ, Smith SC Jr, Sperling L, Virani SS, Yeboah J. 2018 AHA/ACC/AACVPR/AAPA/ABC/ACPM/ADA/AGS/APhA/ASPC/NLA/PCNA guideline on the management of blood cholesterol: a report of the American College of Cardiology/American Heart Association Task Force on Clinical Practice Guidelines. Circulation. 2019;139:e1082–143.
3. Arnett DK, Blumenthal RS, Albert MA, Buroker AB, Goldberger ZD, Hahn EJ, Himmelfarb CD, Khera A, Lloyd-Jones D, McEvoy JW, Michos ED, Miedema MD, Muñoz D, Smith SC Jr, Virani SS, Williams KA Sr, Yeboah J, Ziaeian B. 2019 ACC/AHA guideline on the primary prevention of cardiovascular disease: a report of the American College of Cardiology/American Heart Association Task Force on Clinical Practice Guidelines. Circulation. 2019 Sep 10;140(11):e596–646.
4. Keith F, Annemarie A. Cardiovascular disease in racial and ethnic minorities. Dordrecht: Humana Press; 2010.
5. Divens LL, Chatmon BN. Cardiovascular disease management in minority women: special considerations. Crit Care Nurs Clin North Am. 2019 Mar;31(1):39–47.
6. Pool LR, Ning H, Lloyd-Jones DM, Allen NB. Trends in racial/ethnic disparities in cardiovascular health among US adults from 1999–2012. J Am Heart Assoc. 2017 Sep 22;6(9):e006027.
7. Glasser SP, Judd S, Basile J, Lackland D, Halanych J, Cushman M, Prineas R, Howard V, Howard G. Prehypertension, racial prevalence and its association with risk factors: analysis of the REasons for Geographic And Racial Differences in Stroke (REGARDS) Study. Am J Hypertens. 2011 Feb;24(2):194–9.
8. Sorlie PD, Allison MA, Avilés-Santa ML, Cai J, Daviglus ML, Howard AG, Kaplan R, LaVange LM, Raij L, Schneiderman N, Wassertheil-Smoller S, Talavera GA. Prevalence of hypertension, awareness, treatment, and control in the Hispanic Community Health Study/Study of Latinos. Am J Hypertens. June 2014;27(6):793–800.
9. Lamar M, Durazo-Arvizu R, Rodriguez C, Kaplan R, Perera M, Cai J, et al. Associations of lipid levels and cognition: findings from the Hispanic Community Health Study/Study of Latinos. J Int Neuropsychol Soc. n.d.:1–12.
10. Rubin J, Aggarwal SR, Swett KR, Kirtane AJ, Kodali SK, Nazif TM, Pu M, Dadhania R, Kaplan RC, Rodriguez CJ. Burden of valvular heart diseases in Hispanic/Latino Individuals in the United States: the Echocardiographic Study of Latinos. Mayo Clin Proc. 2019 Aug;94(8):1488–98.
11. Dominguez K, Penman-Aguilar A, Chang MH, Moonesinghe R, Castellanos T, Rodriguez-Lainz A, Schieber R. Vital signs: leading causes of death, prevalence of diseases and risk factors, and use of health services among Hispanics in the United States – 2009-2013. MMWR Morb Mortal Wkly Rep. 2015 May 8;64(17):469–78.
12. Heidenreich PA, Trogdon JG, Khavjou OA, Butler J, Dracup K, Ezekowitz MD, Finkelstein EA, Hong Y, Johnston SC, Khera A, Lloyd-Jones DM, Nelson SA, Nichol G, Orenstein D, Wilson PW, Woo YJ. Forecasting the future of cardiovascular disease in the United States: a policy statement from the American Heart Association. Circulation. 2011 Mar 1;123(8):933–44.
13. Durstenfeld MS, Ogedegbe O, Katz SD, Park H, Blecker S. Racial and ethnic differences in heart failure readmissions and mortality in a large municipal healthcare system. JACC Heart Fail. 2016 Nov;4(11):885–93. https://doi.org/10.1016/j.jchf.2016.05.008. Epub 2016 Jul 6.
14. Raghavan S, Ho Y-L, Kini V, Rhee MK, Vassy JL, Gagnon DR, Cho K, Wilson PWF, Phillips LS. Association between early hypertension control and cardiovascular disease incidence in veterans with diabetes. Diabetes Care. 2019 Oct;42(10):1995–2003.
15. Peprah E, Xu H, Tekola-Ayele F, Royal CD. Genome-wide association studies in Africans and African Americans: expanding the framework of the genomics of human traits and disease. Public Health Genomics. 2015;18:40–51.
16. Landry LG, Ali N, Williams DR, Rehm HL, Bonham VL. Lack of diversity in genomic databases is a barrier to translating precision medicine research into practice. Health Aff (Millwood). 2018 May;37(5):780–5.
17. Mensah GA, Jaquish C, Srinivas P, Papanicolaou GJ, Wei GS, Redmond N, Roberts MC, Nelson C,

Aviles-Santa L, Puggal M, Green Parker MC, Minear MA, Barfield W, Fenton KN, Boyce CA, Engelgau MM, Khoury MJ. Emerging concepts in precision medicine and cardiovascular diseases in racial and ethnic minority populations. Circ Res. 2019 June 21;125(1):7–13.

18. Friedman PN, Shaazuddin M, Gong L, Grossman RL, Harralson AF, Klein TE, Lee NH, Miller DC, Nutescu EA, O'Brien TJ, O'Donnell PH, O'Leary KJ, Tuck M, Meltzer DO, Perera MA. The ACCOuNT consortium: a model for the discovery, translation, and implementation of precision medicine in African Americans. Clin Transl Sci. 2019 May;12(3):209–17.

19. Kumanyika S. Obesity treatment in minorities. In: Wadden TA, Stunkard AJ, editors. Handbook of obesity treatment. New York: The Guilford Press; 2002. p. 416–46.

20. Morris AA, Ko YA, Hutcheson SH, Quyyumi A. Race/ethnic and sex differences in the association of atherosclerotic cardiovascular disease risk and healthy lifestyle behaviors. J Am Heart Assoc. 2018;7(10):e008250.

21. Virani SS, Alonso A, Benjamin EJ, Bittencourt MS, Callaway CW, Carson AP, Chamberlain AM, Chang AR, Cheng S, Delling FN, Djousse L, Elkind MSV, Ferguson JF, Fornage M, Khan SS, Kissela BM, Knutson KL, Kwan TW, Lackland DT, Lewis TT, Lichtman JH, Longenecker CT, Loop MS, Lutsey PL, Martin SS, Matsushita K, Moran AE, Mussolino ME, Perak AM, Rosamond WD, Roth GA, Sampson UKA, Satou GM, Schroeder EB, Shah SH, Shay CM, Spartano NL, Stokes A, Tirschwell DL, VanWagner LB, Tsao CW. Heart disease and stroke statistics-2020 update: a report from the American Heart Association. Circulation. 2020 Jan 29;141:CIR0000000000000757.

22. Amrock SM, Duell PB, Knickelbine T, Martin SS, O'Brien EC, Watson KE, Mitri J, Kindt I, Shrader P, Baum SJ, Hemphill LC, Ahmed CD, Andersen RL, Kullo IJ, McCann D, Larry JA, Murray MF, Fishberg R, Guyton JR, Wilemon K, Roe MT, Rader DJ, Ballantyne CM, Underberg JA, Thompson P, Duffy D, Linton MF, Shapiro MD, Moriarty PM, Knowles JW, Ahmad ZS. Health disparities among adult patients with a phenotypic diagnosis of familial hypercholesterolemia in the CASCADE-FH™ patient registry. Atherosclerosis. 2017 Dec;267:19–26.

23. Ference BA, Bhatt DL, Catapano AL, Packard CJ, Graham I, Kaptoge S, Ference TB, Guo Q, Laufs U, Ruff CT, Cupido A, Hovingh GK, Danesh J, Holmes MV, Smith GD, Ray KK, Nicholls SJ, Sabatine MS. Association of genetic variants related to combined exposure to lower low-density lipoproteins and lower systolic blood pressure with lifetime risk of cardiovascular disease. JAMA. 2019 Sep 2;322:1381–91.

24. Anderson WA, Greene GW, Forse RA, Apovian CM, Istfan NW. Weight loss and health outcomes in African Americans and Whites after gastric bypass surgery. Obesity (Silver Spring). 2007 June;15(6):1455–63.

25. Amirian H, Torquati A, Omotosho P. Racial disparity in 30-day outcomes of metabolic and bariatric surgery. Obes Surg. 2019 Nov 19;30(3):1011–20.

26. Clark D 3rd, Colantonio LD, Min YI, Hall ME, Zhao H, Mentz RJ, Shimbo D, Ogedegbe G, Howard G, Levitan EB, Jones DW, Correa A, Muntner P. Population-attributable risk for cardiovascular disease associated with hypertension in black adults. JAMA Cardiol. 2019 Oct 23;4:1–9.

27. Shah KB, Mankad AK, Castano A, Akinboboye OO, Duncan PB, Fergus IV, Maurer MS. Transthyretin cardiac amyloidosis in black Americans. Circ Heart Fail. 2016;9(6):e002558.

28. Maurer MS, Schwartz JH, Gundapaneni B, Elliott PM, Merlini G, Waddington-Cruz M, Kristen AV, Grogan M, Witteles R, Damy T, Drachman BM, Shah SJ, Hanna M, Judge DP, Barsdorf AI, Huber P, Patterson TA, Riley S, Schumacher J, Stewart M, Sultan MB, Rapezzi C. Tafamidis treatment for patients with transthyretin amyloid cardiomyopathy. N Engl J Med. 2018 Sep 13;379(11):1007–16.

29. Duncan L, Shen H, Gelaye B, Meijsen J, Ressler K, Feldman M, Peterson R, Domingue B. Analysis of polygenic risk score usage and performance in diverse human populations. Nat Commun. 2019 July 25;10(1):3328.

30. Martin AR, Kanai M, Kamatani Y, Okada Y, Neale BM, Daly MJ. Clinical use of current polygenic risk scores may exacerbate health disparities. Nat Genet. 2019 Apr;51(4):584–91.

31. Investigators TA of URP. The "all of us" research program. N Engl J Med [Internet]. 2019 Aug 15;381(7):668–76. Available from: https://www.nejm.org/doi/full/10.1056/NEJMsr1809937.

32. Shahu A, Herrin J, Dhruva SS, Desai NR, Davis BR, Krumholz HM, Spatz ES. Disparities in socioeconomic context and association with blood pressure control and cardiovascular outcomes in ALLHAT. J Am Heart Assoc. 2019 Aug 6;8(15):e012277.

33. Schwalm JD, McCready T, Lopez-Jaramillo P, Yusoff K, Attaran A, Lamelas P, Camacho PA, Majid F, Bangdiwala SI, Thabane L, Islam S, McKee M, Yusuf S. A community-based comprehensive intervention to reduce cardiovascular risk in hypertension (HOPE 4): a cluster-randomised controlled trial. Lancet. 2019 Oct 5;394(10205):1231–42.

34. Glynn P, Lloyd-Jones DM, Feinstein MJ, Carnethon M, Khan SS. Disparities in cardiovascular mortality related to heart failure in the United States. J Am Coll Cardiol. 2019 May 14;73(18):2354–5.

35. Alexander KM, Orav J, Singh A, Jacob SA, Menon A, Padera RF, Kijewski MF, Liao R, Di Carli MF, Laubach JP, Falk RH, Dorbala S. Geographic disparities in reported US amyloidosis mortality from 1979 to 2015: potential underdetection of cardiac amyloidosis. JAMA Cardiol. 2018 Sep 1;3(9):865–70.

36. Andersson C, Vasan RS. Epidemiology of cardiovascular disease in young individuals. Nat Rev Cardiol. 2018 Apr;15(4):230–40.

37. Mensah GA, Cooper RS, Siega-Riz AM, Cooper LA, Smith JD, Brown CH, Westfall JM, Ofili EO, Price LN, Arteaga S, Green Parker MC, Nelson CR, Newsome BJ, Redmond N, Roper RA, Beech BM, Brooks JL, Furr-Holden D, Gebreab SY, Giles WH, James RS, Lewis TT, Mokdad AH, Moore KD, Ravenell JE, Richmond A, Schoenberg NE, Sims M, Singh GK, Sumner AE, Treviño RP, Watson KS, Avilés-Santa ML, Reis JP, Pratt CA, Engelgau MM, Goff DC Jr, Pérez-Stable EJ. Reducing cardiovascular disparities through community-engaged implementation research: a National Heart, Lung, and Blood Institute workshop report. Circ Res. 2018 Jan 19;122(2):213–30.

38. Pandey A, Keshvani N, Ayers C, Correa A, Drazner MH, Lewis A, Rodriguez CJ, Hall ME, Fox ER, Mentz RJ, de Filippi C, Seliger SL, Ballantyne CM, Neeland IJ, de Lemos JA, Berry JD. Association of cardiac injury and malignant left ventricular hypertrophy with risk of heart failure in African Americans: the Jackson Heart Study. JAMA Cardiol. 2019 Jan 1;4(1):51–8.

39. Ferdinand KC, Nasser SA. African-American COVID-19 mortality: a sentinel event. J Am Coll Cardiol. 2020;75(21):2746–8.

Introduction to Precision Medicine: Minority Populations and Cardiovascular Health

2

Latrice Landry

The Perils of Underrepresentation—Contemplating the Impact of Lack of Representation in Research in Precision Care for Minority Patients (a Narrative Case)

"It was a celebration of community engagement for a study of African American Health. After the presentations, she [an audience member] stood up from the back of the audience--- her voice quivered. She shared that she was a young [Black] woman who had recently been diagnosed with a hereditary form of heart disease. As I heard her story, I wondered if she had received genetic testing to identify the cause of her hereditary heart condition or if she had received genetic counseling. Although any diagnosis can be difficult, hereditary diseases have special considerations and should include genetic services. However, research shows minorities are less likely to receive genetic services [3, 32] and less likely to be included in genetic research including clinical trials [16, 28]. As medicine moves towards precision many are concerned that precision medicine will only exacerbate existing disparities [18, 29]. A pretty dire concern if you consider the current state of disparities in the U.S. [25]."

An Introduction to Genomic Testing

Molecular diagnostic genetic testing is a hallmark of genomic medicine. Advances in technology have revolutionized molecular diagnostics.

L. Landry (✉)
Harvard Medical School/Harvard School of Public Health, Brigham and Women's Hospital and Dana Farber Cancer Institute, Boston, MA, USA
e-mail: Latrice_Landry@hms.harvard.edu

These technologies include whole exome sequencing, whole genome sequencing, and complex computational systems that process, filter, and annotate molecular data. Additionally, growth in data storage capacity, as well as information systems which synthesize new knowledge from molecular and clinical data, has further enhanced the field. Fueling this revolution is the development of therapy that targets molecular entities, the potential for gene editing, and increasing knowledge about molecular differences in metabolism. These advances do not only improve care for patients with rare diseases, but also improve care for somatic conditions such as cancer, and potential advances for complex conditions such as heart disease.

Many genetic tests focus on coding single nucleotide variants, which are single variants in coding regions of a gene (exons) which can result in malformed, truncated, or absent proteins causing the indicated condition. However, there are an increasing number of tests focused on non-coding variants (introns), as well as structural variants (copy number variants, deletions, insertions, translocations, and other complex variants). Technological innovations are providing for increased detection of all variants in regions of the genome, which are difficult to sequence.

Furthermore, polygenic scores are transforming genetic testing from individual variants with known biology to cumulative scores of variants of unknown biologic cause. Together this

© Springer Nature Switzerland AG 2021
K. C. Ferdinand et al. (eds.), *Cardiovascular Disease in Racial and Ethnic Minority Populations*, Contemporary Cardiology, https://doi.org/10.1007/978-3-030-81034-4_2

enhancement of diagnostic ability, therapeutic specificity and the increasing ability to predict genetic risk have resulted in a transformative shift in medicine—precision medicine. Therefore, as we approach precision medicine, it is imperative that we carefully consider its impact on minority health. Through exploring (1) the state of genetic research in minority populations, (2) issues around translation, specifically the validity and utility of genetic biomarkers in minority populations, (3) the implications of increasing use of artificial intelligence in healthcare for minority patients, and (4) the strategies for successful implementation of precision medicine and potential for impact on minority health.

Diagnostic Genetic Testing for Heart Disease

Traditionally genomic medicine has focused on rare monogenic and digenic conditions. In testing for cardiovascular disease (Fig. 2.1), these include aortopathies, cardiomyopathies, cardiac channelopathies, and familial hypercholesterolemia in addition to syndromic conditions with cardiac features [12]. In some of these conditions for example 22q11.2, also referred to as DiGeorge's syndrome, the cardiac features are key features in the disorder. In other conditions like Turner's syndrome, which presents with coarctation of the aorta in one-third of patients, the heart defect presents in a smaller portion of those with the syndrome. In many of these examples of rare disease, a broad array of genetic testing strategies are employed and aimed at identifying a single cause. In these cases, the genetic test is carefully designed around what is known. For example, the genes included in a test for an indicated heart condition would center around the genes that have been demonstrated as associated with disease in the literature [33]. In the case where one or two variants in a single gene cause a disease, for example achondroplasia, a genetic test will look for the presence of those two variants. If a disease is caused by one of many variants in a single gene, for example cystic fibrosis, the test may be designed around

capturing a larger number of variants (the most common variants) or may focus on sequencing the entire gene. However, if the disease is known to have many genes involved, panel testing, where multiple genes are included in a single test, is often chosen. This is known as indication-based testing, where a physician orders a genetic test to clarify diagnosis, prognosis, or carrier status.

Advances in Genetic Testing

Therapeutic advances have propelled the development of genetic testing for companion diagnostics and genetic metabolism differences. Additionally, targeted therapies such as gene editing and gene therapy may use genetic testing to monitor disease levels by quantifying the level of a variant remaining. As molecular diagnostics move to include genetic tests for complex conditions (Fig. 2.1), like coronary heart disease, polygenic tests are increasingly being developed. The premise of the polygenic test is slightly different as it does not center around detection of a known variant, but instead examines the aggregated computed risk for disease from multiple variants across the genome. Unlike the diagnostic, prognostic and carrier tests previously described, these polygenic risk scores are focused on determining risk for disease. These risk-based tests are being discussed in a public health context as a first-line screening tests designed to identify high risk patients for disease or those with minimal to low risk for a specific disease [21].

Development of Genetic Tests as an Evidence-Based Process

Together the diagnostic, prognostic, treatment predictive and risk-based genetic tests are a major component of precision medicine. However, as an evidence-based practice, precision medicine requires sufficient research for translation of molecular discoveries into clinical medicine. Over the past few decades, we have seen tremendous growth in both genetic discovery and health

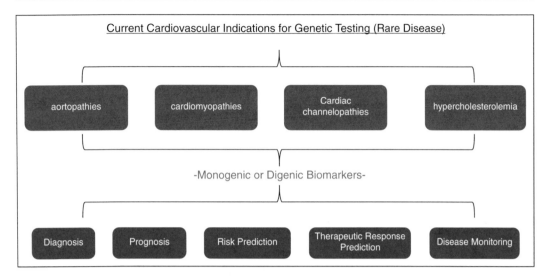

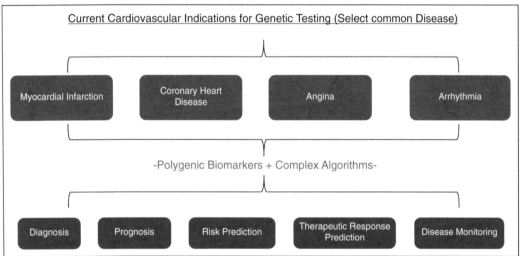

Fig. 2.1 Genetic testing landscape for cardiovascular disease. Genetic testing includes options for diagnostic testing, prognostic testing, risk-based testing, testing for therapeutic response, and testing to monitor disease. Cardiovascular disease indication can be separated into two groups A. Rare Disease and B. Common/Complex Disease. Genetic testing includes options for diagnostic testing, prognostic testing, risk-based testing, testing for therapeutic response, and testing to monitor disease. Each cardiovascular disease indication, some of which are highlighted above (aortopathies, cardiomyopathies, cardiac channelopathies, hypercholesterolemia, myocardial infarction, coronary heart disease, angina, and arrhythmia) may have options for some or all genetic testing options (diagnosis, prognosis, risk prediction, therapeutic response, and disease monitoring). The genetic testing options are based on the scientific knowledge base for the specific biomarker(s) and disease

technology. These successes have been evident by the completion of the human genome project, the 1000 genomes project, the transition of high-throughput targeted sequencing, as well as whole genome sequencing in the clinic. Advances in bioinformatics and clinical informatics, which allow for the processing of large amounts of data through the development of tools and pipelines, have proven pivotal for the integration of precision services as clinical decision support [8]. Technology development is expanding to include health-related applications or software apps, crowd sourcing, and direct-to-consumer health products, including direct-to-consumer genetic services. This growth in discovery and technology has also contributed to an increase in targeted therapies, immunotherapy, pharmacogenomics, gene therapy, gene editing, and other specialized therapies. The combination of translation of molecular discoveries into [diagnostic, prognostic, risk predictive, and treatment predictive] molecular tests in combination with the infrastructure investment in health technology and decision support is revolutionizing care. The result is 'precision medicine'. However, there is a growing concern regarding the impact of a lack of inclusion of diverse populations in genetic research. The concern is that as an evidence-based practice, generalizability has not been established for many of these advances resulting in the potential bias and in the foundation for this healthcare transformation.

Lack of Diversity in Genetic Research and the Missing Evidence Supporting Generalizability of Genetic Tests

This concern was documented in a series of publications going back over a decade. In 2009, Anna Need and David Goldstein reported that 96% of all genome-wide association studies were in people of European descent [26]. These numbers were highlighted before the precision medicine initiative in an article in *Nature* in 2011 by Carlos Bustamante [6], which called for genomic medicine to focus on other ethnic groups to ensure more people would benefit. In his article, Bustamante specifically called for the following: "that those most in need must not be the last to benefit from genetic research; that reviewers and granting bodies demand racial and ethnic diversity in genomic studies; and for financial support of governments and non-profits for global genomics." Bustamante's paper was followed by a call to action in 2012 by Edward Ramos, Shawneequa Callier, and Charles Rotimi entitled "*Why personalized medicine will fail if we stay the course.*" This article continued to raise concern regarding the lack of diversity in genomic research and highlighted opportunities for improving our understanding of genomic diversity in diverse populations by (a) moving beyond race to guide

individualized treatment, (b) informing research with ethnically diverse cohorts, and (c) engaging underrepresented populations in genetic research.

Following the launch of the precision medicine initiative in a 2016 *Nature* article entitled "*Genomics is failing on diversity*," Alice B. Popejoy and Stephanie M. Fullerton highlighted populations are still being left behind on the road to precision medicine. They went on to show that since 2009 where 96% of participants in GWAS studies were of European ancestry, there have been only modest improvements with 81% of participants in GWAS studies being of European ancestry in 2016. Popejoy et al. reported that of the 19% non-European ancestry study participants, 14% were Asian. Continuing this discussion in a 2018 publication in *Health Affairs*, Landry et al. examined the lack of inclusion by disease area—a clear consistent pattern of disparities in research was evident. Furthermore, inclusion in research was not consistent with burden of disease (morbidity or mortality) in underrepresented populations. Moving forward it was suggested that tracking inclusion of diverse populations in research be facilitated by the documentation of ancestral groups in publication and study databases. Landry et al. further suggest that monitoring include information on disease prevalence, disparities in disease morbidity or mortality, pertinent genetic factors such as penetrance, expressivity, as well as frequency of specific genetic factors across ancestral populations. Authors concluded with a call for Americans to make a commitment to the equitable diffusion of precision medicine into clinical care through a variety of activities including funding, scientific engagement in diverse research, creation of policies and guidance to promote inclusion in research, major initiatives to increase genetic education for patients and providers, and investment in the genomic and precision medicine infrastructure needs of diverse communities.

Impaired Discovery of Genetic Causes in Minority Populations

As we think about the importance of the lack of diverse data, it is important to consider the applications to heart disease. Landry et al. reported that underrepresented minorities (URMs) represented 27% of all dbGaP sequencing studies and only 12% of GWAS studies focused on heart disease. This is in contrast to minority groups like African Americans who have higher mortality rates for heart disease, higher prevalence rates of risk factors like hypertension and African Americans and Hispanics who have higher rates of both obesity and diabetes compared to White Americans. As previously mentioned, genetic testing is an evidence-based practice. Subsequently, the lack of this diversity in research can impact the translation of genetic research into genetic testing and precision medicine by impeding discovery of variants at a higher frequency in minority populations resulting in lower test detection rates.

Highlighting this issue, Buxbaum et al. reported a founder mutation in African Americans resulting in transthyretin cardiac amyloidosis where both the variant and the condition have almost exclusively been found in persons of African ancestry [7]. Auer et al. reported that genetic diversity in African Americans' genomes can be harnessed for uncovering rare variation associations. They further report that several variants not significant for complex trait association when using European American genomes were significant when using African American genomes—findings that were only possible with the large-scale sequencing of African American genomes provided by the NHLBI Exome Sequencing Project [4]. Similar findings were echoed by Wright et al. in discussing the discovery of variants related to familial hypercholesterolemia in African Americans.

Misdiagnosis of Genetic Conditions in Minority Populations

Another result of the lack of diversity in human genetic research is that variants may be determined to be causative of disease purely on their rarity in European populations. It is important to understand that frequency of a variant is an important consideration in determining the pathogenicity in rare disease. Lack of diversity in

genomic datasets is important in this context because in a non-diverse literature landscape, the frequency of a variant in non-European populations is unknown. If a variant is presumed to be rare, because of its frequency in European populations, but is in fact more common in non-European populations, the variant may erroneously be classified as disease causing resulting in misdiagnosis of disease [37]. In a 2015 special article in the *New England Journal of Medicine*, Manrai et al. reported misclassification of benign variants as pathogenic resulting in a misdiagnosis of cardiomyopathy, which disproportionately affected African Americans who had a higher frequency of the benign variants. In this article, Manrai exampled the importance of diverse genomes in research and databases and called for the development of an information commons and agile clinical system availing information in real time [22]. Such resources would greatly improve variant classification and improve the clinical utility of genetic tests for underrepresented populations. In a 2018 JAMA cardiology article, Landry et al. demonstrated clinical utility for cardiomyopathy testing was lower in underrepresented minorities compared to their White counterparts. These differences in utility resulted from lower detection rates and higher rates of inconclusive results [variants of uncertain significance]. Authors surmised the higher rate of inconclusive results was the result of the lack of evidence from research and clinical report [19].

Unclear Treatment Response in Minority Populations

While these reports all show the impact of the lack of research on genetic testing, additional evidence shows the lack of genetic research in diverse populations also affects molecular-based treatments and treatment plans, resulting in inaccurate dosing in pharmacogenomic prescriptions [5]. This impact was demonstrated in the case of Warfarin pharmacogenomics dosing studies of African Americans. In these studies, pharmacogenomics dosing algorithms failed to yield the same efficacy in African Americans compared to other population groups. Further research showed the presence of additional variants in the relevant genes in some African American patients who were not included in the original algorithms. These variants, primarily associated with African ancestry, affected the metabolism of the drug necessitating a change in the required dosing [13, 27]. Recent studies suggest additional genetic differences may be associated with Warfarin associated bleeding in African Americans [9]. Other cardiovascular relevant drugs presented by the Clinical Pharmacogenomics Implementation Consortium (CPIC) with implications for diverse populations include Clopidogrel which shows a higher frequency of the null allele in Asians resulting in a higher frequency of non-responders in that population [27]. Additional novel variants in African Americans impacting drug efficacy and metabolism have also been identified [35].

Unclear Validity and Utility of Individual Genetic Tests in Minority Populations

The decreased clinical utility of genetic testing in non-European populations is not limited to diagnostic and predictive testing, but also extends to a critical deficiency in the validity of polygenic risk scores for non-European populations [23]. One of the most striking impacts of the lack of diversity in research on genetic testing is the impact of polygenic risk scores. As previously mentioned, polygenic risk scores differ from other clinical genetic tests because the genetic exposure is not a "known entity." Additionally, the individual variants on their own are not risk factors for disease. The development of polygenic risk scores can be classified as artificial intelligence (AI) driven by machine learning where a "training" dataset is used to develop the algorithm or risk score and a test set is used to validate it. In this sense, the resulting risk score is evaluated in a separate test-set to ensure validity [10]. Assuring clinical validity and utility of polygenic risk scores is an important area of research [36]. In the case of polygenic risk scores, generalizability or reproducibility in other popu-

lations is often not demonstrated because both the training and tests-sets are in populations of predominantly European ancestry. This is a stated limitation of all AI, which are vulnerable to the bias in training and test-sets. In genetics, this vulnerability is exacerbated by the increased heterogeneity (higher level of variation) in African ancestry genomes as compared to European genomes. The result has been that polygenic risk scores developed in European populations may have reduced accuracy in non-European ancestry groups [11]. Clinically, the approach to handling this has been varied. Currently, there is insufficient data across diverse population groups to have polygenic risk scores for all populations with similar performance levels. As such, there are some commercial algorithms, which have been developed in European ancestry individuals, that are not offered to individuals of other demographic groups. This translates to race limited testing, where members of one population may be offered a test, but members of another population are not. Without alternative algorithms for these groups, this concludes in seemingly accurate risk prediction for certain conditions in those of European ancestry with no alternative for other groups. Also of concern is the alternative approach of offering the score to all consumers or patients with a statement of limitations in the fine print. Both approaches have their limitations and demonstrate the necessity of larger numbers of diverse cohorts in genetics research and development of polygenic algorithms.

Understanding the Personal Utility of Genetic Tests in Minority Populations

In addition to both the validity and clinical utility of genetic tests on precision medicine, we also need to consider the personal utility of genetic testing. In addition to the impact of genetic testing on clinical care, there is also the value patients and providers perceive from having done the test. Research on the concept of personal utility has demonstrated that patients can perceive affective, cognitive, behavioral and social value from genetic testing [2, 15]. This aspect of testing, personal utility, can be included in the pre-test counseling associated with genetic testing. The demonstrated lack of diversity in genetic research extends to a limit in information regarding personal utility of genetic testing across population groups. In a 2017 publication of direct-to-consumer (DTC) genetic testing which included questions of importance and interests in DTC genetic testing, African American participants showed similar interests as other population groups. Authors noted limited sample size with African American participants but discussed the results may suggest an interest in ancestry and other non-clinical traits as very important in the decision to purchase DTC testing by African Americans [20]. As genetic testing becomes more widespread with clinical and non-clinical genetic testing available, it is important that more research be done to understand personal utility of genetic testing across diverse populations.

Access to Precision Medicine and the Health Disparities

Equally important as both the clinical and personal utility of genetic testing is access. While the costs of DTC genetic tests are driven by consumer demand and may be considered relatively affordable, the costs of clinical tests vary greatly. Clinical genetic testing varies according to the complexity and size of the test—where single variant tests are on the lower end and whole genome sequencing on the higher end. While the limiting factor for DTC genetic tests is often the cost and digital access, clinical tests have more barriers. Cost can be critically important to = clinically indicated testing where the costs are subjected to usual healthcare paradigms including a patient's insurance. Coverage of testing is of particular interest to health equity in precision medicine as some genetic tests including panel testing, whole exome and whole genome testing can be cost prohibitive for most patients. This gives payers a tremendous amount of power as to the tests a patient receives. Additionally,

another key factor in testing is the provider knowledge or preference regarding genetic services. As a subspecialty, genetic services including genetic testing have been shown to be underutilized by primary care providers. In a 2008 study by Shields et al. it was reported that minority serving providers were less likely to order genetic testing including BRCA 1 and 2 testing. This study showed genetic service usage for minority serving providers in some cases was even lower than providers whose patient populations were primarily uninsured or those who served mostly non-English speakers. Shah et al. found similarly that African Americans were more likely to present with more severe forms of hereditary transthyretin amyloidosis, a condition associated with African ancestry, compared to their White counterparts with the wild-type non-inherited form of the disease. They went on to report that this occurred, despite the existence of a non-invasive genetic test that was available for early detection and a potential therapy for disease. They concluded the findings suggest that genetic testing was not being ordered for these patients. Similar questions regarding access have been raised for familial hypercholesterolemia as well, where differences in stage of diagnosis and aggressiveness of treatment were noted [30]. There is a clear concern regarding the access to genomic testing and precision medicine. Access is such an important issue, that in 2018, Rep. Swalwell introduced the "Advancing Access to Precision Medicine Act" in congress. This bill places a responsibility on the Department of Health and Human Services to work with the National Academy of Medicine to evaluate usage of genetic and genomic testing including barriers to use.

On the Horizon

In 2015, the precision medicine initiative was announced by President Barack Obama as a transformation of healthcare from the "generic" to the "personalized." We are only at the beginning stages of this transformation. The current catalogue of testing is likely to rapidly increase in the coming decades. These increases are evident by the increasing number of "precision medicine studies," research programs on early detection and early intervention, and the increasing size of the commercial market for molecular therapy. Included in the precision medicine initiative is a NIH-funded diverse cohort called the "All of Us" research study. The All of Us study is designed to be a national cohort or biobank resource with biomarker and disease information from 1 million Americans from diverse backgrounds [1]. The All of Us study is a signature feature of the approach to diversifying our genomic data. However, other key initiatives including a NIH workforce diversity initiative, several initiatives to diversify clinical trials, and academic and industry collaborations focused on both workforce diversity and diversity in research have been announced.

These initiatives focused on equity and diversity are long overdue and are critically important at this juncture as the landscape for precision medicine and precision cardiovascular medicine is rapidly increasing. In 2019, the outcomes and progress of the first US patient to receive gene therapy for sickle cell disease were announced [31]. Gene therapies for coronary artery disease, heart failure, and arrhythmias are in various stages of development [14, 38]. Likewise, polygenic risk scores for Mendelian disease as well as complex conditions are being developed [24, 34].

Potentially even more exciting than the new developments in precision cardiovascular medicine that we aware of are the potential applications that we have yet to imagine. Potential developments which include expanding routine testing beyond DNA biomarkers to include RNA, protein, and metabolite markers which may improve resolution, temporality, and provide for testing of more complex conditions. In addition to the expansion of testing to include biomarkers of various molecular monomer analytes, there is also the potential for inclusion of health technology applications collecting survey data for social determinants of health and wearables which can provide precise measurements of environmental exposures. Perhaps the real potential of precision medicine is not the ever-expanding catalogue of potential tests and tools for individual determinants but the development of knowledge bases, information systems, and clinical decision support which are imagined to integrate the individual datapoints and provide information at the point of care.

The Road Forward

Precision medicine is upon us. The transformation of medicine brought by molecular biomarkers, targeted therapies, and artificial intelligence algorithms is already evident in both cancer and rare disease. We are starting to see that penetrance of precision medicine in cardiovascular disease as well. However, learning from the lessons of the past, it is important that minority patients and the principles and strategies around diversity inclusion be clearly stated priorities of the foundation and infrastructure investment in precision medicine. This investment includes evaluation of existing and future tests for generalizability across populations, identification of barriers to access of precision services as well as education regarding the importance of precision medicine. This latter point is important as with the exception of direct-to-consumer testing, precision services are physician mediated. Therefore, education of physicians regarding genetics, genetic services available to patients, and interpretation of genetic findings are critically important. To this point the American Heart Association has put forth a statement regarding the need for sub-specialty training programs in cardiovascular genetics [17]. However, given the importance of potential cardiovascular genetic testing for hypertension, coronary artery disease, and other risk factors, it is imperative that broad-based training for these services be available to primary care physicians as well. Initiatives to train a wide variety of physicians and patients are underway by various groups including the American Medical Association.

Given the transformative nature of precision medicine, equitable integration in our US healthcare system requires partnerships between academia, government, industry, and communities.

The ability of precision medicine to penetrate our entire healthcare system relies upon the depth and strength of these partnerships. In the end, the tools we develop in this era are only as good as their implementation, bringing a key focus on implementation science as a fundamental component of the translation of precision medicine. In 2012, Edward Ramos' article entitled "Why personalized medicine will fail if we stay the course" was a warning to the potential exacerbation of health disparities possible in a molecular enhanced medicine paradigm with a biased evidence base. It is the hope that the transformation and infrastructure captured in precision medicine helps us not only reverse the course but provides new insights to disparities providing the tools to eliminate disparities and provide more equitable care through precision medicine.

References

1. AOU. The "all of us" research program. N Engl J Med. 2019;381(19):1883–5.
2. Kohler JN, Turbitt E, Biesecker BB. Personal utility in genomic testing: a systematic literature review. Eur J Hum Genet. 2017a;25(6):662–8.
3. Armstrong K, Micco E, Carney A, Stopfer J, Putt M. Racial differences in the use of BRCA1/2 testing among women with a family history of breast or ovarian cancer. JAMA. 2005;293:1729–36.
4. Auer PL, Reiner AP, Wang G, Kang HM, Abecasis GR, Altshuler D, et al. Guidelines for large-scale sequence-based complex trait association studies: lessons learned from the NHLBI exome sequencing project. Am J Hum Genet. 2016;99(4):791–801. https://doi.org/10.1016/j.ajhg.2016.08.012.
5. Bachtiar M, Ooi B, Wang J, Jin Y, Tan TW, Chong SS, Lee C. Towards precision medicine: interrogating the human genome to identify drug pathways associated with potentially functional, population-differentiated polymorphisms. Pharm J. 2019;19(6):516–27. https://doi.org/10.1038/s41397-019-0096-y.
6. Bustamante CD, Burchard EG, De la Vega FM. Genomics for the world. Nature. 2011;475:163–5. https://doi.org/10.1038/475163a.
7. Buxbaum JN, Ruberg FL. Transthyretin V122I (pV142I)* cardiac amyloidosis: an age-dependent autosomal dominant cardiomyopathy too common to be overlooked as a cause of significant heart disease in elderly African Americans. Genet Med. 2017;19:733–42.
8. Chow N, Gallo L, Busse JW. Evidence-based medicine and precision medicine: complementary approaches to clinical decision-making. Precis Clin Med. 2018 Sep;1(2):60–4. https://doi.org/10.1093/pcmedi/pby009.
9. De T, Alarcon C, Hernandez W, et al. Association of genetic variants with Warfarin-associated bleeding among patients of African descent. JAMA. 2018;320(16):1670–7. https://doi.org/10.1001/jama.2018.14955.
10. Dias R, Torkamani A. Artificial intelligence in clinical and genomic diagnostics. Genome Med. 2019;11(1):70. https://doi.org/10.1186/s13073-019-0689-8.
11. Duncan L, Shen H, Gelaye B, Meijsen J, Ressler K, Feldman M, Domingue B. Analysis of polygenic risk score usage and performance in diverse human populations. Nat Commun. 2019;10(1):3328. https://doi.org/10.1038/s41467-019-11112-0.
12. Giudicessi JR, Kullo IJ, Ackerman MJ. Precision cardiovascular medicine: state of genetic testing. Mayo Clin Proc. 2017;92:642–62.
13. Johnson JA, Caudle KE, Gong L, Whirl-Carrillo M, Stein CM, Scott SA, Wadelius M. Clinical Pharmacogenetics Implementation Consortium (CPIC) guideline for pharmacogenetics-guided warfarin dosing: 2017 update. Clin Pharmacol Ther. 2017;102(3):397–404. https://doi.org/10.1002/cpt.668.
14. Kieserman JM, Myers VD, Dubey P, Cheung JY, Feldman AM. Current landscape of heart failure gene therapy. J Am Heart Assoc. 2019;8(10):e012239. https://doi.org/10.1161/JAHA.119.012239.
15. Kohler JN, Turbitt E, Lewis KL, Wilfond BS, Jamal L, Peay HL, et al. Defining personal utility in genomics: a Delphi study. Clin Genet 2017b;92(3):290–297. pmid:28218387.
16. Knepper TC, McLeod HL. When will clinical trials finally reflect diversity? Nature. 2018;557:157–9. https://doi.org/10.1038/d41586-018-05049-5.
17. Kullo IJ, et al. Establishment of specialized clinical cardiovascular genetics programs: recognizing the need and meeting standards: a scientific statement from the American Heart Association. Circ Genom Precis Med. 2019;12:e000054.
18. Landry LG, et al. Lack of diversity in genomic databases is a barrier to translating precision medicine research into practice. Health Aff (Millwood). 2018;37:780–5. https://doi.org/10.1377/hlthaff.2017.1595.
19. Landry LG, Rehm HL. Association of racial/ethnic categories with the ability of genetic tests to detect a cause of cardiomyopathy. JAMA Cardiol. 2018;3(4):341–5. https://doi.org/10.1001/jamacardio.2017.5333.
20. Landry L, Nielsen DE, Carere DA, Roberts JS, Green RC, PGen Study Group. Racial minority group interest in direct-to-consumer genetic testing: findings from the PGen study. J Community Genet. 2017;8:293–301.
21. Lewis CM, Vassos E. Prospects for using risk scores in polygenic medicine. Genome Med. 2017;9:96. https://doi.org/10.1186/s13073-017-0489-y.

22. Manrai AK, Funke BH, Rehm HL, et al. Genetic misdiagnoses and the potential for health disparities. N Engl J Med. 2016;375(7):655–65. https://doi.org/10.1056/NEJMsa1507092.

23. Martin AR, Kanai M, Kamatani Y, et al. Clinical use of current polygenic risk scores may exacerbate health disparities. Nat Genet. 2019;51:584–91. https://doi.org/10.1038/s41588-019-0379-x.

24. Natarajan P. Polygenic risk scoring for coronary heart disease: the first risk factor. J Am Coll Cardiol. 2018;72(16):1894–7. https://doi.org/10.1016/j.jacc.2018.08.1041.

25. National Academies of Sciences, Engineering, and Medicine; Health and Medicine Division; Board on Population Health and Public Health Practice; Committee on Community-Based Solutions to Promote Health Equity in the United States; Baciu A, Negussie Y, Geller A, et al., editors. Communities in Action: Pathways to Health Equity. Washington (DC): National Academies Press (US); 2017 Jan 11. 2, The State of Health Disparities in the United States. Available from: https://www.ncbi.nlm.nih.gov/books/NBK425844/

26. Peloso GM, Lange LA, Varga TV, Nickerson DA, Smith JD, Griswold ME, Musani S, Polfus LM, Mei H, Gabriel S, et al. Association of exome sequences with cardiovascular traits among Blacks in the Jackson Heart Study. Circ Cardiovasc Genet. 2016;9:368–74.

27. Perera MA, Cavallari LH, Limdi NA, Gamazon ER, Konkashbaev A, Daneshjou R, Johnson JA. Genetic variants associated with warfarin dose in African-American individuals: a genome-wide association study. Lancet (London, England). 2013;382(9894):790–6. https://doi.org/10.1016/S0140-6736(13)60681-9.

28. Popejoy AB, Fullerton SM. Genomics is failing on diversity. Nature. 2016;538:161–4. https://doi.org/10.1038/538161a.

29. Ramos E, Callier SL, Rotimi CN. Why personalized medicine will fail if we stay the course. Pers Med. 2012;9:839–47. https://doi.org/10.2217/pme.12.100.

30. Raygor V, Knowles J. JACC. What have the recent registry-related studies told us about familial hypercholesterolemia care? 2018 Feb 7. https://www.acc.org/latest-in-cardiology/articles/2018/02/07/13/27/what-have-the-recent-registry-related-studies-told-us-about-fh-care

31. Ribeil J-A, Hacein-Bey-Abina S, Payen E, Magnani A, Semeraro M, Magrin E, Caccavelli L, Neven B, Bourget P, El Nemer W. Gene therapy in a patient with sickle cell disease. N Engl J Med. 2017;376(9):848–55.

32. Shah KB, Mankad AK, Castano A, et al. Transthyretin cardiac amyloidosis in black Americans. Circ Heart Fail. 2016;9(6):e002558. https://doi.org/10.1161/CIRCHEARTFAILURE.115.002558.

33. Shields AE, Burke W, Levy DE. Differential use of available genetic tests among primary care physicians in the United States: results of a national survey. Genet Med. 2008;10:404–14.

34. Strande NT, Riggs ER, Buchanan AH, Ceyhan-Birsoy O, DiStefano M, Dwight SS, et al. Evaluating the clinical validity of gene-disease associations: an evidence-based framework developed by the clinical genome resource. Am J Hum Genet. 2017;100:895–906. https://doi.org/10.1016/j.ajhg.2017.04.015.

35. Sugrue LP, Desikan RS. What are polygenic scores and why are they important? JAMA. 2019;321(18):1820–1. https://doi.org/10.1001/jama.2019.3893.

36. Topol EJ. Cholesterol, racial variation and targeted medicines. Nat Med. 2005;11:122–3.

37. Torkamani A, Wineinger NE, Topol EJ. The personal and clinical utility of polygenic risk scores. Nat Rev Genet. 2018;19:581–90. https://doi.org/10.1038/s41576-018-0018-x.

38. Walsh R, Thomson K, Ware J, et al. Reassessment of Mendelian gene pathogenicity using 7,855 cardiomyopathy cases and 60,706 reference samples. Genet Med. 2017;19:192–203. https://doi.org/10.1038/gim.2016.90.

Lipoprotein(a): A Cardiovascular Risk Factor Affecting Ethnic Minorities

Ronald R. Nelson Jr, Karol Watson, and Gissette Reyes-Soffer

Introduction to Lipoprotein(a)

In 1963, geneticist, Dr. Kare Berg, looking to define lipoprotein differences observed in human serum, discovered Lipoprotein(a) [Lp(a)]. He showed that the new antigen was a genetic trait and called it Lp(a). "Lp" referred to the lipoprotein and "a" was the accepted terminology for naming antigens in human immunogenetics [1]. Lipoprotein(a) is an apoB100 containing protein made unique by its disulfide linkage with glycoprotein apolipoprotein(a) [apo(a)] [2]. It is encoded by the apo(a) gene (*LPA*) located on chromosome 6q26-27 in humans. In 70–90% of cases, serum Lp(a) concentrations are determined by the *LPA* gene [3]. As with many genetic determinants, ethnic differences affect the heritability of apo(a), with Black Americans from African descent having a lower heritability when compared to White populations [4].

A majority of people have two distinct apo(a) isoforms on each of the two alleles that are both expressed at varying concentrations [5]. Apo(a)

is mainly composed of large autonomous looping protein domains known as kringle domains. Having evolved from plasminogen through a series of deletions, duplications, gene conversions, and point mutations, apo(a) retains these kringle domains, which play important roles in the coagulation pathway and therefore in atherogenic processes [6]. One type of kringle domain, kringle-IV type 2 (KIV-2), represents one of the most studied genetic variations in the *LPA* gene, and is a significant determinant of apo(a) size in White and Black subjects [7–9].

Despite its discovery in 1963, there has been an increased focus on Lp(a) in clinical and scientific communities driven by recent findings from genome wide association studies (GWAS) and Mendelian randomization studies that highlight its role as a causal risk factor in coronary, valvular, and atherogenic vascular disease [10–13]. Approximately one in five individuals has Lp(a) plasma concentrations greater than 50 mg/dl and is at increased risk for development of cardiovascular disease (CVD) and aortic stenosis [10], the latter in studies completed in mostly White cohorts. Lp(a) particles have been identified in human atheroma dissections [14, 15] indicating that the molecule is involved in atherogenic mechanisms. The putative mechanisms are a combination of intimal deposition in the arterial wall leading to atherogenesis as well as a potential net prothrombotic effect of apolipoprotein(a) which is a competitive binder of its structural

R. R. Nelson Jr · G. Reyes-Soffer (✉)
Columbia University Medical Center-College of Physicians and Surgeons, New York City, NY, USA
e-mail: rrn2117@cumc.columbia.edu;
gr2104@cumc.columbia.edu

K. Watson
David Geffen School of Medicine at UCLA, Los Angeles, CA, USA
e-mail: KWatson@mednet.ucla.edu

© Springer Nature Switzerland AG 2021
K. C. Ferdinand et al. (eds.), *Cardiovascular Disease in Racial and Ethnic Minority Populations*,
Contemporary Cardiology, https://doi.org/10.1007/978-3-030-81034-4_3

homologue, plasminogen [16]. In addition, genetic studies have provided convincing evidence that *LPA* is associated with various pathways that lead to coronary heart disease (CHD) [11, 13, 17–20]. Finally, targeted therapies toward the apo(a) moiety of Lp(a) are in phase 2–3 development [21–24]. Despite lower heritability, absolute Lp(a) levels are highest in people of African ancestry [4]. In multi-ethic studies, Lp(a) has been found to be higher in Black Americans of African descent when compared to Hispanic Americans, Chinese Americans, or White Americans [25–27]. In the MESA study associations of Lp(a) with calcific aortic [28] disease and heart failure [29] were found but these were not limited to Black subjects. There is a need for prospective studies addressing if high levels of Lp(a) place Black Americans and Hispanic individuals at higher risk and phase 2 studies of novel treatments have low enrollments of these underrepresented populations.

Current ongoing efforts are underway to standardize Lp(a) measurements via validated assays [30–32]. The latter has been a barrier in widespread uptake of Lp(a) testing for assessing cardiovascular risk. A recent review of Lp(a) literature from the last decade highlights the lack of data of studies in diverse populations; a total of only 51 studies were found to involve non-White populations compared to a large number of studies (>200 studies) in White populations. In addition, these studies show a large discrepancy in the assays used to assess serum Lp(a) levels including **a.** enzyme-linked immunosorbent assay ($n = 17$), **b.** immunonephelometric assay ($n = 12$), **c.** immunoturbidimetric assay ($n = 19$), and **d.** unspecified assays ($n = 4$). Consistent with previous literature, both mean and median serum Lp(a) concentrations tend to be elevated in Black individuals compared to their White and East Asian counterparts; however, there exists considerable variation in these data, with mean concentrations ranging between 43 mg/dL and 99 mg/dL (71–132 nmol/L), and median concentrations ranging between 27.11 mg/dL and 46 mg/dL (60–79 nmol/L), with wide IQRs. Hispanic participants tend to have relatively low mean (14.9 mg/dL, $n = 2073$) and median serum Lp(a)

levels (14.7–24 nmol/L); it is necessary to acknowledge that data on this group are limited, and only five studies [33–37] examining serum Lp(a) in Hispanic patients were discovered in the review of the literature from the last 10 years. Most preliminary literature suggests that East Asian populations tend to have lower mean and median serum Lp(a) concentrations compared to their White, and especially Black and South Asian counterparts. East Asian median Lp(a) concentrations range between 1.11 mg/dL and 12.9 mg/dL (22–38 nmol/L). There are recommendations from leaders in the field to adapt the use of molar measurements as part of standardizing assays. The current use of conversion factors from mg/dl to nmol/dl does not provide exact levels due to the variability in apo(a) sizes that exist in various study populations [38].

Inflammatory pathways play a large role in the development and outcomes of cardiovascular disease (CVD). Elevated levels of plasma interleukins (IL-6 and IL-18) are associated with CVD risk in humans [39]. There are convincing data illustrating that blockage of known inflammatory signaling pathways has an inverse effect on Lp(a) plasma levels. Blockade of the interleukin-6 (IL-6) receptors by tocilizumab has resulted in decreased serum Lp(a) concentrations [40], and meta-analyses and Mendelian randomization studies have implicated the IL-6 receptor in CVD [41, 42]. More recently, the canakinumab anti-inflammatory thrombosis outcomes study (CANTOS) trial for the first time has provided conclusive evidence that inflammation enhances CVD in humans [43]. While C-reactive protein (CRP) is the preferred inflammatory biomarker for CVD risk stratification [44], Lp(a) also enhances vascular inflammation in humans [45]. Much of the published literature classifies oxidized phospholipids and oxidized low-density lipoprotein (OxPL and OxLDL) as pro-atherogenic biomarkers. Additionally, Lp(a) is identified as the preferential carrier of OxPL. Interestingly, carriers of an IL-1 haplotype associated with increased inflammation showed increased cardiovascular mortality when Lp(a)-associated OxPL levels were elevated [22]. Studies in mice and humans have described the role of cholesterol, and OxPL within the isolated Lp(a) particles, establishing that binding of OxPL and Lp(a) promotes atherosclerosis [38, 39]. Many inflammatory markers appear in the previously published proteomic data [46]. Studying inflammatory pathways does not only provide insights into the detrimental effects of high serum Lp(a) concentrations. Moreover, the current COVID-19 pandemic has highlighted the importance of understanding inflammatory pathways of disease, especially in populations at risk, as patients with known CVD have exhibited worse outcomes [47]. Additionally, increases in strokes and myocardial infarction (MI) in previously "healthy" young individuals have been reported as disease presenting signs [48, 49].

Though population studies have shown differences in serum Lp(a) levels and CVD risk among different ethnicities [50], the majority of existing data focuses on predominantly White and male populations and cohorts. Studies that have examined Lp(a) concentrations in underrepresented groups with minority population sample sizes greater than 500 are severely limited compared to available sample sizes for White groups. The inclusion of larger sample sizes will not eliminate disparity; however, it will provide greater precision for serum levels per race/ethnicity. Importantly, to predict cardiovascular risk, guidelines and clinicians often use race. More robust analyses of Lp(a) levels by race can likely yield a more quantifiable basis for cardiovascular risk in addition to that conferred by race alone, a relatively indiscrete metric. A recent study using the UK Biobank dataset has enrolled a large amount of Blacks, however Hispanics population were not represented [27]. In this study, using a risk threshold of per 50nmol/L increase in Lp(a), they found similiar hazard ratios for CVD between Blacks, Whites and South Asians.

Largely genetically determined, Lp(a) levels are not easily modifiable. Recent review of dietary studies points to a potential role of dietary fat in modifying Lp(a) plasma levels, but the responses to usual LDL-C lowering effects of low saturated fat are less evident with modifying Lp(a) [51]. In some European countries, apheresis [52] is the only available and approved treatment modality. Apheresis is part of ongoing clinical investigation in the USA [53] and outcome studies in Europe (NCT02791802). However, there are many limitations to the approval of this modality as standard of care. The proprotein convertase subtilisin/kexin type 9 (PCSK9) inhibitors have shown promise in decreasing Lp(a) and therefore the incidence of CV mortality in clinical trials [29]. As PSCK9 inhibitors also decrease LDL cholesterol, the mortality benefit associated with this intervention is not exclusively linked to its effect on Lp(a). Additional studies have demonstrated a favorable relationship between niacin (nicotinic acid) therapy and cardiovascular risk reduction [54]. While niacin primarily achieves this effect by broadly modifying serum lipoprotein concentrations, high doses of the drug are required before any significant changes in serum Lp(a) levels are observed, indicating its preferential activity with other lipoproteins [36].

Contrarily, statins have been cited as a therapy that increases Lp(a) levels. A meta-analysis of published statin therapy studies over the past decade ($n = 11$) has shown significant increases in mean patient-level Lp(a) levels following treatment [4]. It must be noted that these conclusions follow a collection of previous studies that have shown variability in the relationship between Lp(a) levels and statin use, much of which is attributed to genetic makeup, assay selection, and smaller sample sizes [21].

There are multiple programs developing treatments targeting the apo(a) component of Lp(a) to lower its plasma concentrations (NCT04606602 and NCT0423552) [55]. These therapies include anti-sense mRNA silencing via oligonucleotides (ASO) [56] and siRNAs [57]. An ASO is a single strand of deoxynucleotides that bind to a complimentary mRNA target, shutting off its translation; in siRNA-mediated gene silencing, multiprotein RNA-induced silencing complexes (RISC) are recruited that complementarily bind to and cleave target mRNA. The targets of ASOs are the primary mRNA transcripts of apo(a). Complexing of ASO and apo(a) mRNA blocks translation of the nascent proteins, resulting in decreased serum Lp(a).

Significant evidence points to Lp(a) levels as a highly useful markers of CVD and CHD risk; however, much work still remains in terms of investigating differences in Lp(a) levels stratified by race and ethnicity. Though existing studies primarily identify Black and South Asian patients as populations with elevated Lp(a) (despite lower heritability), available sample sizes and assay variability certainly pose limitations on the generalizability of these findings. Furthermore, researchers hypothesize that apo(a) isoform size plays a significant role in the pro-atherogenic properties of Lp(a), warranting further examination of the relationship between the particle and cardiovascular risk stratified by race and isoform size. Accordingly, though Lp(a)-lowering therapies are in their infancy in terms of establishing long-term CVD mortality, the representative inclusion of minority populations in clinical trials for these treatments is essential for ensuring an effective therapeutic agent for all groups. The latter will surely yield an expanded understanding of the association between Lp(a) levels and CVD in these groups compared to White individuals.

References

1. Berg K. A new serum type system in man-the LP system. Acta Pathol Microbiol Scand. 1963;59:369–82.
2. Lawn RM, Schwartz K, Patthy L. Convergent evolution of apolipoprotein(a) in primates and hedgehog. Proc Natl Acad Sci U S A. 1997;94:11992–7.
3. Boerwinkle E, Leffert CC, Lin J, Lackner C, Chiesa G, Hobbs HH. Apolipoprotein(a) gene accounts for greater than 90% of the variation in plasma lipoprotein(a) concentrations. J Clin Invest. 1992;90:52–60.
4. Enkhmaa B, Anuurad E, Zhang W, Kim K, Berglund L. Heritability of apolipoprotein (a) traits in two-generational African-American and Caucasian families. J Lipid Res. 2019;60:1603–9.
5. Lackner C, Boerwinkle E, Leffert CC, Rahmig T, Hobbs HH. Molecular basis of apolipoprotein (a) isoform size heterogeneity as revealed by pulsed-field gel electrophoresis. J Clin Invest. 1991;87:2153–61.
6. McLean JW, Tomlinson JE, Kuang WJ, Eaton DL, Chen EY, Fless GM, Scanu AM, Lawn RM. cDNA sequence of human apolipoprotein(a) is homologous to plasminogen. Nature. 1987;330:132–7.
7. Gencer BKF, Stroes ES, Mach F. Lipoprotein(a): the revenant. Eur Heart J. 2017;38(20):1553–60.
8. Marcovina SM, Albers JJ, Wijsman E, Zhang Z, Chapman NH, Kennedy H. Differences in Lp[a] concentrations and apo[a] polymorphs between black and white Americans. J Lipid Res. 1996;37:2569–85.
9. Coassin S, Schonherr S, Weissensteiner H, Erhart G, Forer L, Losso JL, Lamina C, Haun M, Utermann G, Paulweber B, Specht G, Kronenberg F. A comprehensive map of single-base polymorphisms in the hypervariable LPA kringle IV type 2 copy number variation region. J Lipid Res. 2019;60:186–99.
10. Afshar M, Kamstrup PR, Williams K, Sniderman AD, Nordestgaard BG, Thanassoulis G. Estimating the population impact of Lp(a) lowering on the incidence of myocardial infarction and aortic stenosis-brief report. Arterioscler Thromb Vasc Biol. 2016;36:2421–3.
11. Saleheen DHP, Zhao W, Rasheed A, Taleb A, Imran A, Abbas S, Majeed F, Akhtar S, Qamar N, Zaman KS, Yaqoob Z, Saghir T, Rizvi SN, Memon A, Mallick NH, Ishaq M, Rasheed SZ, Memon FU, Mahmood K, Ahmed N, Frossard P, Tsimikas S, Witztum JL, Marcovina S, Sandhu M, Rader DJ, Danesh J. Apolipoprotein(a) isoform size, lipoprotein(a) concentration, and coronary artery disease: a mendelian randomisation analysis. Lancet Diabetes Endocrinol. 2017;5(7):524–33.
12. Mack S, Coassin S, Rueedi R, Yousri NA, Seppala I, Gieger C, Schonherr S, Forer L, Erhart G, Marques-Vidal P, Ried JS, Waeber G, Bergmann S, Dahnhardt D, Stockl A, Raitakari OT, Kahonen M, Peters A, Meitinger T, Strauch K, Kedenko L, Paulweber B, Lehtimaki T, Hunt SC, Vollenweider P, Lamina C, Kronenberg F. A genome-wide association meta-analysis on lipoprotein (a) concentrations adjusted for apolipoprotein (a) isoforms. J Lipid Res. 2017;58:1834–44.
13. Larsson SC, Gill D, Mason AM, Jiang T, Bäck M, Butterworth AS, Burgess S. Lipoprotein(a) in Alzheimer, atherosclerotic, cerebrovascular, thrombotic, and valvular disease: mendelian randomization investigation. Circulation. 2020;141:1826–8.
14. Pepin JM, O'Neil JA, Hoff HF. Quantification of apo[a] and apoB in human atherosclerotic lesions. J Lipid Res. 1991;32:317–27.
15. Hoff HF, O'Neil J, Yashiro A. Partial characterization of lipoproteins containing apo[a] in human atherosclerotic lesions. J Lipid Res. 1993;34:789–98.
16. Wilson DPJT, Jones PH, Koschinsky ML, McNeal CJ, Nordestgaard BG, Orringer CE. Use of lipoprotein(a) in clinical practice: a biomarker whose time has come. A scientific statement from the National Lipid Association. J Clin Lipidol. 2019;13:374–92.
17. Clarke R, Peden JF, Hopewell JC, Kyriakou T, Goel A, Heath SC, Parish S, Barlera S, Franzosi MG, Rust S, Bennett D, Silveira A, Malarstig A, Green FR, Lathrop M, Gigante B, Leander K, de Faire U, Seedorf U, Hamsten A, Collins R, Watkins H, Farrall M. Genetic variants associated with Lp(a) lipoprotein level and coronary disease. N Engl J Med. 2009;361:2518–28.

18. Kamstrup PR, Tybjaerg-Hansen A, Nordestgaard BG. Genetic evidence that lipoprotein(a) associates with atherosclerotic stenosis rather than venous thrombosis. Arterioscler Thromb Vasc Biol. 2012;32:1732–41.
19. Thanassoulis GCC, Owens DS, Smith JG, Smith AV, Peloso GM, Kerr KF, Pechlivanis S, Budoff MJ, Harris TB, Malhotra R, O'Brien KD, Kamstrup PR, Nordestgaard BG, Tybjaerg-Hansen A, Allison MA, Aspelund T, Criqui MH, Heckbert SR, Hwang SJ, Liu Y, Sjogren M, van der Pals J, Kälsch H, Mühleisen TW, Nöthen MM, Cupples LA, Caslake M, Di Angelantonio E, Danesh J, Rotter JI, Sigurdsson S, Wong Q, Erbel R, Kathiresan S, Melander O, Gudnason V, O'Donnell CJ, Post WS, CHARGE Extracoronary Calcium Working Group. Genetic associations with valvular calcification and aortic stenosis. N Engl J Med. 2013;368:503–12.
20. Kamstrup PRT-HA, Nordestgaard BG. Elevated lipoprotein(a) and risk of aortic valve stenosis in the general population. J Am Coll Cardiol. 2014;63:470–7.
21. Tsimikas S. A test in context: lipoprotein(a): diagnosis, prognosis, controversies, and emerging therapies. J Am Coll Cardiol. 2017;69:692–711.
22. Tsimikas S. Potential causality and emerging medical therapies for lipoprotein(a) and its associated oxidized phospholipids in calcific aortic valve stenosis. Circ Res. 2019;124:405–15.
23. van Capelleveen JC, van der Valk FM, Stroes ES. Current therapies for lowering lipoprotein (a). J Lipid Res. 2016;57:1612–8.
24. Borrelli MJ, Youssef A, Boffa MB, Koschinsky ML. New frontiers in Lp(a)-targeted therapies. Trends Pharmacol Sci. 2019;40:212–25.
25. Guan WCJ, Steffen BT, et al. Race is a key variable in assigning lipoprotein(a) cutoff values for coronary heart disease risk assessment: the Multi-Ethnic Study of Atherosclerosis. Arterioscler Thromb Vasc Biol. 2015;35:996–1001.
26. Virani SSBA, Davis BC, et al. Associations between lipoprotein(a) levels and cardiovascular outcomes in black and white subjects: the Atherosclerosis Risk in Communities (ARIC) Study. Circulation. 2012;125:241–9.
27. Patel AP, Wang M, Pirruccello JP, Ellinor, PT, Ng K, Kathiresan S, & Khera AV. (2020). Lp(a) (lipoprotein[a]) concentrations and incident atherosclerotic cardiovascular disease. Arteriosclerosis, Thrombosis, and Vascular Biology. 2021;41:465–74.
28. Cao J, Steffen BT, Budoff M, Post WS, Thanassoulis G, Kestenbaum B, McConnell JP, Warnick R, Guan W, Tsai MY. Lipoprotein(a) levels are associated with subclinical calcific aortic valve disease in white and black individuals: the multi-ethnic study of atherosclerosis. Arterioscler Thromb Vasc Biol. 2016;36:1003–9.
29. Steffen BT, Duprez D, Bertoni AG, Guan W, Tsai MY. Lp(a) [lipoprotein(a)]-related risk of heart failure is evident in whites but not in other racial/

ethnic groups. Arterioscler Thromb Vasc Biol. 2018;38:2498–504.
30. Tsimikas S, Fazio S, Viney NJ, Xia S, Witztum JL, Marcovina SM. Relationship of lipoprotein(a) molar concentrations and mass according to lipoprotein(a) thresholds and apolipoprotein(a) isoform size. J Clin Lipidol. 2018;12(5):1313–23.
31. Wieringa G, Toogood AA, Ryder WD, Anderson JM, Mackness M, Shalet SM. Changes in lipoprotein(a) levels measured by six kit methods during growth hormone treatment of growth hormone-deficient adults. Growth Hormon IGF Res. 2000;10:14–9.
32. Dembinski T, Nixon P, Shen G, Mymin D, Choy PC. Evaluation of a new apolipoprotein(a) isoform-independent assay for serum lipoprotein(a). Mol Cell Biochem. 2000;207:149–55.
33. Paré G, Çaku A, McQueen M, Anand SS, Enas E, Clarke R, Boffa MB, Koschinsky M, Wang X, Yusuf S. Lipoprotein(a) levels and the risk of myocardial infarction among 7 ethnic groups. Circulation. 2019;139:1472–82.
34. Lee S-R, Prasad A, Choi Y-S, Xing C, Clopton P, Witztum JL, Tsimikas S. The LPA gene, ethnicity, and cardiovascular events. Circulation. 2016;135(3):251–63.
35. Beheshtian A, Shitole SG, Segal AZ, Leifer D, Tracy RP, Rader DJ, Devereux RB, Kizer JR. Lipoprotein (a) level, apolipoprotein (a) size, and risk of unexplained ischemic stroke in young and middle-aged adults. Atherosclerosis. 2016;253:47–53.
36. Khera AV, Everett BM, Caulfield MP, Hantash FM, Wohlgemuth J, Ridker PM, Mora S. Lipoprotein(a) concentrations, rosuvastatin therapy, and residual vascular risk: an analysis from the JUPITER Trial (Justification for the Use of Statins in Prevention: an Intervention Trial Evaluating Rosuvastatin). Circulation. 2014;129:635–42.
37. Dumitrescu L, Glenn K, Brown-Gentry K, Shephard C, Wong M, Rieder MJ, Smith JD, Nickerson DA, Crawford DC. Variation in LPA is associated with Lp(a) levels in three populations from the Third National Health and Nutrition Examination Survey. PLoS One. 2011;6:e16604.
38. Cegla J, France M, Marcovina SM, Neely RDG. Lp(a): when and how to measure it. Ann Clin Biochem. 2020; https://doi.org/10.1177/0004563220968473.
39. Ridker PM. Anticytokine agents: targeting interleukin signaling pathways for the treatment of atherothrombosis. Circ Res. 2019;124:437–50.
40. Müller N, Schulte DM, Türk K, Freitag-Wolf S, Hampe J, Zeuner R, Schröder JO, Gouni-Berthold I, Berthold HK, Krone W, Rose-John S, Schreiber S, Laudes M. IL-6 blockade by monoclonal antibodies inhibits apolipoprotein (a) expression and lipoprotein (a) synthesis in humans. J Lipid Res. 2015;56:1034–42.
41. Sarwar N, Butterworth AS, Freitag DF, Gregson J, Willeit P, Gorman DN, Gao P, Saleheen D, Rendon A, Nelson CP, Braund PS, Hall AS, Chasman DI, Tybjærg-Hansen A, Chambers JC, Benjamin EJ,

Franks PW, Clarke R, Wilde AA, Trip MD, Steri M, Witteman JC, Qi L, van der Schoot CE, de Faire U, Erdmann J, Stringham HM, Koenig W, Rader DJ, Melzer D, Reich D, Psaty BM, Kleber ME, Panagiotakos DB, Willeit J, Wennberg P, Woodward M, Adamovic S, Rimm EB, Meade TW, Gillum RF, Shaffer JA, Hofman A, Onat A, Sundström J, Wassertheil-Smoller S, Mellström D, Gallacher J, Cushman M, Tracy RP, Kauhanen J, Karlsson M, Salonen JT, Wilhelmsen L, Amouyel P, Cantin B, Best LG, Ben-Shlomo Y, Manson JE, Davey-Smith G, de Bakker PI, O'Donnell CJ, Wilson JF, Wilson AG, Assimes TL, Jansson JO, Ohlsson C, Tivesten Å, Ljunggren Ö, Reilly MP, Hamsten A, Ingelsson E, Cambien F, Hung J, Thomas GN, Boehnke M, Schunkert H, Asselbergs FW, Kastelein JJ, Gudnason V, Salomaa V, Harris TB, Kooner JS, Allin KH, Nordestgaard BG, Hopewell JC, Goodall AH, Ridker PM, Hólm H, Watkins H, Ouwehand WH, Samani NJ, Kaptoge S, Di Angelantonio E, Harari O, Danesh J. Interleukin-6 receptor pathways in coronary heart disease: a collaborative meta-analysis of 82 studies. Lancet (London, England). 2012;379:1205–13.

42. Wensley F, Gao P, Burgess S, Kaptoge S, Di Angelantonio E, Shah T, Engert JC, Clarke R, Davey-Smith G, Nordestgaard BG, Saleheen D, Samani NJ, Sandhu M, Anand S, Pepys MB, Smeeth L, Whittaker J, Casas JP, Thompson SG, Hingorani AD, Danesh J. Association between C reactive protein and coronary heart disease: mendelian randomisation analysis based on individual participant data. BMJ (Clin Res Ed). 2011;342:d548.

43. Ridker PM, Everett BM, Thuren T, MacFadyen JG, Chang WH, Ballantyne C, Fonseca F, Nicolau J, Koenig W, Anker SD, Kastelein JJP, Cornel JH, Pais P, Pella D, Genest J, Cifkova R, Lorenzatti A, Forster T, Kobalava Z, Vida-Simiti L, Flather M, Shimokawa H, Ogawa H, Dellborg M, Rossi PRF, Troquay RPT, Libby P, Glynn RJ. Antiinflammatory therapy with canakinumab for atherosclerotic disease. N Engl J Med. 2017;377:1119–31.

44. Sperling LS, Mechanick JI, Neeland IJ, Herrick CJ, Despres JP, Ndumele CE, Vijayaraghavan K, Handelsman Y, Puckrein GA, Araneta MR, Blum QK, Collins KK, Cook S, Dhurandhar NV, Dixon DL, Egan BM, Ferdinand DP, Herman LM, Hessen SE, Jacobson TA, Pate RR, Ratner RE, Brinton EA, Forker AD, Ritzenthaler LL, Grundy SM. The CardioMetabolic Health Alliance: working toward a new care model for the metabolic syndrome. J Am Coll Cardiol. 2015;66:1050–67.

45. van der Valk FM, Bekkering S, Kroon J, Yeang C, Van den Bossche J, van Buul JD, Ravandi A, Nederveen AJ, Verberne HJ, Scipione C, Nieuwdorp M, Joosten LA, Netea MG, Koschinsky ML, Witztum JL, Tsimikas S, Riksen NP, Stroes ES. Oxidized phospholipids on lipoprotein(a) elicit arterial wall inflam-

mation and an inflammatory monocyte response in humans. Circulation. 2016;134:611–24.

46. von Zychlinski A, Williams M, McCormick S, Kleffmann T. Absolute quantification of apolipoproteins and associated proteins on human plasma lipoproteins. J Proteome. 2014;106:181–90.

47. Guo T, Fan Y, Chen M, Wu X, Zhang L, He T, Wang H, Wan J, Wang X, Lu Z. Cardiovascular implications of fatal outcomes of patients with coronavirus disease 2019 (COVID-19). JAMA Cardiol. 2020;5(7):811–8.

48. Baracchini C, Pieroni A, Viaro F, Cianci V, Cattelan AM, Tiberio I, Munari M, Causin F. Acute stroke management pathway during Coronavirus-19 pandemic. Neurol Sci. 2020;41:1003–5.

49. Khot UN, Reimer AP, Brown A, Hustey FM, Hussain MS, Kapadia SR, Svensson LG. Impact of COVID-19 pandemic on critical care transfers for ST-elevation myocardial infarction, stroke, and aortic emergencies. Circ Cardiovasc Qual Outcomes. 2020;13(8):e006938.

50. Pearson K, Rodriguez F. Lipoprotein(a) and cardiovascular disease prevention across diverse populations. Cardiol Ther. 2020;9(2):275–92.

51. Enkhmaa B, Petersen KS, Kris-Etherton PM, Berglund L. Diet and Lp(a): does dietary change modify residual cardiovascular risk conferred by Lp(a)? Nutrients. 2020;12:2024.

52. Khan TZ, Gorog DA, Arachchillage DJ, Ahnström J, Rhodes S, Donovan J, Banya W, Pottle A, Barbir M, Pennell DJ. Impact of lipoprotein apheresis on thrombotic parameters in patients with refractory angina and raised lipoprotein(a): findings from a randomized controlled cross-over trial. J Clin Lipidol. 2019;13:788–96.

53. Moriarty PM, Hemphill L. Lipoprotein apheresis. Endocrinol Metab Clin N Am. 2016;45:39–54.

54. Warden BA, Minnier J, Watts GF, Fazio S, Shapiro MD. Impact of PCSK9 inhibitors on plasma lipoprotein(a) concentrations with or without a background of niacin therapy. J Clin Lipidol. 2019;13:580–5.

55. Rehberger Likozar A, Zavrtanik M, Šebeštjen M. Lipoprotein(a) in atherosclerosis: from pathophysiology to clinical relevance and treatment options. Ann Med. 2020;52:1–16.

56. Stiekema LCA, Prange KHM, Hoogeveen RM, Verweij SL, Kroon J, Schnitzler JG, Dzobo KE, Cupido AJ, Tsimikas S, Stroes ESG, de Winther MPJ, Bahjat M. Potent lipoprotein(a) lowering following apolipoprotein(a) antisense treatment reduces the pro-inflammatory activation of circulating monocytes in patients with elevated lipoprotein(a). Eur Heart J. 2020;41(24):2262–71.

57. Tadin-Strapps MRM, Le Voci L, Andrews L, Yendluri S, Williams S, Bartz S, Johns DG. Development of lipoprotein(a) siRNAs for mechanism of action studies in non-human primate models of atherosclerosis. J Cardiovasc Transl Res. 2015;8:44–53.

Emerging Precision Medicine Concepts and Cardiovascular Health in African Americans and Hispanics

4

George A. Mensah and Muin J. Khoury

Introduction

The launch of the Precision Medicine Initiative in 2015 created an exciting opportunity and great potential for improving the health of all Americans [1]. This initiative, now renamed the *All of Us* Research Program [2], leverages recent advances in large-scale genomic databases and powerful computational tools and methods for characterizing individual biologic variation in order to personalize the prevention, detection, evaluation, and treatment of human diseases [1]. Although the near-term focus of precision medicine research has been on cancers, there is a clear longer-term aim to generate new knowledge that will be applicable to all diseases including cardiovascular diseases (CVD) and the promotion of cardiovascular health.

The promise of a new era of precision prevention and treatment for CVD is especially relevant to African Americans because of the excess car-

diovascular mortality in this population group [3]. It is also highly relevant to African Americans, Mexican Americans, and other racial and ethnic minority populations with very low prevalences of ideal cardiovascular health metrics [4]. Because of this promise of accelerating health improvements in all Americans, several emerging concepts in precision medicine that have relevance to African Americans, Hispanics, and other racial and ethnic minority populations deserve attention. This chapter reviews several of these emerging concepts beginning with the renewed emphasis on race and ethnicity as social—and not—biological constructs. This chapter concludes with the central issue of trust and the importance of active community engagement as a strategy to increase diversity and inclusion in biomedical research participation as well as to facilitate the translation and implementation of precision medicine discoveries into health impact at the individual and population levels and the promotion of health equity.

Race, Ethnicity, and Genetic Ancestry

The promise of precision medicine and the *All of Us* Research Program have rekindled interest in, and examination of how race, ethnicity, and genetic ancestry are used in biomedical research

G. A. Mensah (✉)
Center for Translation Research and Implementation Science (CTRIS), National Heart, Lung, and Blood Institute, National Institutes of Health, Bethesda, MD, USA
e-mail: George.Mensah@nih.gov

M. J. Khoury
Office of Genomics and Precision Public Health, Centers for Disease Control and Prevention, Atlanta, GA, USA
e-mail: muk1@cdc.gov

© This is a U.S. government work and not under copyright protection in the U.S.; foreign copyright protection may apply 2021
K. C. Ferdinand et al. (eds.), *Cardiovascular Disease in Racial and Ethnic Minority Populations*, Contemporary Cardiology, https://doi.org/10.1007/978-3-030-81034-4_4

[5–7]. Race and ethnicity are important categories in clinical medicine and public health practice and research. However, they are social, political, and cultural constructs and not biological variables [5, 6, 8]. Nevertheless, there are substantial biological determinants that differ among people of different self-identified race or ethnicity. Many of these differences are driven by population history and relevant geographic ancestral markers while others are influenced by other mechanisms that are incompletely understood (epigenetics, metabolic pathways, microbiome, circulating RNA) and in continuous interaction with individual, social, environmental and structural factors [5].

Unlike race and ethnicity, genetic ancestry is a biological construct that reflects the architecture of genome variation between populations [9, 10]. Using a set of ancestry informative markers, which are genetic loci with alleles demonstrating significant frequency differences between populations, ancestry can be determined at the individual and population level [9–11]. For example, in their study of the genetic ancestry of 5269 self-described African Americans, 8663 Latinos, and 148,789 European Americans, Bryc et al. demonstrated the presence of "pervasive mixed ancestry" in all groups studied [11]. They showed that persons who self-identified as Latinos encompassed nearly all possible combinations of African, Native American, and European ancestries, with the exception of individuals who have a mix of African and Native American ancestry without European ancestry [11]. Thus, self-reported race/ethnicity is less reliable for the Hispanic-American population when compared to ancestry-informative genetic markers [11].

These new findings call for increased collaboration between research investigators, research funding agencies, medical and scientific journal editors, and the general public to advance the development of best practices in research study design, data collection, data interpretation, and more precision in the appropriate use of race, ethnicity, and genetic ancestry information. Within this emerging concept, it is important to emphasize that although race and ethnicity are not biological or genetic constructs, they remain very important in clinical and public health practice and research, especially as we undertake efforts to advance health equity.

The Lack of Diversity in Genomics Research Resources

There is a well-recognized Eurocentric bias in extant genome-wide association studies (GWAS) and genomic biorepositories that has tremendous implications for precision medicine and the prediction of disease risk in African Americans, Hispanics, and racial and ethnic populations worldwide. For example, in their recent report on "the missing diversity" in genomic studies, Sirugo et al. [12] demonstrated that, as of 2018, the majority of GWAS participants, based on self-identified race/ethnicity, have been European (78%) or Asians (10%) while Africans, Hispanics, and all other ethnicities make up only 2%, 1%, and less than 1%, respectively [12].

Citing examples from sickle cell disease, cystic fibrosis, and transthyretin amyloid cardiomyopathy—an important and underdiagnosed cause of heart failure in African Americans—Sirugo et al. [12] make a compelling case for why the continued lack of diversity in genomics research impedes our progress in fully understanding the genetic architecture of human disease [12]. In addition, the lack of diversity and inclusion in genomics studies creates challenges for replication of findings across different ancestry populations and barriers for dissemination and implementation of research findings. In response to this research gap, several NIH-funded large genomics studies such as the Trans-Omics for Precision Medicine (TOPMed) program [13], the Human Health and Heredity in Africa (H3Africa) [14], and Population Architecture using Genomics and Epidemiology (PAGE) [15] have large participant representation from non-European ancestry populations. For example, currently, nearly 60% of the 155,000 sequenced participants in the TOPMed program are of predominantly non-European ancestry (Fig. 4.1) [13].

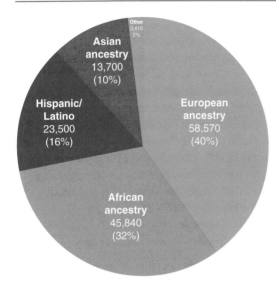

Fig. 4.1 Participant diversity in the Trans-Omics for Precision Medicine (TOPMed) Program. Currently, nearly 60% of the 155,000 sequenced participants in TOPMed are of predominantly non-European ancestry. Being Hispanic/Latino can correspond with either European, African, Amerindian and/or Asian ancestry. A significant proportion of Hispanics will have predominant European ancestry. (Source: National Heart, Lung, and Blood Institute. https://www.nhlbiwgs.org/)

Misclassification of Benign Variants as Genetic Misdiagnosis

Another important emerging concept is the potential for misclassification of benign variants as pathogenic that could lead to genetic misdiagnoses in African Americans, Hispanics, and other racial and ethnic populations currently underrepresented in GWAS and genomics databases. Manrai and colleagues use the example of hypertrophic cardiomyopathy to illustrate this concept [16]. Hypertrophic cardiomyopathy, defined by the presence of increased left ventricular wall thickness that is unexplained by abnormal left ventricular loading conditions, is the most common inherited cardiovascular disease with a complex and heterogeneous clinical presentation [17, 18]. Among its most serious clinical presentations are ventricular arrhythmias, heart failure, left ventricular outflow tract obstruction, and sudden cardiac death [17]. Although previously considered a disease attributed to sarcomeric protein gene mutations [18], recent studies suggest that pathogenic sarcomere mutations may be absent in up to 70% of patients [19]; and other genetic and non-genetic causes have been established [17]. Additionally, more than 2000 variants in at least 11 genes encoding proteins of the cardiac sarcomere or related structures have been reported in clinical genetic testing of probands with hypertrophic cardiomyopathy [20].

Manrai et al. showed that five high-frequency variants out of 94 identified mutations accounted for nearly 75% of the overall genotype prevalence signal in their study and that all five high-frequency variants associated with hypertrophic cardiomyopathy had significantly greater frequencies among African Americans than among white Americans [16]. Significant differences in allele frequencies between groups may lead to misdiagnosis and contribute to health disparities because of the lack of racial and ethnic diversity in control populations. They hypothesized that genetic variants that are common in African Americans had previously been misclassified in patients undergoing genetic testing for hypertrophic cardiomyopathy [16]. They point out that this phenomenon could contribute to health disparities independent of access to care but simply a result of "historical dearth of control populations that include persons of diverse racial and ethnic backgrounds." [16]

Polygenic Risk Scores and the Potential to Exacerbate Health Disparities

Polygenic risk scores, derived from the combination of a large number of genetic variants each associated with a small increase in disease risk, are gaining increased clinical and public health attention because of their potential to identify individuals at significantly increased risk from specific common diseases and even offer insights on appropriate screening, evaluation, prevention, and treatment strategies [21, 22]. However, an important emerging concept of considerable concern is the notion that clinical use of tools, strategies, and applications such as the polygenic risk score that are predominantly based on the current Eurocentric GWAS information has the real potential to exacerbate health disparities [21–23].

The basis for this concern includes the fact that allele frequencies and effect sizes of common polymorphisms used in polygenic risk scores vary substantially with population ancestry. Nevertheless, the proportion of individuals of non-European ancestry in GWAS has stagnated and may have declined since 2014 [24]. Thus, polygenic risk scores derived from GWAS from participants of mostly European ancestry will not have optimal risk prediction in populations of a different ancestry [21–24]. For example, Martin et al. [24] examined how prediction accuracy deteriorated across globally diverse populations for 17 anthropometric and blood-panel traits in the UK Biobank when European-derived summary statistics were used and demonstrated that prediction accuracy (relative to Europeans) was substantially lower in Hispanic/Latino Americans and South Asians (1.6-fold lower), East Asians (2.0-fold lower), and 4.5-fold lower in Africans [24]. Solutions proposed to address this challenge include diversifying the ancestry populations in GWAS studies and ensuring diversity and inclusion in related clinical trials [21–24]. In addition, Martin et al. [24] have called on existing multi-ancestral GWAS projects and consortia to consider releasing finer-scale continental ancestries and phenotypes to enable ancestry-matched analyses that are not possible with current summary statistics, and to increase data access and data sharing.

Trust and Patient Engagement

There are substantial benefits for diversifying ancestral populations in genomics studies, and in sustaining active participation of African Americans, Hispanics, and other racial and ethnic minority populations currently underrepresented in genomics research. Without such diversification, many of the emerging concepts raised in this chapter cannot be addressed. In particular, the misclassification of benign variants as pathogenic in underrepresented ancestry populations and the relatively lower predictive accuracy of polygenic risk scores compared to European Americans cannot be ameliorated without vastly

diversifying the underlying GWAS data upon which these applications are built.

In the African American population, an important challenge to diversity in genomic studies is distrust in biomedical research, research organizations, and investigators because of the historical legacy of the Tuskegee study of untreated syphilis and other unethical human experimentation [25–27]. There is also a perception of potential use of research findings to stigmatize or discriminate at the individual, community and population levels [27, 28].

The extensive systematic review by Scherr et al. [27] documented that the overarching theme of distrust was present in most studies; however, African Americans were not uniformly distrustful of biomedical research and research investigators, and that some studies found that African American participants trusted medical research and were favorable to research participation [27]. Similarly, Sankaré et al. [26] found high levels of research participation in African Americans and Latino community residents when recruitment strategies emerged from the community itself. Active outreach efforts and engagement of African American and Hispanic/Latino communities based on mutual respect, transparency, and a sustained commitment to clarify the benefits and harms of research will be necessary. Equally importantly, a commitment to honor the established principles of participant privacy and protections as well as the ethical, legal and social implications of genomics research will go a long way to rebuild trust and engagement in genomics research to support precision medicine [26–29].

Conclusion

Although the genetic contributions to various diseases will be increasingly leveraged to advance precision prevention and treatment of CVD, a major unresolved issue is whether these advances will improve or worsen current CVD disparities in racial and ethnic minority populations. The emerging concepts discussed in this chapter suggest that the lack of diversity in genomics studies risk exacerbating existing disparities.

Strategies that directly address diversity and inclusion will need to explore ancestry-matched controls, as well as cultural, social, and environmental determinants. Current NIH efforts such as TOPMed and the *All of Us* Research Program will go a long way to ensure diversification of precision medicine efforts. Another major challenge is that of unequal healthcare access and delivery. Designing interventions for a broad reach in racial and ethnic minority populations will be needed to ensure the success of precision medicine.

Disclaimer The views expressed in this chapter are those of the authors and do not necessarily represent the views of the National Institutes of Health, Centers for Disease Control and Prevention, or the U.S. Department of Health and Human Services.

Conflict of Interest Disclosure None

References

1. Collins FS, Varmus H. A new initiative on precision medicine. N Engl J Med. 2015;372(9):793–5.
2. National Institutes of Health. All of Us Research Program. 2016. https://www.nih.gov/research-training/allofus-research-program. Published 2016. Accessed 15 July 2019.
3. National Center for Health Statistics. Health, United States, 2017: with special feature on mortality. Hyattsville: U.S. Department of Health and Human Services; 2018.
4. Brown AF, Liang LJ, Vassar SD, et al. Trends in racial/ethnic and nativity disparities in cardiovascular health among adults without prevalent cardiovascular disease in the United States, 1988 to 2014. Ann Intern Med. 2018;168(8):541–9.
5. Bonham VL, Green ED, Perez-Stable EJ. Examining how race, ethnicity, and ancestry data are used in biomedical research. JAMA. 2018;320(15):1533–4.
6. Bonham VL, Green ED, Perez-Stable EJ. Race and ethnicity data in research-reply. JAMA. 2019;321(12):1218.
7. Caulfield T, Fullerton SM, Ali-Khan SE, et al. Race and ancestry in biomedical research: exploring the challenges. Genome Med. 2009;1(1):8.
8. Burchard EG, Ziv E, Coyle N, et al. The importance of race and ethnic background in biomedical research and clinical practice. N Engl J Med. 2003;348(12):1170–5.
9. Kittles RA, Weiss KM. Race, ancestry, and genes: implications for defining disease risk. Annu Rev Genomics Hum Genet. 2003;4:33–67.
10. Dries DL. Genetic ancestry, population admixture, and the genetic epidemiology of complex disease. Circ Cardiovasc Genet. 2009;2(6):540–3.
11. Bryc K, Durand EY, Macpherson JM, Reich D, Mountain JL. The genetic ancestry of African Americans, Latinos, and European Americans across the United States. Am J Hum Genet. 2015;96(1):37–53.
12. Sirugo G, Williams SM, Tishkoff SA. The missing diversity in human genetic studies. Cell. 2019;177(1):26–31.
13. National Heart, Lung, and Blood Institute. Trans-Omics for Precision Medicine (TOPMed) Program. NHLBI. 2016. https://www.nhlbi.nih.gov/research/resources/nhlbi-precision-medicine-initiative/topmed. Published 2016.
14. Human Heredity and health in Africa. H3Africa Vision. https://h3africa.org/index.php/about/vision/. Accessed 8 Dec 2018.
15. Matise TC, Ambite JL, Buyske S, et al. The Next PAGE in understanding complex traits: design for the analysis of Population Architecture Using Genetics and Epidemiology (PAGE) Study. Am J Epidemiol. 2011;174(7):849–59.
16. Manrai AK, Funke BH, Rehm HL, et al. Genetic misdiagnoses and the potential for health disparities. N Engl J Med. 2016;375(7):655–65.
17. Elliott PM, Anastasakis A, Borger MA, et al. 2014 ESC Guidelines on diagnosis and management of hypertrophic cardiomyopathy: the Task Force for the Diagnosis and Management of Hypertrophic Cardiomyopathy of the European Society of Cardiology (ESC). Eur Heart J. 2014;35(39):2733–79.
18. Sabater-Molina M, Perez-Sanchez I, Hernandez Del Rincon JP, Gimeno JR. Genetics of hypertrophic cardiomyopathy: a review of current state. Clin Genet. 2018;93(1):3–14.
19. Maron BJ, Maron MS, Maron BA, Loscalzo J. Moving beyond the sarcomere to explain heterogeneity in hypertrophic cardiomyopathy: JACC review topic of the week. J Am Coll Cardiol. 2019;73(15):1978–86.
20. Alfares AA, Kelly MA, McDermott G, et al. Results of clinical genetic testing of 2,912 probands with hypertrophic cardiomyopathy: expanded panels offer limited additional sensitivity. Genet Med. 2015;17(11):880–8.
21. Natarajan P, Young R, Stitziel NO, et al. Polygenic risk score identifies subgroup with higher burden of atherosclerosis and greater relative benefit from statin therapy in the primary prevention setting. Circulation. 2017;135(22):2091–101.
22. Khera AV, Chaffin M, Aragam KG, et al. Genome-wide polygenic scores for common diseases identify individuals with risk equivalent to monogenic mutations. Nat Genet. 2018;50(9):1219–24.
23. Roberts MC, Khoury MJ, Mensah GA. Perspective: the clinical use of polygenic risk scores: race, ethnicity, and health disparities. Ethn Dis. 2019;29(3):513–6.

24. Martin AR, Kanai M, Kamatani Y, Okada Y, Neale BM, Daly MJ. Clinical use of current polygenic risk scores may exacerbate health disparities. Nat Genet. 2019;51(4):584–91.

25. White RM. Misinformation and misbeliefs in the Tuskegee Study of Untreated Syphilis fuel mistrust in the healthcare system. J Natl Med Assoc. 2005;97(11):1566–73.

26. Sankare IC, Bross R, Brown AF, et al. Strategies to build trust and recruit African American and Latino Community Residents for Health Research: a Cohort Study. Clin Transl Sci. 2015;8(5):10.

27. Scherr CL, Ramesh S, Marshall-Fricker C, Perera MA. A review of African Americans' beliefs and attitudes about genomic studies: opportunities for message design. Front Genet. 2019;10:548.

28. Clayton EW. Ethical, legal, and social implications of genomic medicine. N Engl J Med. 2003;349(6):562–9.

29. Ceballos RM, Knerr S, Scott MA, et al. Latino beliefs about biomedical research participation: a qualitative study on the U.S.-Mexico border. J Empir Res Hum Res Ethics. 2014;9(4):10–21.

The Implementation Frontier: Impact on Cardiovascular Health in Racial and Ethnic Minority Populations

5

George A. Mensah

Introduction

The dramatic declines in the death rate from cardiovascular diseases (CVD), principally heart disease and stroke, represent one of the greatest public health achievements of the twentieth century [1, 2]. For example, from 1950 to 2017, the age-adjusted death rate declined 72% for heart disease and nearly 79% for stroke [3]. Although these remarkable improvements were seen in both men and women and in all racial-ethnic groups at the national level, the national data mask important differences at the sub-national level. This is particularly true for population groups defined by race, ethnicity, gender, geography, income, education, and other social and environmental determinants of health [3, 4]. In essence, cardiovascular disparities remain pervasive despite remarkable national progress in cardiovascular health.

The reasons for these disparities are numerous and include important differences in the quality of healthcare delivered to different groups as documented in the Institute for Medicine report: *"Unequal Treatment: Confronting Racial and Ethnic Disparities in Health Care."* [5] As correctly pointed out in the report, unequal treatment reflects a myriad factors including access to care, adverse socioeconomic conditions, communication and other cross-cultural challenges, and mismatched patient and provider attitudes and expectations. Nevertheless, even after adjusting for these factors, race and ethnicity remain significant predictors of the quality of healthcare received [5]. In fact, for the 15th year in a row, the Agency for Healthcare Research and Quality's comprehensive overview of the quality of healthcare received by the general US population and disparities in care experienced by different racial and socioeconomic groups demonstrates that racial and ethnic disparities remain pervasive [6].

This chapter explores one aspect of unequal treatment—the failure to accelerate and optimize the implementation of evidence-based, proven-effective interventions in African American and Hispanic patients at high risk for cardiovascular morbidity and mortality. This chapter first explores the challenges inherent in this "implementation frontier" and a framework for exploring strategies to address these challenges. It then provides selected examples of "underuse" of evidence-based guideline recommendations as well as overuse of ineffective or low-value interventions in African American and Hispanic patients [7, 8]. These examples are discussed as scenarios where accelerated adoption, scale-up, and increased adherence to

G. A. Mensah (✉)
Center for Translation Research and Implementation Science (CTRIS), National Heart, Lung, and Blood Institute, National Institutes of Health, Bethesda, MD, USA
e-mail: George.Mensah@nih.gov

K. C. Ferdinand et al. (eds.), *Cardiovascular Disease in Racial and Ethnic Minority Populations*, Contemporary Cardiology, https://doi.org/10.1007/978-3-030-81034-4_5

35

guideline-recommended treatment can contribute significantly to reducing documented cardiovascular disparities. This chapter concludes with examples of roles that implementors such as healthcare providers, health systems, and policymakers can play, as well as the implications for clinical practice and research.

Implementation Challenges

Within the context of best practices for high-quality healthcare, "implementation" represents the successful adoption, adaptation, and sustained adherence to evidence-based, guideline-recommended practices for the prevention, detection, evaluation, treatment, and control of diseases and the promotion of health. In essence, implementation is the successful translation of research evidence into routine clinical and public health practice; and implementation science represents the broad field of scientific inquiry that seeks to accelerate the adoption and integration of evidence-based interventions, tools, strategies, and policies into routine clinical and public health practice [9].

For the general population, implementation challenges are numerous. For example, Balas and Boren estimated that it takes an average of 17 years for only 15% of scientific discovery to enter routine practice [10]. Several studies have also shown that Americans, on average, receive only half of guideline-recommended preventive and treatment interventions for quality healthcare [11, 12]. For African Americans and Hispanics, the implementation challenges are even greater. They have a higher prevalence of socioeconomic challenges, lack of health insurance, lower access to care, lower educational attainment, and greater linguistic barriers in the healthcare environment. In fact, some African American, Hispanic, and other racial and ethnic minority groups are at an increased risk of what has been described in the literature as "double jeopardy"—where instances of underuse of high-value interventions coexist with clinical overuse of ineffective or low-value interventions [7, 8]. Other implementation challenges include implicit bias [13, 14], as well as institutional and structural racism [5, 15, 16].

Figure 5.1 shows the major stakeholders in the implementation context with the patient at the center of the implementation ecosystem. Healthcare providers, health systems, the community, and policymakers all play crucial roles as implementors in helping traverse the implementation frontier in addressing underuse and

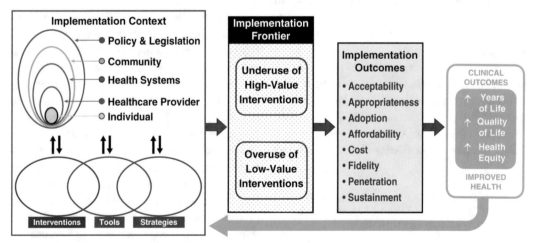

Fig. 5.1 The implementation frontier. Underuse of high-value interventions and overuse of ineffective or low-value interventions constitute important challenges in efforts to maximize the years and quality of life and achieve health equity

overuse. The primary challenges in the implementation frontier are underuse of high-value interventions and overuse of ineffective or low-value interventions. Fortunately, several validated implementation research frameworks are available to guide the development and testing of strategies to address underuse and overuse [17–23]. Important are the implementation research outcomes of acceptability, affordability, adoption, costs, reach, sustainability, fidelity, and sustainment of interventions, tools, and strategies [24]. Reducing disparities and improving health equity in this effort are as important as improving overall years and quality of life. Several examples are provided in subsequent sections of this chapter to highlight specific clinical settings where traversing this implementation frontier presents unique opportunities for reducing disparities in cardiovascular care for racial and ethnic minorities.

Hypertension Treatment and Control

The treatment and control of hypertension presents excellent examples of the substantial successes made over the last four decades in the United States [25–31], as well as the significant concerns regarding implementation challenges in racial and ethnic minorities [26, 31]. For example, in 1976–1980, the National Health and Nutrition Examination Surveys (NHANES II) showed that hypertension awareness (using blood pressure partition values of 140 mmHg and 90 mmHg diastolic) was only 50% in black men with corresponding treatment and control rates of 24% and 5%, respectively [25]. In black women, the awareness, treatment, and control rates were 77%, 49%, and 17%, respectively [25]. Awareness rates have improved dramatically in black men and women to the current levels of 80% or greater with corresponding treatment rates of 68.4% and 81.2% in black men and women, respectively [32]. Importantly, awareness and treatment levels are lowest among Mexican American men (68.5% and 57.7%) and Mexican American women (80.8% and 73.1%).

These data represent important progress; however, considering that hypertension control rates of 80–90% are achievable today [28–30], the control rates of 37%, 41.6%, and 49.2% in Mexican American men, non-Hispanic black men, and Mexican American women, respectively, represent important implementation challenges [32]. After all, the Kaiser Permanente Southern California (KPSC) health system with a large ethnically diverse population of more than 3.6 million (39% Hispanic, 8% Black, 9% Asian/Pacific Islander, 19% others/Unknown) achieved hypertension control rates over 85% in 6 years [30]. Similarly, Jaffe et al. successfully improved hypertension control in the Kaiser Permanente Northern California health system from 44% to 90% in 13 years [29]. A recent analysis of 8.8 million veterans of whom 3.2 million were hypertensive showed that hypertension control rates improved from 46% in 2000 to 81% in 2010, although control rates subsequently declined to 76% in 2014 [33]. Blacks had higher systolic blood pressure (by 2.1 mm Hg) and lower control rates (by 5.6%) than Whites for all age groups [33]. The Veterans Affairs study is an excellent example of the use of electronic health record data (containing more than 241 million blood pressure readings in this example) to examine implementation challenges in hypertension management.

In their analysis of elderly enrollees in Medicare Advantage health plans in 2011 who had hypertension, cardiovascular disease, or diabetes, Ayanian et al. compared successful control of these conditions in 2011 to control rates in 2006 as well as to control rates at the national level and within regions and health plans [34]. They demonstrated that black enrollees in 2006 and 2011 were substantially less likely than white enrollees to have successful control of blood pressure, cholesterol, or glycated hemoglobin; Hispanic enrollees were less likely than whites to have adequate control of all three measures in 2011; and Asians and Pacific Islanders were more likely than whites to have adequate control of blood pressure and cholesterol but had similar control of glycated hemoglobin [34]. The study noted that differing distribution of enrollees among health plans was responsible for 39%–59% of observed disparities in 2011; but most importantly, although the disparities persisted in 2011 in the Northeast, Midwest, and South, they were eliminated in the West for all three measures suggesting that these disparities can be eliminated [34].

Cardiac Catheterization and Invasive Coronary Procedures

The evidence for the pervasiveness of racial and ethnic disparities in cardiac catherization and invasive coronary interventions is extensive [35–39]. In their classic study of the effect of race and sex on physicians' recommendations for cardiac catheterization, Schulman et al. [37] elegantly demonstrated that a patient's race and sex independently influenced how physicians manage chest pain. In that study, blacks were 40% less likely to be referred for cardiac catheterization than men and whites; and black women, in particular, were significantly (60%) less likely to be referred for catheterization than white men. This study is believed to have played an important role in the genesis of the Institute of Medicine report *"Unequal Treatment"* published in 2002 [5].

To examine the impact of the IOM report and related national initiatives to reduce disparities in cardiovascular interventions, Bolorunduro et al. conducted a retrospective analysis of data on two million patients managed for acute ST elevation myocardial infarction (STEMI) from 1998 to 2007 using the National Inpatient Sample [40]. The analysis adjusted for gender, insurance status, comorbidities, hospital bed size, as well as hospital location and teaching status. The main study findings were that racial and ethnic disparities persisted; and that the receipt of primary percutaneous coronary intervention (PCI) after STEMI was 29.1% in Caucasians, 23.3% in African Americans, and 28.3% in Hispanics. Compared to Caucasians, African Americans and Hispanics were 26% and 16% less likely to receive primary PCI [40].

Racial and ethnic disparities that also persist in the use and outcomes of drug-eluting stents [41–44] are considered superior to bare metal stents for preventing repeat revascularization and stent thrombosis in patients receiving coronary stents [45]. Hannan and colleagues used the New York State's Percutaneous Coronary Interventions Reporting System (PCIRS), which contains detailed clinical and demographic information on patients as well as data on the type and brand of stent used, to examine disparities in the use of drug-eluting stents and the relative contribution of hospital practice pattern variation in comparison with patient characteristics [41]. The study concluded that disparities by race, ethnicity, and insurance status persist in the use of DES in patients receiving coronary stents; and that African Americans and Hispanics were 30% and 20% less likely, to receive DES than their white counterparts [41].

Utilization of Structural Heart Disease Interventions

Compared with coronary interventions, much less is known about disparities in the utilization and outcomes of interventions for structural heart diseases such as the repair and replacement of heart valves. To study this, Alkhouli et al. [46] used the 2011–2016 National Inpatient Sample to examine racial and ethnic differences in the utilization, in-hospital outcomes, and cost of hospitalizations for transcatheter aortic valve replacement (TAVR), transcatheter mitral valve repair (TMVr), and left atrial appendage occlusion (LAAO). To minimize the impact of a lack of health insurance as a confounding factor, the study included only patients aged 65 years or older; most of whom are eligible for health insurance coverage under the Centers of Medicare & Medicaid Services. The in-hospital morbidity, mortality, and cost of these common structural heart disease interventions were comparable white, black, and Hispanic patients. However, there were statistically significantly higher utilization rates in whites compared with blacks and Hispanics for TAVR (43.1 vs. 18.0 vs. 21.1), TMVR (5.0 vs. 3.2 vs. 3.2), and LAAO (6.6 versus 2.1 versus 3.5), respectively [46]. Although blacks and Hispanics constitute 11% and 7%, respectively, of the overall elderly population in the United States, they made up only 4% of the patients receiving these interventions in the period of 2011–2016 [46].

Prevention and Treatment of Heart Failure

The health and economic burden of heart failure continues to rise in the United States fueled in large part by the aging population. This trend is projected to exacerbate heart failure disparities in part because African Americans have early onset of the disease, greater incidence, are more likely to be hospitalized with heart failure, and have a 34% greater risk-adjusted mortality rate in comparison to white counterparts [47]. Additionally, racial and ethnic disparities in overall clinical presentation, hospitalization, treatment, quality of care, and clinical outcomes remain pervasive [48, 49]. For example, black men have the highest proportion of heart failure presentations with reduced ejection fraction (approximately 70%), while white women have the highest proportion of clinical presentations as hospitalizations with preserved ejection fraction (approximately 60%) [32].

Using a nationally representative prospective cohort of adults aged 45 years and older, Dupre et al. examined racial and ethnic differences in trajectories of hospitalization in men and women with heart failure in the United States [50]. Although no racial and ethnic differences were noted for men at hospitalization, Hispanic men had significant declines in hospitalizations after diagnosis followed by a substantial increase in hospitalizations at later stages of heart failure [50]. However, in women, hospitalizations were consistently high for black women at diagnosis and throughout the follow-up period in comparison with white women. The study also demonstrated that racial and ethnic disparities varied by place of residence and disparities persisted after adjusting for multiple factors including psychosocial, behavioral, and physiological factors [50].

Patients with severe, refractory, or advanced heart failure have a very poor prognosis and typically require care by teams that include a cardiologist with expertise in heart failure to offer potential options such as mechanical circulatory support, cardiac transplantation, and palliative care to improve quality of life and prognosis. For example, several studies have shown that among patients hospitalized for heart failure, in-patient care by a cardiologist is associated with clinical practice guideline-recommended treatments, reduced readmissions, and improved survival [51–53]. Nevertheless, African Americans hospitalized with heart failure [54], including those admitted to the intensive care unit with a primary diagnosis of heart failure [55], were less likely than Caucasians to receive primary care by a cardiologist.

Similarly, despite compelling evidence that African American patients eligible for left ventricular assist device (LVAD) implantation derive similar benefits as Caucasians [56], they remain less likely to receive an LVAD [56, 57]. For example, although LVAD implantations increased the fastest among African American Medicare beneficiaries over the period of 2004–2011, they constituted only 7.7% of the 612 patients who received the device in 2011 [56]; and Asian, Hispanic, North American Native, and all other race-ethnic groups other than black or white constituted only 4.7% of Medicare beneficiaries who received LVADs in 2011. A similar level of systematic racial/ethnic underutilization has been demonstrated for the use of cardiac resynchronization therapy (CRT) for advanced heart failure [58, 59]. For example, Farmer et al. [59] showed that black and Hispanic patients who were eligible for implantation of CRT with defibrillator were less likely to receive therapy compared with white patients; and Sridhar et al. demonstrated that gender and racial disparities favoring men (71.4%) and white patients (79.6%) remain significant and pervasive [58].

Anticoagulation in Atrial Fibrillation

The recent focused update of the guideline-recommended management of patients with atrial fibrillation from the American College of Cardiology, American Heart Association, and the

Heart Rhythm Society calls for extending the indications for the use of novel direct-acting oral anticoagulants (DOACs) and eliminating aspirin as an alternative antithrombotic strategy for patients with atrial fibrillation [60]. Although racial, ethnic, and socioeconomic disparities exist in the use of anticoagulation for the prevention of ischemic stroke in patients with atrial fibrillation [61, 62], it is not known whether these disparities will also be present in the use of the novel DOACs and what impact the updated guideline recommendations would have. Understanding the implementation challenges would be invaluable for improving adherence to this guideline recommendation as well as overall quality care and reducing the known disparities in anticoagulation in atrial fibrillation.

The findings from the Outcomes Registry for Better Informed Treatment of Atrial Fibrillation II (ORBIT-AF II) provide some important lessons. This prospective, US-based registry included 12,417 outpatients (5.2% black and 5.4% Hispanic) aged 21 years and older who had non-transient atrial fibrillation enrolled and followed up from February 2013 to July 2016. The study examined the type of anticoagulation used, as well as the quality of anticoagulation management [63]. Receipt of DOACs in the setting of CHA2DS2-VASc scores of 2 or more was lower in both black patients (67.5%) and Hispanic patients (69.9%) compared to white patients (77.0%) [63]. Importantly, disparities in the receipt of DOACs were seen between blacks and whites but not between whites and Hispanics when CHA2DS2-VASc scores were less than 2 [63]. Overall, black patients were 25% less likely to receive oral anticoagulation in accordance with guideline recommendation for stroke prevention and nearly 40% less likely to receive DOACs [63]. Importantly, the quality of anticoagulation therapy in black and Hispanic patients was noted to be inferior to that in white patients, with lower time spent in guideline-recommended therapeutic range (for patients on warfarin) and substantially greater underdosing in patients taking DOACs [63]. Adjustment for socioeconomic factors reduced black–white disparities in DOAC use, but the race effect remained significant [63].

The Florida Puerto Rico Atrial Fibrillation (FLiPER-AF) Stroke Study provides information on patients with ischemic stroke secondary to atrial fibrillation who were anticoagulated as a secondary prevention strategy. The 24,040 patients included 10% black, 12% Florida-Hispanics, and 4% Puerto Rico-Hispanic patients. Black patients had the highest rate of being discharged on aspirin and warfarin and the lowest rate of DOACs at time of discharge [64]. In fact, even after adjustment for age, insurance status, stroke severity, stroke risk, renal function, and hospital academic status, black patients had a 22% greater chance of being prescribed warfarin, rather than DOACs, in comparison with white patients at discharge [64]. The causes of these disparities are complex and uncertain; however, the authors emphasized the "possible influence of unconscious bias or lack of awareness of existing treatment disparities in practitioner decision-making" [64]. Of note, DOAC underuse was not noted in Hispanic patients from Puerto Rico.

The Role for Diverse Actors in the Implementation Context

Although the patient is central to all aspects of healthcare delivery, the challenges of underuse and overuse in the implementation frontier cannot be addressed by patients. These challenges fall on healthcare providers, the health systems within which they operate, the community at large, and policy and legislation that impact the delivery of healthcare. Importantly, no single actor in the implementation context shown in Fig. 5.1 can successfully address these challenges on their own. However, multiple actors acting with the common vision of providing the highest quality care for all patients are likely to be successful. Dissemination and implementation research in health to identify strategies for accelerating the sustained adoption of evidence-based, high-value, guideline-recommended practices in racial and ethnic populations that manifest cardiovascular disparities is invaluable.

For example, healthcare providers need ready access to trustworthy guidelines with appropriate tools for decision support at the point-of-care that take into account known underuse of high-value diagnostic and therapeutic at the local practice level [65]. In one systematic review, routine audit and feedback, as well as educational outreach visits with providers, were generally effective, while the use of provider incentives had, at best, mixed effectiveness in both process-of-care outcomes and clinical effectiveness outcomes in guideline adherence [66]. In this systematic review, the use of reminders for providers had mixed effectiveness for process-of-care outcomes and was generally ineffective for clinical outcomes [66]. Strategies targeting guideline adherence are important but will not be enough. We also need programs that directly address implicit provider bias, cultural competency, medical mistrust, and help improve provider–patient communication in cardiovascular care delivery, as well as medical training [67–70]. The full support of the clinics, hospitals, health systems, and communities within which healthcare is delivered is needed for this to be successful (Fig. 5.1).

There is an important role for policy and legislation in addressing the challenges inherent in the implementation frontier. Policy and legislation can create incentives that reward quality healthcare delivery and withdraw support or levy penalties for medical overuse. A detailed discussion of this concept is beyond the scope of this chapter; however, as an example, a brief overview of current national efforts in hospital cardiovascular outcome measures in federal pay-for-reporting and pay-for-performance programs has been provided by Spivack et al. [71] Other important recent publications highlight caveats and lessons learned [72–78]. It should be noted that the potential for policies to have the unintended consequence of exacerbating disparities has been reported [79, 80].

Research Implications

The implementation frontier challenges of overuse and underuse present unique opportunities for social science and biomedical research to help chart an agenda for reducing cardiovascular health disparities evident in the care that African Americans, Hispanics, and other racial and ethnic minorities receive. There are many gaps in our fundamental understanding of the why, when, and the scope of overuse in racial and ethnic minorities, as well as its primary drivers and sustaining factors [81]. The National Heart, Lung, and Blood Institute and other Institutes and Centers at the National Institutes of Health remain committed to supporting dissemination and implementation research to address health disparities [82–85]. The good news is that there are examples of programs that have been successful in reducing or eliminating disparities in cardiovascular care [86–89]. Research that helps replicate these successes, as well as identify the primary drivers of success, will be invaluable. Equally important will be efforts to scale up and spread successful programs, as well as learn from programs that fail.

Conclusion

From the perspective of healthcare providers, policymakers, and health systems, the implementation frontier embodies the impediments that stand in the way of turning discovery science into maximum health impact at the individual and population levels. It represents underuse of high-value, proven-effective interventions, and overuse of low-value and ineffective interventions—a scenario termed "double jeopardy" that is often seen in African American and Hispanic populations and an important contributor to pervasive racial and ethnic disparities in cardiovascular health. Selected examples used to demonstrate the challenges at the frontier include disparities in the treatment and control of hypertension; referrals for cardiac catheterization and invasive coronary procedures; utilization of structural heart disease interventions; prevention and treatment of heart failure; and the quality of anticoagulation for the primary and secondary prevention of ischemic stroke in atrial fibrillation.

A framework that articulates the elements of the implementation context, as well as the implementation outcomes that need to be addressed in order to traverse the implementation frontier, has been presented. Healthcare professionals and multiple stakeholders have important roles to play in addressing the adverse impact of the implementation frontier by actively disseminating and implementing best practices in African American and Hispanic communities where the double jeopardy is common and contributes to pervasive disparities in cardiovascular health.

The National Heart, Lung, and Blood Institute remains committed to working with other Institutes and Centers at the National Institutes of Health and with other research funding agencies to support the development and testing of strategies to reduce and eliminate cardiovascular health disparities [83, 90]. We also recognize that the implementation frontier is only one part of a complex set of structural and institutional systems and factors that perpetuate health disparities. Sustainable success in eliminating these disparities will come from a truly comprehensive approach that engages all stakeholders including cardiovascular specialists, other healthcare providers, health systems, and policymakers, in strategic partnerships with patients, their families, and whole communities on a common mission to achieve health equity for all.

Conflict of Interest Disclosure None

Disclaimer The views expressed in this chapter are those of the author and do not necessarily represent the views of the National Heart, Lung, and Blood Institute, the National Institutes of Health, or the United States Department of Health and Human Services.

References

1. Mensah GA, Wei GS, Sorlie PD, et al. Decline in Cardiovascular Mortality: Possible Causes and Implications. Circ Res. 2017;120(2):366–80.
2. Centers for Disease Control and Prevention. Achievements in Public Health, 1900–1999: Decline in Deaths from Heart Disease and Stroke – United States, 1900–1999. MMWR Morb Mortal Wkly Rep. 1999;48(30):649–656.
3. National Center for Health Statistics. Health, United States. 2017: with special feature on mortality. Hyattsville, MD: U.S. Department of Health and Human Services; 2018.
4. Murray CJ, Kulkarni SC, Michaud C, et al. Eight Americas: investigating mortality disparities across races, counties, and race-counties in the United States. PLoS Med. 2006;3(9):e260.
5. Institute of Medicine. Unequal treatment: confronting racial and ethnic disparities in health care. National Academies Press; 2003.
6. Agency for Healthcare Research and Quality. 2017 National healthcare quality and disparities report, September, 2018. AHRQ Pub. No. 18-0033-EF. Rockville: AHRQ; 2018.
7. Schpero WL, Morden NE, Sequist TD, Rosenthal MB, Gottlieb DJ, Colla CH. For selected services, blacks and hispanics more likely to receive low-value care than whites. Health Aff (Millwood). 2017;36(6):1065–9.
8. Kressin NR, Groeneveld PW. Race/ethnicity and overuse of care: a systematic review. Milbank Q. 2015;93(1):112–38.
9. Mensah GA, Boyce CA, Price LN, Mishoe HO, Engelgau MM. Perspective: late-stage (T4) translation research and implementation science: the National Heart, Lung, and Blood Institute strategic vision. Ethn Dis. 2017;27(4):367–70.
10. Balas EA, Boren SA. Managing clinical knowledge for health care improvement. In: Bemmel J, McCray AT, editors. Yearbook of medical informatics 2000: patient-centered systems. Stuttgart, Germany: Schattauer Verlagsgesellschaft mbH; 2000. p. 65–70.
11. McGlynn EA, Asch SM, Adams J, et al. The quality of health care delivered to adults in the United States. N Engl J Med. 2003;348(26):2635–45.
12. Levine DM, Linder JA, Landon BE. The quality of outpatient care delivered to adults in the United States, 2002 to 2013. JAMA Int Med. 2016;176(12):1778–90.
13. FitzGerald C, Hurst S. Implicit bias in healthcare professionals: a systematic review. BMC Med Ethics. 2017;18(1):19.
14. Green AR, Carney DR, Pallin DJ, et al. Implicit bias among physicians and its prediction of thrombolysis decisions for black and white patients. J Gen Intern Med. 2007;22(9):1231–8.
15. Lukachko A, Hatzenbuehler ML, Keyes KM. Structural racism and myocardial infarction in the United States. Soc Sci Med. 2014;103:42–50.
16. Pallok K, De Maio F, Ansell DA. Structural racism – a 60-year-old black woman with breast cancer. N Engl J Med. 2019;380(16):1489–93.
17. Whittington MD, Ho PM, Helfrich CD. Recommendations for the use of audit and feedback to de-implement low-value care. Am J Med Qual. 2019;1062860618824153
18. Helfrich CD, Hartmann CW, Parikh TJ, Au DH. Promoting health equity through de-implementation research. Ethn Dis. 2019;29(Suppl 1):93–6.
19. McKay VR, Morshed AB, Brownson RC, Proctor EK, Prusaczyk B. Letting go: conceptualizing intervention

de-implementation in public health and social service settings. Am J Community Psychol. 2018;

20. Davidson KW, Ye S, Mensah GA. Commentary: De-implementation science: a virtuous cycle of ceasing and desisting low-value care before implementing new high value care. Ethn Dis. 2017;27(4):463–8.

21. Prasad V, Ioannidis JP. Evidence-based de-implementation for contradicted, unproven, and aspiring healthcare practices. Implement Sci. 2014;9(1):1–9. https://doi.org/10.1186/1748-5908-9-1.

22. Glasgow RE, McKay HG, Piette JD, Reynolds KD. The RE-AIM framework for evaluating interventions: what can it tell us about approaches to chronic illness management? Patient Educ Couns. 2001;44(2):119–27.

23. O'Gara PT, Oetgen WJ. Innovation and implementation in cardiovascular medicine: challenges in the face of opportunity. JAMA. 2015;313(10):1007–8.

24. Proctor E, Silmere H, Raghavan R, et al. Outcomes for implementation research: conceptual distinctions, measurement challenges, and research agenda. Admin Pol Ment Health. 2011;38(2):65–76.

25. Burt VL, Cutler JA, Higgins M, et al. Trends in the prevalence, awareness, treatment, and control of hypertension in the adult US population. Data from the health examination surveys, 1960 to 1991. Hypertension. 1995;26(1):60–9.

26. Fryar CD, Ostchega Y, Hales CM, Zhang G, Kruszon-Moran D. Hypertension prevalence and control among adults: United States, 2015–2016. NCHS Data Brief. 2017;(289):1–8.

27. Sripipatana A, Pourat N, Chen X, Zhou W, Lu C. Exploring racial/ethnic disparities in hypertension care among patients served by health centers in the United States. J Clin Hyper (Greenwich, Conn). 2019;21(4):489–98.

28. Victor RG, Lynch K, Li N, et al. A cluster-randomized trial of blood-pressure reduction in black barbershops. N Engl J Med. 2018;378(14):1291–301.

29. Jaffe MG, Young JD. The Kaiser Permanente Northern California story: improving hypertension control from 44% to 90% in 13 years (2000 to 2013). J Clin Hyper (Greenwich, Conn). 2016;18(4):260–1.

30. Sim JJ, Handler J, Jacobsen SJ, Kanter MH. Systemic implementation strategies to improve hypertension: the Kaiser Permanente Southern California experience. Can J Cardiol. 2014;30(5):544–52.

31. Dorans KS, Mills KT, Liu Y, He J. Trends in prevalence and control of hypertension according to the 2017 American College of Cardiology/American Heart Association (ACC/AHA) Guideline. J Am Heart Assoc. 2018;7(11)

32. Benjamin EJ, Muntner P, Alonso A, et al. heart disease and stroke statistics-2019 update: a report from the American Heart Association. Circulation. 2019;139(10):e56–e528.

33. Fletcher R, Maron D, Jones R, et al. Better blood pressure control among white than black veteran patients from 2000 to 2014. J Am Coll Cardiol. 2019;73(9 Suppl 1):1822.

34. Ayanian JZ, Landon BE, Newhouse JP, Zaslavsky AM. Racial and ethnic disparities among enrollees in medicare advantage plans. N Engl J Med. 2014;371(24):2288–97.

35. Lillie-Blanton M, Maddox TM, Rushing O, Mensah GA. Disparities in cardiac care: rising to the challenge of Healthy People 2010. J Am Coll Cardiol. 2004;44(3):503–8.

36. Lillie-Blanton M, Rushing OE, Ruiz S, Mayberry R, Boone L. Racial/ethnic differences in cardiac care: the weight of the evidence. Washington, DC: Henry J Kaiser Family Foundation; 2004.

37. Schulman KA, Berlin JA, Harless W, et al. The effect of race and sex on physicians' recommendations for cardiac catheterization. N Engl J Med. 1999;340(8):618–26.

38. Ayanian JZ. Determinants of racial and ethnic disparities in surgical care. World J Surg. 2008;32(4):509–15.

39. Schneider EC, Leape LL, Weissman JS, Piana RN, Gatsonis C, Epstein AM. Racial differences in cardiac revascularization rates: does "overuse" explain higher rates among white patients? Ann Intern Med. 2001;135(5):328–37.

40. Bolorunduro OB, Kiladejo AV, Animashaun IB, Akinboboye OO. Disparities in revascularization after ST elevation myocardial infarction (STEMI) before and after the 2002 IOM report. J Natl Med Assoc. 2016;108(2):119–23.

41. Hannan EL, Racz MJ, Walford G, et al. Disparities in the use of drug-eluting coronary stents by race, ethnicity, payer, and hospital. Can J Cardiol. 2016;32(8):e925–31.

42. Mohamad T, Panaich SS, Alani A, et al. Racial disparities in left main stenting: insights from a real world inner city population. J Interv Cardiol. 2013;26(1):43–8.

43. Freund KM, Jacobs AK, Pechacek JA, White HF, Ash AS. Disparities by race, ethnicity, and sex in treating acute coronary syndromes. J Women's Health. 2002;21(2):126–32.

44. Gaglia MA Jr, Steinberg DH, Pinto Slottow TL, et al. Racial disparities in outcomes following percutaneous coronary intervention with drug-eluting stents. Am J Cardiol. 2009;103(5):653–8.

45. Bonaa KH, Mannsverk J, Wiseth R, et al. Drug-eluting or bare-metal stents for coronary artery disease. N Engl J Med. 2016;375(13):1242–52.

46. Alkhouli M, Alqahtani F, Holmes DR, Berzingi C. Racial disparities in the utilization and outcomes of structural heart disease interventions in the united states. J Am Heart Assoc. 2019;8(15):e012125.

47. Van Nuys KE, Xie Z, Tysinger B, Hlatky MA, Goldman DP. Innovation in heart failure treatment: life expectancy, disability, and health disparities. JACC Heart failure. 2018;6(5):401–9.

48. Lee WC, Serag H, Ohsfeldt RL, et al. Racial disparities in type of heart failure and hospitalization. J Immigr Minor Health. 2019;21(1):98–104.

49. Casper M, Nwaise I, Croft JB, Hong Y, Fang J, Greer S. Geographic disparities in heart failure hospitaliza-

tion rates among medicare beneficiaries. J Am Coll Cardiol. 2010;55(4):294–9.

50. Dupre ME, Gu D, Xu H, Willis J, Curtis LH, Peterson ED. Racial and ethnic differences in trajectories of hospitalization in US men and women with heart failure. J Am Heart Assoc. 2017;6(11)

51. Selim AM, Mazurek JA, Iqbal M, Wang D, Negassa A, Zolty R. Mortality and readmission rates in patients hospitalized for acute decompensated heart failure: a comparison between cardiology and general-medicine service outcomes in an underserved population. Clin Cardiol. 2015;38(3):131–8.

52. Uthamalingam S, Kandala J, Selvaraj V, et al. Outcomes of patients with acute decompensated heart failure managed by cardiologists versus noncardiologists. Am J Cardiol. 2015;115(4):466–71.

53. Kociol RD, Hammill BG, Fonarow GC, et al. Associations between use of the hospitalist model and quality of care and outcomes of older patients hospitalized for heart failure. JACC Heart Failure. 2013;1(5):445–53.

54. Auerbach AD, Hamel MB, Califf RM, et al. Patient characteristics associated with care by a cardiologist among adults hospitalized with severe congestive heart failure. SUPPORT investigators. Study to understand prognoses and preferences for outcomes and risks of treatments. J Am Coll Cardiol. 2000;36(7):2119–25.

55. Breathett K, Liu WG, Allen LA, et al. African Americans are less likely to receive care by a cardiologist during an intensive care unit admission for Heart failure. JACC Heart Failure. 2018;6(5):413–20.

56. Lampropulos JF, Kim N, Wang Y, et al. Trends in left ventricular assist device use and outcomes among Medicare beneficiaries, 2004–2011. Open Heart. 2014;1(1):e000109.

57. Joyce DL, Conte JV, Russell SD, Joyce LD, Chang DC. Disparities in access to left ventricular assist device therapy. J Surg Res. 2009;152(1):111–7.

58. Sridhar AR, Yarlagadda V, Parasa S, et al. Cardiac resynchronization therapy: US trends and disparities in utilization and outcomes. Circ Arrhythm Electrophysiol. 2016;9(3):e003108.

59. Farmer SA, Kirkpatrick JN, Heidenreich PA, Curtis JP, Wang Y, Groeneveld PW. Ethnic and racial disparities in cardiac resynchronization therapy. Heart Rhythm. 2009;6(3):325–31.

60. January CT, Wann LS, Calkins H, et al. AHA/ACC/HRS focused update of the 2014 AHA/ACC/HRS guideline for the Management of Patients with Atrial Fibrillation: a report of the American College of Cardiology/American Heart Association task force on clinical practice guidelines and the Heart Rhythm Society. J Am Coll Cardiol. 2019;74(1):104–32.

61. Birman-Deych E, Radford MJ, Nilasena DS, Gage BF. Use and effectiveness of warfarin in Medicare beneficiaries with atrial fibrillation. Stroke. 2006;37(4):1070–4.

62. Shen AY, Yao JF, Brar SS, Jorgensen MB, Wang X, Chen W. Racial/ethnic differences in ischemic stroke rates and the efficacy of warfarin among patients with atrial fibrillation. Stroke. 2008;39(10):2736–43.

63. Essien UR, Holmes DN, Jackson LR 2nd, et al. Association of race/ethnicity with oral anticoagulant use in patients with atrial fibrillation: findings from the outcomes registry for better informed treatment of atrial fibrillation II. JAMA Cardiol. 2018;

64. Sur NB, Wang K, Di Tullio MR, et al. Disparities and temporal trends in the use of anticoagulation in patients with ischemic stroke and atrial fibrillation. Stroke. 2019;50(6):1452–9.

65. Institute of Medicine. Clinical practice guidelines we can trust. Washington, DC: National Academy Press; 2013.

66. Chan WV, Pearson TA, Bennett GC, et al. ACC/AHA special report: clinical practice guideline implementation strategies: a summary of systematic reviews by the NHLBI Implementation Science Work Group: a report of the American College of Cardiology/American Heart Association Task Force on Clinical Practice Guidelines. J Am Coll Cardiol. 2017;69(8):1076–92.

67. Zeidan AJ, Khatri UG, Aysola J, et al. Implicit Bias education and emergency medicine training: step one? Awareness. AEM Educ Train. 2019;3(1):81–5.

68. Gonzalez CM, Kim MY, Marantz PR. Implicit bias and its relation to health disparities: a teaching program and survey of medical students. Teach Learn Med. 2014;26(1):64–71.

69. Karcher R, Berman AE, Gross H, et al. Addressing disparities in stroke prevention for atrial fibrillation: educational opportunities. Am J Med Qual. 2016;31(4):337–48.

70. Beach MC, Cooper LA, Robinson KA, et al. Strategies for improving minority healthcare quality. Summary, evidence report/technology assessment no. 90. (prepared by the Johns Hopkins University Evidencebased practice center, Baltimore, MD). AHRQ publication no. 04-E008–01. Agency for Healthcare Research and Quality: Rockville; 2004.

71. Spivack SB, Bernheim SM, Forman HP, Drye EE, Krumholz HM. Hospital cardiovascular outcome measures in federal pay-for-reporting and pay-for-performance programs: a brief overview of current efforts. Circulation Cardiovascular Quality and Outcomes. 2014;7(5):627–33.

72. Kaplan CM, Thompson MP, Waters TM. How have 30-day readmission penalties affected racial disparities in readmissions?: an analysis from 2007 to 2014 in five US States. J Gen Intern Med. 2019;34(6):878–83.

73. Joynt Maddox KE, Reidhead M, Hu J, et al. Adjusting for social risk factors impacts performance and penalties in the hospital readmissions reduction program. Health Serv Res. 2019;54(2):327–36.

74. Gaskin DJ, Zare H, Delarmente BA. The supply of hospital care to minority and low-income communities and the hospital readmission reduction program. Med Care Res Rev. 2019:1077558719861242.

75. Gaskin DJ, Zare H, Vazin R, Love D, Steinwachs D. Racial and ethnic composition of hospitals' service

areas and the likelihood of being penalized for excess readmissions by the medicare program. Med Care. 2018;56(11):934–43.

76. Figueroa JF, Zheng J, Orav EJ, Epstein AM, Jha AK. Medicare program associated with narrowing hospital readmission disparities between black and white patients. Health Aff (Millwood). 2018;37(4):654–61.

77. Chaiyachati KH, Qi M, Werner RM. Changes to racial disparities in readmission rates after medicare's hospital readmissions reduction program within safety-net and non-safety-net hospitals. JAMA Netw Open. 2018;1(7):e184154.

78. Hawn MT. Unintended consequences of the hospital readmission reduction program. Ann Surg. 2015;261(6):1032–3.

79. Rubin R. How value-based medicare payments exacerbate health care disparities. JAMA. 2018;319(10):968–70.

80. Joynt Maddox KE. Financial incentives and vulnerable populations – will alternative payment models help or hurt? N Engl J Med. 2018;378(11):977–9.

81. Morgan DJ, Brownlee S, Leppin AL, et al. Setting a research agenda for medical overuse. BMJ. 2015;351:h4534.

82. Mensah GA. Embracing dissemination and implementation research in cardiac critical care. Glob Heart. 2014;9(4):363–6.

83. Mensah GA, Stoney CM, Freemer MM, et al. The National Heart, Lung, and Blood Institute strategic vision implementation for health equity research. Ethn Dis. 2019;29(Suppl 1):57–64.

84. Norton WE, Kennedy AE, Chambers DA. Studying de-implementation in health: an analysis of funded research grants. Implementation Sci IS. 2017;12(1):144.

85. Perez-Stable EJ, Collins FS. Science visioning in minority health and health disparities. Am J Public Health. 2019;109(S1):S5.

86. Yancy CW, Wang TY, Ventura HO, et al. The coalition to reduce racial and ethnic disparities in cardiovascular disease outcomes (credo): why credo matters to cardiologists. J Am Coll Cardiol. 2011;57(3):245–52.

87. Betancourt JR, Tan-McGrory A, Kenst KS, Phan TH, Lopez L. Organizational change management for health equity: perspectives from the disparities leadership program. Health Aff (Millwood). 2017;36(6):1095–101.

88. Hisam B, Zogg CK, Chaudhary MA, et al. From understanding to action: interventions for surgical disparities. J Surg Res. 2016;200(2):560–78.

89. Cohen MG, Fonarow GC, Peterson ED, et al. Racial and ethnic differences in the treatment of acute myocardial infarction: findings from the Get With the Guidelines-Coronary Artery Disease program. Circulation. 2010;121(21):2294–301.

90. National Heart, Lung, and Blood Institute. Charting the Future Together: The NHLBI Strategic Vision. 2016. https://www.nhlbi.nih.gov/sites/default/files/2017-11/NHLBI-Strategic-Vision-2016_FF.pdf. Accessed 16 May 2021.

Genomic Approaches to Hypertension

Nnamdi Uche and Ivor J. Benjamin

Introduction

Hypertension (HTN) is the leading cause of cardiovascular morbidity and mortality worldwide [1–3] affecting more than a third of the US adult population [4, 5]. In both personal and societal terms, blood pressure (BP) control has emerged as an important health indicator in the US population with a disproportionate burden in underrepresented racial and ethnic groups (URGs) such as Black or African Americans and Hispanic or Latinx populations [6]. Among the American Heart Association Strategy Impact Goals to improve cardiovascular health of all Americans by 2020 and beyond, an ideal BP target (<120/80 mmHg) ranks among the seven leading indicators of cardiovascular health for general population health, including Black Americans [7]. As a significant medical and public health problem, HTN remains the major risk factor of heart

N. Uche
Cardiovascular Center, Department of Physiology,
Medical College of Wisconsin, Milwaukee, WI, USA
e-mail: nuche@mcw.edu

I. J. Benjamin (✉)
Cardiovascular Center, Department of Physiology,
Medical College of Wisconsin, Milwaukee, WI, USA

Cardiovascular Center, Division of Cardiovascular
Medicine, Department of Medicine, Medical College
of Wisconsin, Milwaukee, WI, USA
e-mail: ibenjamin@mcw.edu

failure, coronary artery disease (CAD), and atrial fibrillation with one of the highest disease burdens on global health [8]. In fact, an earlier publication by Lawes et al. concluded that 13.5% of premature deaths, 54% of stroke, and 47% of ischemic heart disease worldwide are attributable to uncontrolled HTN [2]. These authors further concluded that about 80% of the attributable burden occurred in low- and middle-income economies.

Significant recent epidemiological factors and demographic trends—whose timing coincides with the global COVID-19 pandemic—have created a toxic admixture and fueled devastating consequences, especially for US communities of color [9]. During the past two decades, for example, cross-sectional data from the National Health and Nutrition Examination Survey (NHANES) have revealed an increased prevalence of obesity in children and adults [10], and decreased control of HTN [6], especially among vulnerable and underserved communities. Obesity, along with changes in inflammatory state, contributes to multiorgan afflictions including cardiovascular disease, chronic kidney disease, type 2 diabetes, nonalcoholic fatty liver disease, and certain types of cancer [11]. Additionally, HTN is the leading risk factor for heart disease, stroke, and chronic kidney disease [12].

Although the etiology of HTN remains partially understood, both genetic and environmental factors play important roles in its pathophysio-

K. C. Ferdinand et al. (eds.), *Cardiovascular Disease in Racial and Ethnic Minority Populations*, Contemporary Cardiology, https://doi.org/10.1007/978-3-030-81034-4_6

logical mechanisms [13]. As a quantitative physiological trait, there is emerging evidence that the distribution and variability of BP in the general population is significantly influenced by environmental factors. In epidemiological studies, Poulter and colleagues have highlighted the increasing prevalence of HTN among members of the Luo tribe in Kenya who had lower BP in their traditional rural environment compared with the urban center of Nairobi where their urinary sodium concentration was higher and urinary potassium concentration was lower [14]. Clinical and experimental observations have strongly supported a key role of the kidney but the underlying mechanism for development of HTN involves the interaction of multiple organ systems and both dependent and/or independent pathways [15]. In support of the hypothesis that a sodium-deprived environment favors sodium conservation as the default phenotype, the renin-angiotensin-aldosterone system (RAAS) has emerged to play a pivotal role in the pathogenesis of HTN, especially in modern societies with high intake of dietary salt [15]. While the important effects of behavioral and environmental factors are being addressed elsewhere [16], this chapter will emphasize how applications of genetics and genomics, linked to mutations of renal salt reabsorption, have fundamentally advanced our understanding of underlying hypertensive disorders in humans.

Primer on Genomic Approaches of HTN

Genetic mapping provides a powerful approach for the study of inherited diseases in humans [17]. Genes can be localized by linkage analysis, then cloned based onto chromosomal positions [18]. This approach has been proven successful for a variety of human diseases that have simple Mendelian inheritance [19]. However, this approach is more problematic for HTN, which has polygenic inheritance [20]. In addition, it may be impossible to study a homogeneous population for polygenic traits since different families may segregate for different loci [17]. The idea that polygenic inheritance of qualitative and quantitative traits could be genetically dissected into discrete

Mendelian factors came about as early as the 1900s [21, 22]. Both practicality and implementation of this idea were accelerated by the development of genetic linkage maps that consist of highly polymorphic, phenotypically neutral genetic markers whose patterns of inheritance could be followed in a cross [17]. In the late 1980s, scientists shifted focus onto the genetic dissection of complex traits with the use of animal models as a means of identifying important genes that had potential relevance in human patients. Methodological advances included the crossing of inbred strains to mitigate concerns of genetic heterogeneity and the strategic use of sufficient numbers of animals in order to achieve the statistical power to detect genes affecting a quantitative trait such as BP [23]. Rats had long been the favored animal model for the study of HTN as exemplified by the spontaneously hypertensive rat (SHR) and the stroke-prone spontaneously hypertensive rat (SHRSP), which were among the best genetically characterized hypertensive lines [24]. In turn, genetic linkage studies took advantage of the proximity between two genetic markers to co-segregate, thereby lowering their chances of a recombination event and an increased likelihood for inheritence [25]. These studies had been applied only for two candidate genes in these rat models at the time; namely, renin and kallikrein [26–28]. As a result, Jacob and colleagues pioneered a large collection of polymorphic DNA markers to study their inheritance in a cross between the SHRSP rat and the normotensive control line, Wistar-Kyoto (WKY), becoming among the first to report the partial genetic dissection of the purely quantitative trait, HTN, in the SHRSP rat [17, 25]. Such foundational efforts, which have significantly advanced preclinical studies of HTN, have coincided with applications of the human genome project to usher in the modern era of genomic medicine [29].

The Genomic Variants in Blood Pressure Regulation Cause Rare Familial Hypertensive Syndromes

The aforementioned genomic approaches and techniques provide an important means to investigate the remaining inheritability of

BP. Following the completion of the human genome project, efforts have steadily progressed to identify specific genetic variations of BP inheritance using linkage analysis, candidate gene, and genome-wide association studies (GWAS)[30]. Both family and twin research suggest that BP is moderately heritable and influences the inheritability of arterial function (30–50%) [31, 32].

Along with traditional cardiovascular risks factors, two broad groups of genomic variants have been proposed to influence the development of HTN. These are (i) genomic variants of rare familial syndromes that lead to monogenic HTN and (ii) the single nucleotide variants (SNVs) underlying common essential HTN. Familial genomic variants of monogenic HTN with large effect sizes are typically rare and either involve the RAAS and/or the adrenal glucocorticoid pathways. In many of these familial hypertensive syndromes, the clinical spectrum of patients who develop HTN at an early age might have effect sizes as large as 10 mmHg in systolic BP, astronomically high BP, hypertensive crises, and severe cardiovascular morbidity and mortality [33, 34].

Also, rare mutations segregating in families can cause secondary HTN, even in the absence of other risk factors [35]. Once a monogenic form of HTN is identified, such cases should be correctly labeled as secondary rather than primary HTN [36]. This distinction is especially important when diagnosing HTN in children as the younger the child, the more likely that their HTN is due to a secondary cause [37, 38]. In addition to rare variants that are associated with secondary HTN, there also exist rare mutations that lower BP and, therefore, protect against the development of HTN. [36] One example is Gitelman syndrome, an autosomal recessive kidney disorder, where loss-of-function mutations in the thiazide-sensitive Na–Cl cotransporter in the distal tubule are associated with lower BPs than in individuals without this defect. [39, 40]

These monogenic variants, which have been identified either to modulate and/or influence distinct rare familial hypertensive syndromes, are now known to be inherited via the Mendelian mode of inheritance. [41, 42] For example, two of the four genes known to cause Gordon syndrome were identified [43, 44]. Other Mendelian HTN syndromes have been mapped to a genomic region and their specific defects are yet to be demonstrated. These conditions remain active areas of exploration and intense research.

Key Features of Monogenic HTN

Monogenic forms of HTN include a group of conditions that are characterized by insults to the normal regulation of BP by the kidney and adrenal gland. Monogenic HTN is driven by volume expansion including excessive sodium ion reabsorption by hyperactive channels, hyperstimulation of mineralocorticoid receptors due to alterations in steroid synthesis, and excess mineralocorticoid synthesis causing volume expansion [16, 45, 46]. The monogenic HTN genes follow the rules of the classical Mendelian mode of inheritance, thus may be inherited as autosomal dominant and recessive disorders. Single mutations can lead to maladaptive overabsorption of electrolytes, which result in fluid shift into the vasculature and HTN. [16] Phenotypic features, electrolyte, and hormonal disturbance may therefore contribute clinically to distinguish these familial monogenic hypertensive syndromes [47]. The serum concentration of potassium may provide a good indication of these Mendelian forms of HTN, but this may be misleading. A more precise phenotypic analysis is done by biochemical analysis including dosing of aldosterone, renin, and additional hormones. These syndromes often lead to severe hypertensive crises in one of two ways: either a reduction of an inhibitory effect on BP or by a positive feedback loop that leads to an increase in BP. The identification of the genetic basis of these hypertensive disease states may be important in our request for therapeutic approaches to these rare disease entities. Along with the increasing availability of genetic testing [48, 49], it is recommended that these patients with suspected monogenic HTN syndrome be referred to an advanced specialized center.

Mechanistic Pathways of the Monogenic HTN Genes

It is now well-established that multiple genes are members of two groups of pathways outlined in the pathogenesis of monogenic HTN; namely, renal sodium homeostasis and steroid hormone metabolism, as well as mineralocorticoid receptor activity.

Other known monogenic defects include PPAR gamma mutations in the pathogenesis of diabetes and HTN21 or RET gene mutations underlying the manifestation of pheochromocytoma, HTN, and other malignancies [50, 51]. The finding that genetic defects in HTN syndromes localize to proteins of the kidney and to steroid hormone activity suggested that similar mechanisms also contribute to the genetic origin of essential HTN. Of note, there is also the partial overlap between the pathways of monogenic HTN and commonly used anti-hypertensive drugs used to treat essential HTN (e.g. diuretics, aldosterone receptor antagonists).

Genome-Wide Association Studies and HTN

Beyond monogenic disorders of HTN, linkage analysis has been an extremely powerful tool used to identify genomic loci of high penetrance. The majority of common single nucleotide variants (SNVs) with minor allele frequency (MAF) > 0.5 underlying increased BP are individually associated with small effect sizes [52]. Along with more recent exome-array-wide association studies (EAWAS) and GWAS, these approaches have successfully identified >1000 BP-related SNVs affecting BP [52]. The application of GWAS in populations requires large and well-characterized populations as well as the capacity to accurately type very large numbers of SNVs in these individuals [30, 53]. The first large-scale attempt to identify HTN variants by GWAS was carried out by the Welcome Trust Case Control Consortium in 2007 [54] and several consortia have been successful at replicating and validating in independent samples, although having diverse cohorts for race and ethnicity remain challenging [55, 56].

Most investigative endeavors have been carried out using the samples of European origin such as the CHARGE (Cohorts for Heart and Aging Research in Genomic Epidemiology) consortium, the Global BP Gen (Global BP Genetics) consortium, and the ICBP (International Consortium for BP GWAS) [57]. Those involving Non-European samples, particularly, cohorts of Asian origin, include the studies by the Korea Association Resource consortium and the Asian Genetic Epidemiology Network [58]. The study using participants of African origin is the CARe (Candidate-gene Association Resource) consortium [59].

Perspectives from the Discovery of Genetic Variants for Essential HTN by GWAS

Earlier studies of the International Consortium for Blood Pressure (ICBP) considered GWAS data involving 69,395 individuals, further replication genotyping/lookups used up to 133,661 subjects and genomic loci to discover SNPs with genome-wide significance for SBP, DBP, and HTN [13]. Several other overlapping studies have contributed additional variants [60, 61]. From over three decades of research on the genetics of essential HTN, several interesting lessons have emerged on SNVs numbering over 1000, which were identified by the GWAS and other similar linkage analyses thus far [62]. The BP effect sizes of individual genetic variants are small, typically 1 mmHg for SBP and 0.5 mm Hg for DBP (subset of SNPs). Collectively, all variants tested in one experiment account for only 1–2% of SBP and DBP variance [13]. It had been previously observed that, perhaps, only little of the total heritability of HTN can currently be explained by the GWAS, which has led to the term "missing heritability" [63].

Exome Arrays for Discovery of Rare Variants Contributing to BP Regulation

Besides association studies of common variants, the recent most extensive analysis of rare variants has identified SNVs significantly associated with

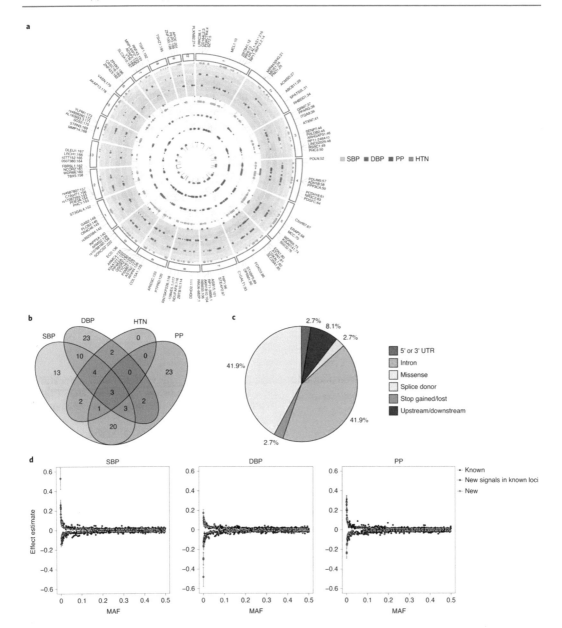

Fig. 6.1 (**a**) Fuji plot of the genome-wide-significant BP-associated SNVs from stage 2 EAWAS and stage 2 RV-GWAS. The first four circles (from inside to outside) and the last circle (locus annotation) summarize pleiotropic effects, while circles 5–8 summarize the genome-wide-significant associations. Every dot or square represents a BP-associated locus; large dots represent new BP-associated loci, while small dots represent loci containing new variants identified in this study, which are in LD with a variant reported by Evangelou et al. [20] and/or Giri et al. [21] All loci are independent of each other, but due to the scale of the plot, dots for loci in close proximity overlap. Asterisks denote loci with rare-variant associations. (**b**) Venn diagram showing the overlap of the 106 new BP loci across the analyzed BP traits. (**c**) Functional annotation from VEP of all the identified rare variants in known and new regions. (**d**) Plots of MAF against effect estimates on the transformed scale for the BP-associated SNVs. Blue squares are new BP-associated SNVs, black dots represent SNVs at known loci and red dots are newly identified distinct BP-associated SNVs at known loci. Effect estimates and standard errors for the new loci are taken from the stage 2 EUR analyses (up to 1,164,961 participants), while those for the known loci are from stage 1 analyses (up to 810,865 participants). Results are from EAWAS where available and from the GWAS (up to 670,472 participants) if the known variants were not on the exome array. (Reprinted with permission from *Surendran, P., et al. (2020). "Discovery of rare variants associated with blood pressure regulation through meta-analysis of 1.3 million individuals." Nat Genet 52* [12]: *1314–1332*)

SBP, DBP, and HTN outlined in Fig. 6.1 [52]. In this meta-analysis of 1.3 million participants, 106 new genomic regions and 87 rare variants of which 32 loci were discovered to be associated with known BP regions, whereas the remaining 55 variants were BP-independent SNVs found within known regions for BP. Of interest, this study identified for the first time that rare variants using exome arrays had oversized effects on BP compared with common variants, suggesting not only the identification of new causal genes but the potential localization at both new and known loci [52]. Among the most revealing insights that exome array has identified are novel biological pathways such as regions of active remodeling of chromatin during fetal development, which has been implicated in post-natal manifestations for BP regulation over the lifespan [52]. By design, an exome array facilitates the analysis of whether rare variants have functional consequences (minor allele frequency [MAF] ≤ 0.01). To date, researchers have applied this approach with considerable success to identify predominantly missense mutations (*RBM47, COL21A1, RRAS,* etc.) and new non-sense mutation (*ENPEP*) as causal genes associated with BP regulation [64, 65]. Of interest, these rare variants appear to have large effect size on BP (~1.5 mm Hg per minor allele) compared with common variants (~0.5 mm Hg per minor allele). Since the majority of variants identified were predominantly from individuals of European decent, there is compelling rationale for further validation especially among cohorts of either Asian and/or African ancestry [66]. This lends credence to the fact that, although genomic analysis in multiple ethnicities is far from complete, many of these variants identified may have significant impact across ethnicities, a subject of intense investigations using genetic ancestry [66, 67].

Conclusion

Genomic insights and analyses of Mendelian HTN syndromes and GWAS on essential HTN have contributed significantly to our understanding of the genetic origins of HTN. These rare hypertensive syndromes are infrequently encountered in clinical practice, yet this heterogeneous category of essential HTN requires a high index of suspicion in order for most physicians to seek medical and genetic consultation. Mendelian syndromes are important to recognize because such knowledge might lead to specific forms of pharmacotherapy for the affected individual. Further, both findings of GWAS and new approaches such as exome array studies of rare variants are constantly evolving while affording insights of therapeutic target of HTN. Comprehensive identification of all genomic variants of HTN, along with their individual associated mechanisms, has implications for the emerging era of precision genomic medicine. Major challenges ahead include how to translate the explosion of scientific discoveries into effective management and prevention strategies of a major public health problem.

Acknowledgments This work has been supported by the **TL1 training award (NU) of the Clinical Translational Sciences Institute (CTSI) of Southeast Wisconsin. IJB serves as Program Director and MPI (contact) for the NHLBI T32 Training grant on** *Training in Signature Transdisciplinary Cardiovascular Sciences.*

Disclosure Statement The authors have no financial or commercial conflicts of interest to declare.

References

1. Hsu CY, McCulloch CE, Darbinian J, Go AS, Iribarren C. Elevated blood pressure and risk of end-stage renal disease in subjects without baseline kidney disease. Arch Intern Med. 2005;165(8):923–8.
2. Lawes CM, Vander Hoorn S, Rodgers A. International Society of H. global burden of blood-pressure-related disease, 2001. Lancet. 2008;371(9623):1513–8.
3. Lewington S, Clarke R, Qizilbash N, Peto R, Collins R, Prospective SC. Age-specific relevance of usual blood pressure to vascular mortality: a meta-analysis of individual data for one million adults in 61 prospective studies. Lancet. 2002;360(9349):1903–13.
4. Burt VL, Cutler JA, Higgins M, et al. Trends in the prevalence, awareness, treatment, and control of hypertension in the adult US population. Data from the health examination surveys, 1960 to 1991. Hypertension. 1995;26(1):60–9.

5. Benjamin EJ, Virani SS, Callaway CW, et al. Heart disease and stroke Statistics-2018 update: a report from the American Heart Association. Circulation. 2018;137(12):e67–e492.

6. Muntner P, Hardy ST, Fine LJ, et al. Trends in blood pressure control among US adults with hypertension, 1999–2000 to 2017–2018. JAMA. 2020;

7. Sims M, Glover LM, Norwood AF, et al. Optimism and cardiovascular health among African Americans in the Jackson Heart Study. Prev Med. 2019;129:105826.

8. Wang Y, Wang JG. Genome-wide association studies of hypertension and several other cardiovascular diseases. Pulse (Basel). 2019;6(3–4):169–86.

9. Moore JT, Ricaldi JN, Rose CE, et al. Disparities in Incidence of COVID-19 Among Underrepresented Racial/Ethnic Groups in Counties Identified as Hotspots During June 5–18, 2020–22 States, February–June 2020. MMWR Morb Mortal Wkly Rep. 2020;69(33):1122–6.

10. Ogden CL, Fryar CD, Martin CB, et al. Trends in obesity prevalence by race and hispanic origin-1999–2000 to 2017–2018. JAMA. 2020;

11. Jensen MD, Ryan DH, Apovian CM, et al. 2013 AHA/ACC/TOS guideline for the management of overweight and obesity in adults: a report of the American College of Cardiology/American Heart Association Task Force on Practice Guidelines and The Obesity Society. Circulation. 2014;129(25 Suppl 2):S102–38.

12. Malhotra R, Nguyen HA, Benavente O, et al. Association between more intensive vs less intensive blood pressure lowering and risk of mortality in chronic kidney disease stages 3 to 5: a systematic review and meta-analysis. JAMA Intern Med. 2017;177(10):1498–505.

13. International Consortium for Blood Pressure Genome-Wide Association S, Ehret GB, Munroe PB, et al. Genetic variants in novel pathways influence blood pressure and cardiovascular disease risk. Nature. 2011;478(7367):103–9.

14. Poulter N, Khaw KT, Hopwood BE, et al. Blood pressure and its correlates in an African tribe in urban and rural environments. J Epidemiol Community Health. 1984;38(3):181–5.

15. Hall JE, Granger JP, do Carmo JM, et al. Hypertension: physiology and pathophysiology. Compr Physiol. 2012;2(4):2393–442.

16. Raina R, Krishnappa V, Das A, et al. Overview of monogenic or Mendelian forms of hypertension. Front Pediatr. 2019;7:263.

17. Jacob HJ, Lindpaintner K, Lincoln SE, et al. Genetic mapping of a gene causing hypertension in the stroke-prone spontaneously hypertensive rat. Cell. 1991;67(1):213–24.

18. Botstein D, White RL, Skolnick M, Davis RW. Construction of a genetic linkage map in man using restriction fragment length polymorphisms. Am J Hum Genet. 1980;32(3):314–31.

19. Riordan JR, Rommens JM, Kerem B, et al. Identification of the cystic fibrosis gene: cloning and characterization of complementary DNA. Science (New York, NY). 1989;245(4922):1066–73.

20. Lander ES, Botstein D. Mapping complex genetic traits in humans: new methods using a complete RFLP linkage map. Cold Spring Harb Symp Quant Biol. 1986;51(Pt 1):49–62.

21. East EM. Studies on size inheritance in Nicotiana. Genetics. 1916;1(2):164–76.

22. Thoday JM. Location of polygenes. Nature. 1961;191(4786):368–70.

23. Lander ES, Botstein D. Mapping mendelian factors underlying quantitative traits using RFLP linkage maps. Genetics. 1989;121(1):185–99.

24. Okamoto K, Aoki K. Development of a strain of spontaneously hypertensive rats. Jpn Circ J. 1963;27:282–93.

25. Brown DM, Matise TC, Koike G, et al. An integrated genetic linkage map of the laboratory rat. Mamm Genome. 1998;9(7):521–30.

26. Kurtz TW, Simonet L, Kabra PM, Wolfe S, Chan L, Hjelle BL. Cosegregation of the renin allele of the spontaneously hypertensive rat with an increase in blood pressure. J Clin Invest. 1990;85(4):1328–32.

27. Lindpaintner K, Takahashi S, Ganten D. Structural alterations of the renin gene in stroke-prone spontaneously hypertensive rats: examination of genotype-phenotype correlations. J Hypertens. 1990;8(8):763–73.

28. Pravenec M, Kren V, Kunes J, et al. Cosegregation of blood pressure with a kallikrein gene family polymorphism. Hypertension. 1991;17(2):242–6.

29. Guyer MS, Collins FS. The human genome project and the future of medicine. Am J Dis Child. 1993;147(11):1145–52.

30. Doris PA. The genetics of blood pressure and hypertension: the role of rare variation. Cardiovasc Ther. 2011;29(1):37–45.

31. Miall WE, Oldham PD. The hereditary factor in arterial blood-pressure. Br Med J. 1963;1(5323):75–80.

32. Hayward CS, Benetos A. Hereditary and environmental influences on arterial function. Clin Exp Pharmacol Physiol. 2007;34(7):658–64.

33. Chebib FT, Torres VE. Recent advances in the management of autosomal dominant polycystic kidney disease. Clin J Am Soc Nephrol. 2018;13(11):1765–76.

34. Lip S, Padmanabhan S. Genomics of blood pressure and hypertension: extending the mosaic theory toward stratification. Can J Cardiol. 2020;36(5):694–705.

35. Ji W, Foo JN, O'Roak BJ, et al. Rare independent mutations in renal salt handling genes contribute to blood pressure variation. Nat Genet. 2008;40(5):592–9.

36. Ehret G. Next steps for gene identification in primary hypertension genomics. Hypertension. 2017;70(4):695–7.

37. Lifton RP, Gharavi AG, Geller DS. Molecular mechanisms of human hypertension. Cell. 2001;104(4):545–56.

38. Cakici EK, Yazilitas F, Kurt-Sukur ED, et al. Clinical assessment of primary and secondary hyperten-

sion in children and adolescents. Arch Pediatr. 2020;27(6):286–91.

39. Knoers NV, Levtchenko EN. Gitelman syndrome. Orphanet J Rare Dis. 2008;3:22.

40. Gug C, Mihaescu A, Mozos I. Two mutations in the thiazide-sensitive NaCl co-transporter gene in a Romanian Gitelman syndrome patient: case report. Ther Clin Risk Manag. 2018;14:149–55.

41. Deng AY. Genetic basis of polygenic hypertension. Hum Mol Genet. 2007;16 Spec No. 2:R195–R202.

42. Lifton RP. Molecular genetics of human blood pressure variation. Science. 1996;272(5262):676–80.

43. Boyden LM, Choi M, Choate KA, et al. Mutations in kelch-like 3 and cullin 3 cause hypertension and electrolyte abnormalities. Nature. 2012;482(7383):98–102.

44. Louis-Dit-Picard H, Barc J, Trujillano D, et al. KLHL3 mutations cause familial hyperkalemic hypertension by impairing ion transport in the distal nephron. Nat Genet. 2012;44(4):456–60, S451-453

45. Garovic VD, Hilliard AA, Turner ST. Monogenic forms of low-renin hypertension. Nat Clin Pract Nephrol. 2006;2(11):624–30.

46. Simonetti GD, Mohaupt MG, Bianchetti MG. Monogenic forms of hypertension. Eur J Pediatr. 2012;171(10):1433–9.

47. Lifton RP. Genetic dissection of human blood pressure variation: common pathways from rare phenotypes. Harvey Lect. 2004;100:71–101.

48. Aggarwal A, Rodriguez-Buritica D. Monogenic hypertension in children: a review with emphasis on genetics. Adv Chronic Kidney Dis. 2017;24(6):372–9.

49. Bao M, Li P, Li Q, et al. Genetic screening for monogenic hypertension in hypertensive individuals in a clinical setting. J Med Genet. 2020;57(8):571–80.

50. Usuda D, Kanda T. Peroxisome proliferator-activated receptors for hypertension. World J Cardiol. 2014;6(8):744–54.

51. Pelham CJ, Keen HL, Lentz SR, Sigmund CD. Dominant negative PPARgamma promotes atherosclerosis, vascular dysfunction, and hypertension through distinct effects in endothelium and vascular muscle. Am J Physiol Regul Integr Comp Physiol. 2013;304(9):R690–701.

52. Surendran P, Feofanova EV, Lahrouchi N, et al. Discovery of rare variants associated with blood pressure regulation through meta-analysis of 1.3 million individuals. Nat Genet. 2020;52(12):1314–32.

53. Kato N, Loh M, Takeuchi F, et al. Trans-ancestry genome-wide association study identifies 12 genetic loci influencing blood pressure and implicates a role for DNA methylation. Nat Genet. 2015;47(11):1282–93.

54. Wellcome Trust Case Control C. Genome-wide association study of 14,000 cases of seven common diseases and 3,000 shared controls. Nature. 2007;447(7145):661–78.

55. Evangelou E, Warren HR, Mosen-Ansorena D, et al. Genetic analysis of over 1 million people identifies 535 new loci associated with blood pressure traits. Nat Genet. 2018;50(10):1412–25.

56. Giri A, Hellwege JN, Keaton JM, et al. Trans-ethnic association study of blood pressure determinants in over 750,000 individuals. Nat Genet. 2019;51(1):51–62.

57. Simino J, Kume R, Kraja AT, et al. Linkage analysis incorporating gene-age interactions identifies seven novel lipid loci: the family blood pressure program. Atherosclerosis. 2014;235(1):84–93.

58. Yang X, Gu D, He J, et al. Genome-wide linkage and regional association study of blood pressure response to the cold pressor test in Han Chinese: the genetic epidemiology network of salt sensitivity study. Circ Cardiovasc Genet. 2014;7(4):521–8.

59. Deo R, Nalls MA, Avery CL, et al. Common genetic variation near the connexin-43 gene is associated with resting heart rate in African Americans: a genome-wide association study of 13,372 participants. Heart Rhythm. 2013;10(3):401–8.

60. Newton-Cheh C, Johnson T, Gateva V, et al. Genome-wide association study identifies eight loci associated with blood pressure. Nat Genet. 2009;41(6):666–76.

61. Levy D, Ehret GB, Rice K, et al. Genome-wide association study of blood pressure and hypertension. Nat Genet. 2009;41(6):677–87.

62. Cabrera CP, Ng FL, Nicholls HL, et al. Over 1000 genetic loci influencing blood pressure with multiple systems and tissues implicated. Hum Mol Genet. 2019;28(R2):R151–61.

63. Manolio TA, Collins FS, Cox NJ, et al. Finding the missing heritability of complex diseases. Nature. 2009;461(7265):747–53.

64. Surendran P, Drenos F, Young R, et al. Trans-ancestry meta-analyses identify rare and common variants associated with blood pressure and hypertension. Nat Genet. 2016;48(10):1151–61.

65. Liu C, Kraja AT, Smith JA, et al. Meta-analysis identifies common and rare variants influencing blood pressure and overlapping with metabolic trait loci. Nat Genet. 2016;48(10):1162–70.

66. Borrell LN, Elhawary JR, Fuentes-Afflick E, et al. Race and genetic ancestry in medicine – a time for reckoning with racism. N Engl J Med. 2021;384(5):474–80.

67. Wassel CL, Jacobs DR Jr, Duprez DA, et al. Association of self-reported race/ethnicity and genetic ancestry with arterial elasticity: the multi-ethnic study of atherosclerosis (MESA). J Am Soc Hypertens. 2011;5(6):463–72.

Heart Failure in African Americans and Hispanic Americans: A Persistent and Disproportionate Burden in Underrepresented Minorities

Quentin R. Youmans, Ike S. Okwuosa, and Clyde W. Yancy

Introduction

Heart failure (HF) is estimated to affect approximately 26 million people around the globe [1]. The prevalence in the United States continues to rise with approximately 6.5 million Americans living with HF in 2014; an estimated increase of 800,000 people compared to just 3 years prior [2]. The prevalence of HF is projected to increase dramatically over the next decade. Over eight million adults in the United States will be affected by heart failure by the fourth decade of the millenium [3]. Similarly, the total cost of HF is expected to rise in the United States from $31 billion in 2012 to an astonishing $70 billion by 2030 [3].

As the national burden of HF grows, disparities in care and outcomes persist, particularly for African Americans and Hispanic Americans. These groups remain disproportionately affected by risk factors that lead to the development of HF, especially hypertension, diabetes and obesity. Once developed, minority groups face worse outcomes in treatment, readmissions, and morbidity owing to the social determinants of health and a disproportionate burden of poorly controlled comorbidities that lead to progression of disease.

This chapter will serve as a contemporary exploration of heart failure in African Americans (AAs) and Hispanic Americans, discussing specific considerations related to epidemiology, prevention, heart failure phenotypes, treatment, and heart failure quality metrics in these at-risk patient populations.

Learning Objectives:

1. To understand the disparate incidence and prevalence of HF in AAs and Hispanic Americans.
2. To review the risk factor profiles specific to these patient populations.
3. To learn the evidence for prevention of HF and cardiovascular disease.
4. To discuss the unique treatment considerations for these two groups.
5. To review specific cardiomyopathies that disproportionately affect AA and Hispanic American populations.

Q. R. Youmans · I. S. Okwuosa · C. W. Yancy (✉)
Division of Cardiology, Department of Medicine, Northwestern University, Feinberg School of Medicine, Chicago, IL, USA
e-mail: Quentin-Youmans@northwestern.edu; ike.okwuosa@nm.org; cyancy@nm.org

© Springer Nature Switzerland AG 2021
K. C. Ferdinand et al. (eds.), *Cardiovascular Disease in Racial and Ethnic Minority Populations*, Contemporary Cardiology, https://doi.org/10.1007/978-3-030-81034-4_7

Defining Heart Failure

HF is a clinical syndrome resulting from a structural or functional impairment of ventricular filling and/or ejection of blood [4]. It can be a result of disorders of the pericardium, myocardium, endocardium, or valves of the heart [5]. A cardiomyopathy is specifically a disease of the myocardium that can result in HF. The diagnosis of HF hinges on the history and physical examination. The symptoms are primarily a result of volume overload leading to dyspnea, fatigue, and edema [4]. The clinical signs of pulmonary edema, jugular venous distention, hepatojugular reflux, and lower extremity edema can both help with the diagnosis and serve as signs of response to treatment.

HF is classified by both stages of disease progression and degree of symptoms. The American College of Cardiology (ACC) and American Heart Association (AHA) define the stages and classifications as outlined in Table 7.1. (Adaptation with permission from the ACC/AHA guidelines) [4].

Defining the Populations

Before we explore the landscape of HF for Hispanic Americans and AAs, it is important to define these populations. This begins by recognizing the intergroup variance in ethnicity (Hispanic Americans) and race (African Americans).

Hispanic American

According to the US Census Bureau, the Hispanic population of the United States as of July 2018 was 58.9 million, making people of Hispanic origin the nation's largest ethnic or racial minority [6]. Hispanic American populations are diverse and include heritages from Central America/Caribbean, Cuba, Dominican Republic, Mexico, Puerto Rico, and South America. They are the only ethnic group defined by a common language, Spanish, as opposed to a geographic origin [7]. In turn, studies have shown that these different groups have diverse

Table 7.1 Stages of heart failure

	Stage A	Stage B	Stage C	Stage D
Patients with:	Risk factors for HF including: HTN Atherosclerosis Diabetes Obesity Metabolic syndrome *or* with exposure to cardiotoxic medications or a family history of HF	Structural heart disease without symptoms	Structural heart disease with HF signs/symptoms	Recurrent HF signs/symptoms at rest
Goals of treatment	Prevention of progression, heart healthy lifestyle, prevention of structural abnormalities of the heart	Prevent symptoms and progression	Prevent hospitalization and mortality; improve QOL	Same as stage C with addition of GOC and advanced therapies
Treatments	Statins where appropriate, ACEi or ARB in diabetes	Where appropriate: Beta-blockers, ACEi and ARB, ICD placement, valve surgery, and/or revascularization	GDMT	GDMT + advanced care including considering MCS, transplantation, ICD, inotropes, palliative care

Yancy et al. [122]

HF heat failure, *HTN* hypertension, *ACEi* angiotensin-converting enzyme inhibitor, *ARB* angiotensin-receptor blocker, *MCS* mechanical circulatory support, *ICD* implantable cardioverter defibrillator, *GDMT* guideline-directed medical therapy health needs and different barriers to accessing care [8]. These difference are likely, in part, owing to diverse social histories and cultural identities [9]. It is often difficult to draw broadly applicable conclusions about Hispanic America given the heterogeneity of the population. Nevertheless, the burden of HF is profound and is expected to be magnified in the Hispanic American population owing to several key factors: (1) The rate of growth of the population may challenge the health care system, (2) The higher prevalence of cardiometabolic risk burden, and (3) The disproportionate burden of health care disparities present within Hispanic American communities [10].

Black/African American

While the self-described designation as "Hispanic American" is an ethnicity, Black/African American is considered a race. Race is quite confounded as there is at best only a loose association with genetic ancestry but a stronger association with a social construct. Thus African American race per se has social, economic, and political ramifications, and may be a unique experience in the United States [11]. The US census Bureau estimates that African Americans make up 13.4% of the US population [6]. Like Hispanic Americans, AAs are also a heterogenous group of descendants coming from the West Indies, Haiti, and miscellaneous parts of Africa [12]. These descendant groups have distinct behaviors, beliefs, and risk profiles that must be acknowledged when grouping in health-related research [13]. One common factor that contributes to poorer health outcomes, including HF, across all AAs are the social determinants of health. In 2015, AAs lagged behind non-Hispanic White individuals in insurance coverage (54.4% privately insured compared to 75.8%, respectively), educational attainment (85.8% of those aged 25 years and older had gained a high school diploma compared to 92.3%, respectively), and economics (median income of $36,515 compared to $61,394, respectively) [14].

Epidemiology

The prevalence of HF is growing likely owing to improved survival of patients with the known antecedent diseases that lead to heart failure, e.g., hypertension and coronary artery disease, and increased prevalence of its associated risk factors [15, 16]. Using National Heart, Lung, and Blood Institute-sponsored cohorts, researchers estimated the lifetime risk of HF to be between 20% and 45% [17]. While the prevalence is certainly increasing, data are mixed regarding incidence, with data from Olmsted County, MN indicating a decline from 315.8 per 1000,000 in the year 2000 to 219.3 per 100,000 in 2010 [18].

While there is a general trend of increased prevalence, there are also racial/ethnic disparities to highlight. The Multi-Ethnic Study of Atherosclerosis (MESA) study showed a step-wise increase in the risk of developing HF for White, Hispanic, and Black participants, respectively (2.4, 3.5, and 4.6 per 1000 person-years) [19]. A more recent analysis of data from the Atherosclerosis Risk in Communities (ARIC) study cohort confirmed that, when age-adjusted, Black males have the *highest annual rate of incident heart failure* (15.7 per 1000), followed closely by Black females at 13.3 per 1000 [20]. This is compared to White males at 12.3 per 1000 and White females 9.9 per 1000 [20]. These differences are likely owing to the differential disease burden of several important comorbidities. An estimated 10.3% of AAs have heart disease, 5.5% have coronary heart disease (CHD) and 33% have hypertension [21]. For Hispanic Americans in comparison, 7.8% have heart disease, 4.9% have CHD and 19.5% have hypertension [21].

Survival with HF has generally improved-attributable to remarkable strides in evidence-based therapies. But the improvements in outcomes have not been uniform among all patient cohorts. The ARIC study determined 30-day, 1-year, and 5-year case fatality rates after hospitalization for HF to be 10.4%, 22%, and 42.3% respectively [22]. Black participants in this study had a greater 5-year case fatality rate than Whites participants [22]. Interestingly, although Hispanic Americans have higher hospitalization and readmission rates for HF than non-Hispanic White Americans, their age- and sex-adjusted in-hospital and short-term mortality rates are lower [10]. This represents an important potential "Hispanic paradox" that is still an area of active research with some data refuting its presence, particularly in Mexican Americans [23, 24].

Risk Factors

Risk factors for HF are myriad and well-defined in the literature. Coronary heart disease, hypertension, diabetes mellitus, obesity, and smoking were estimated to cause 52% of incident HF in one study [25]. A comprehensive list of traditional risk factors can be found in Table 7.2.

Investigators in the Health, Aging, and Body Composition Study identified a 67.8% proportion of HF that was attributable to modifiable risk factors in Black participants compared to 48.9% in White participants [26]. Of those risk factors, the primary drivers for this disparity were a greater than 50% population-attributable risk for smoking, increased heart rate, CHD, left ventricular hypertrophy, uncontrolled blood pressure, and reduced glomerular filtration compared to White participants. For AAs, the cause of HF is predominately related to hypertension contrasted to CHD for the general population [27].

The risk factor profile for Hispanic Americans is similar with disproportionate rates of diabetes mellitus, obesity, dyslipidemia, and hypertension. Age-matched Hispanic Americans are almost twice as likely to have diabetes compared to non-Hispanic White Americans [28]. For tobacco smoke, 16.7% of AAs and 10.1% of Hispanic Americans are current smokers compared with 16.6% of White Americans [29]. According to National Health and Nutrition Examination Study (NHANES) data from 2014, males across the different racial/ethnic groups had a similar age-adjusted prevalence of obesity from 35% to 38%, while Black females had a greater (57.2%) prevalence compared to Asians, Hispanic Americans, and White females (38–

Table 7.2 Prevalence of risk factors for heart failure in African and Hispanic Americans

Risk factors	African Americans	Hispanic Americans
Coronary heart disease	7.2% of males and 6.5% of females	6.0% of males and 6.0% of females
High blood pressure	58.6% of males and 56% of females	47.4% of males and 40.8% of females
High total cholesterol	29.8% of males and 33.1% of females	39.9% of males and 38.9% of females
Smoking	14.9% prevalence in adults 18 years or older	9.9% prevalence in adults 18 years or older
Physical inactivity	High school boys 12.7%, girls 26.6%	High school boys 12.3%, girls 20%
Overweight and obesity	69.1% of males and 79.5% of females overweight or obese	80.8% of males and 77.8% of females overweight or obese
Diabetes mellitus	14.7% of males and 13.4% of females with physician diagnosed diabetes.	15.1% of males and 14.1% of females had physician diagnosed diabetes.
Cardiovascular disease	60.1% of males and 57.1% of females	49.0% of males and 42.6% of females

Data for adults age > or = 20 years unless otherwise specified. High cholesterol = total cholesterol levels of 200 mg/dL or higher

Adapted from 2020 Heart Disease & Stroke Statistical Update Fact Sheet

Blacks & Cardiovascular Diseases and 2020 Heart Disease & Stroke Statistical Update Fact Sheet Hispanics/Latinos & Cardiovascular Diseases (Heart.org/statistics)

47%) [30]. The age-adjusted prevalence of hypertension among AAs was 45% and 46.3% for males and females, respectively, among White Americans was 34.5% and 32.3% for males and females, respectively, and among Hispanic Americans was 28.9% and 30.7% for males and females, respectively [2].

While differences exist in the prevalence and incidence of risk factors for HF, the propensity to develop HF following an insult is also disparate. AAs who suffer a myocardial infarction are more likely than White individuals to develop HF [19].

From a mechanistic standpoint, AAs with mild to moderate left ventricular (LV) systolic dysfunction had previously been found to be more likely than White individuals to progress to HF in the Studies of Left Ventricular Dysfunction (SOLVD) [31].

Diet Types and Risk of Heart Failure

Diet is a well-established component of cardiovascular risk and prevention. The two predominant types of diet that are considered protective against cardiovascular disease are the Mediterranean-type and the Dietary Approaches to Stop Hypertension (DASH) diets. The Mediterranean diet consists of plant-based food consumption, fresh fruit, dairy, fish/poultry, and olive oil as the principal source of fat; while recommending low to moderate consumption of eggs, red meat, and wine [32]. Similarly, the DASH diet emphasizes fruits, vegetables, whole grains, low-fat dairy products and discourages sugary foods and beverages, red meats, and added fats [33].

Studies examining the link between HF and the Mediterranean diet have had mixed results with some showing an association with reduction in incident HF and others not [34]. Two cohort studies evaluating the DASH diet in the Swedish population found a lower rate of HF in patients who adhered to the diet most closely, with women having a relative risk of HF of 0.63 (95% CI 0.48–0.81, p < 0.001) [35] and men having a relative risk of HF of 0.78 (95%, 0.65–0.95, p = 0.006) [36]. For AAs, a link between the DASH diet and sodium intake has also been described. Sacks and colleagues found that decreased sodium intake in addition to the DASH diet leads to a further drop in blood pressure in patients both with and without hypertension [33].

In addition to diet types with protective effect, studies have also identified diet types with increased risk. A study examining data from the REasons for Geographic and Racial Difference in Stroke (REGARDS) cohort found that participants with the greatest adherence to a Southern diet (which included more fried food, processed meats, added fats, and sugary beverages) had a *72% higher risk of HF* [37]. Interestingly, partici-pants in this highest quartile of adherence were more likely to be men, Black and have hypertension and diabetes compared with the lowest quartile of participants who ate a Southern dietary pattern [37]. Conversely, consumption of a plant-based dietary pattern was associated with a 41% lower risk of new HF hospitalizations.

The Curious Case of Hypertension in Black Americans

Hypertension accounts for approximately 20% of HF cases in the general population [25]. Moreover, death from hypertension has been identified as the leading contributor to the racial disparity in potential life-years lost between Black and White individuals [38]. The prevalence of hypertension in AAs is among the highest in the world [2]. Indeed, the MESA study identified discrepant prevalence of hypertension (and diabetes) in Black patients with concurrent increased prevalence and magnitude of left ventricular hypertrophy compared to White participants [19]. Several additional studies have defined the higher prevalence of hypertension in Black participants compared to White participants starting from childhood to older adulthood [39–41].

The exact causes of this disparity are still unknown [42]. Using data from the REGARDS study, researchers sought to identify factors that were associated with increased incidence of hypertension in Black patients. Among men, the Southern dietary pattern, education level of high school or less, and an elevated sodium to potassium intake level were all associated with excess risk of hypertension in Blacks [43]. Among women, the Southern dietary pattern was also the largest mediator of excess risk for Blacks in addition to higher body mass index (BMI), larger waist circumference, less adherence to the DASH diet, income $35,000 or less, a higher dietary ratio of sodium to potassium, and education level of high school or less [43].

Overall, diet types appear to play an important role in the genesis of cardiovascular disease and HF. Efforts to stem the tide of HF should address dietary practices particularly for AAs with a focus on (1) addressing the prevalence of the Southern dietary type in this patient population and (2) recommendation of the DASH diet and decreased sodium intake to decrease the prevalence of hypertension.

American Heart Association 2020 Strategic Plan

With these risk factors in mind, in 2011, the American Heart Association (AHA) recommended seven metrics, four health behaviors and three health factors, termed "Life's Simple 7" to improve health and cardiovascular disease risk by 20% by 2020—Manage Blood Pressure, Control Cholesterol, Reduce blood sugar, Get Active, Eat Better, Lose Weight, and Stop Smoking [44]. The goal of these metrics is to augment primary prevention efforts in HF [2]. It is estimated that 6 in 10 White adults have no more than 3 of 7 metrics at ideal levels while that number is 7 in 10 for AAs and Hispanic Americans [2]. These metrics have been found to be particularly effective in AA and Hispanic American patients. Spahillari and colleagues identified a 61% lower risk of incident heart failure in Black patients with ≥4 ideal cardiovascular health metrics compared to those with 0–2 ideal metrics. [45] In addition, Hispanic Americans have been found to have poorly controlled risk factors, for example target blood glucose, lipids and blood pressure [46], making targeting these components especially important in this patient population.

Heart Failure with Reduced and Preserved Ejection Fractions

The presence of either systolic or diastolic dysfunction commonly predates the clinical syndrome of HF. These clinical entities are frequently dichotomized into heart failure with reduced ejection fraction (HFrEF) and heart failure with preserved ejection fraction (HFpEF). The American College of Cardiology/American Heart Association guidelines define HFrEF as systolic heart failure with an ejection fraction (EF) of less than or equal to 40%, and HFpEF as diastolic heart failure with an EF of greater than or equal to 50% [47]. Incident hospitalized HF for the general population is split evenly between HFrEF and HFpEF. Interestingly, while Black males have the highest proportion of presentations with reduced ejection fraction at approximately 70% [20], the lifetime risk of HFrEF has been estimated to be similar among AAs and non-Blacks [48].

The disease processes that lead to HFpEF versus HFrEF are distinct, contributing to this difference in prevalence. Using data from the MESA study, investigators discovered that asymptomatic LV systolic dysfunction was most prevalent in AAs at 2.7% compared to White, Chinese and Hispanic Americans (1.7% overall) [49]. Incident HF in the young is also more common in AAs. Participants in the Coronary Artery Risk Development in Young Adults (CARDIA) study were Black and White with ages ranging from 18 to 30 years at the time of enrollment [50]. Analysis of CARDIA data determined a cumulative incidence of HF before the age of 50 in Black women of 1.1%, Black men of 0.9%, White women of 0.08%, and White men of 0% [51]. Seventy-five percent of participants who went on to develop heart failure in the cohort had hypertension by the age of 40 [51]. More recently, an analysis using the Multiple Cause of Death data from the Centers for Disease Control and Prevention ascertained an age-adjusted HF-related cardiovascular disease death rate that was 2.6- and 2.97-fold higher for Black individuals aged 35–64 years compared to White men and women, respectively, in 2017 [52].

A study comparing non-Hispanic Americans to Hispanic Americans using the Get with the Guidelines-Heart Failure registry found that Hispanic Americans with HF were more likely to be younger and to have diabetes, hypertension, and be overweight or obese [53]. In addition, Hispanic Americans with HFpEF had an approximate 50% lower odds of in-hospital mortality in multivariate analysis [53].

HFpEF can be considered more complex than HFrEF because of the diverse etiologies and manifestations of the disease. Using the

Nationwide Inpatient Sample, investigators found that AAs with HFpEF were on average 10 years younger than White adults and in turn had a lower comparative prevalence of most comorbidities [54]. AAs, however, did have higher rates of hypertension, diabetes mellitus, anemia, and chronic kidney disease in the study [54]. These may offer plausible mechanistic links with hypertension at a younger age contributing to left ventricular hypertensive remodeling; and diabetes, anemia, and chronic kidney disease being a marker for or direct causative insult resulting in inflammation contributing to HFpEF in this population [54]. Even with these data, the lifetime risk of HFpEF for AAs has been estimated to be lower than for non-Black patients (7.7% vs. 11.2%, respectively) [48].

Hospitalizations and Readmissions

The hospitalization can serve as a sentinel event for patients with HF. Hospitalized patients have a 1-month rehospitalization rate of 25% [4]. Repeated hospitalizations are also associated with a worse prognosis with one study showing median survival having a stepwise decline from 2.4, 1.4, 1.0, to 0.6 years from the first through fourth hospitalizations, respectively [55]. Disparities exist in the space of hospitalization as well. Studies have shown that HF patients who receive care from a cardiologist tend to have better outcomes [56, 57]. However, AAs were found to be less likely to receive care from a cardiologist both on the general wards [58] and in the intensive care unit [59].

Readmission for HF portends a worse prognosis for patients because it is a sign of worsening hemodynamics and/or pump function. For patients aged ≥55 years the average incidence of hospitalized heart failure is 11.6 per 1000 people per year, with 6.6 per 1000 people per year for recurrent hospitalized heart failure [1]. A study of patients enrolled in the Health, Aging, and Body Composition Study had no racial difference in survival in HF; however, rates of rehospitalization for AAs were 62.1 per 100 person-years compared to 30.3 per person-years for White participants [26].

The Hospital Readmission Reductions Program (HRRP) passed as part of the Affordable Care Act in 2010 was a legislative effort to stem readmissions for acute myocardial infarction, pneumonia, and HF. Analysis of readmission rates for HF prior to passage of the ACA showed higher rates for Black compared to White Medicare beneficiaries [60]. Addressing readmissions and the effects of legislation will continue to be an area of active research.

Heart Failure Treatment

The management of HF has evolved over the decades. In the 1960s, standard of care consisted of diuretics, digoxin, and bed rest [61]. By the 1970s, interventions shifted toward augmenting hemodynamic performance specifically by targeting systemic vascular resistance with vasodilator therapies [62]. Studies utilizing intravenous sodium nitroprusside in patients with intractable heart failure showed a reduction in left ventricular filling pressures and augmented cardiac output [62]. Building on the success of afterload reduction with intravenous vasodilator therapy, in 1980 the Veterans Administration Cooperative study (V-HEFT) was launched. V-HEFT was the first study to investigate the role of oral vasodilators and HF mortality [63]. V-HEFT randomized 642 men with an EF <45% who were on background therapy of digoxin and a diuretic in a double-blinded manner to placebo, Prazosin 20 mg daily, or the combination of hydralazine and isosorbide dinitrate. The study showed that the combination of hydralazine and isosorbide dinitrate was associated with a 34% risk reduction in mortality (p≤0.028) compared to placebo. The mortality rate of those treated with prazosin was similar to those treated with placebo [63]. This study ushered in the era of oral vasodilators and suggested that the combination of hydralazine and isosorbide dinitrate in addition to a HF regimen of digoxin and diuretics was associated with favorable survival (see Table 7.3 for complete list of guideline-directed medical therapy).

Table 7.3 Treatment of heart failure with reduced ejection fraction: guideline-directed medical therapy

	NYHA Class I	NYHA Class II	NYHA Class III	NYHA Class IV
Medications	ACEi or ARB and beta-blocker[a]	+Aldosterone antagonist, Ivabradine, consider ARNI	+Hydralazine-nitrates in black patients, Ivabradine, consider ARNI	+Hydralazine-nitrates in black patients, Ivabradine, consider ARNI
Devices	[b]	CRT or CRT-D; ICD	CRT or CRT-D; ICD; LVAD; transplant	CRT or CRT-D; ICD; LVAD; transplant

Yancy et al. [122]
NYHA New York Heart Association, *ACEi* angiotensin-converting enzyme inhibitor, *ARB* angiotensin-receptor blocker, *LVAD* left ventricular assist device, *ICD* implantable cardioverter defibrillator, *ARNI* angiotensin receptor-neprilysin inhibitor
[a]Appropriate for all NYHA Classes
[b]Not Applicable

Angiotensin Converting Enzyme Inhibitors

The renin-angiotensin-aldosterone system is considered one of the most important systems in the regulation of systemic blood pressure and the pathogenesis of HF [64]. Angiotensin converting enzyme inhibitors (ACE-I) are potent vasodilators [65]. The beneficial effect of the ACE-I on HF mortality was first demonstrated on a large scale in 1987 with the Cooperative North Scandinavian Enalapril Survival (CONSENSUS) Study. CONSENSUS included 253 HF patients with New York Heart Association (NYHA) Class IV symptoms. The patients were randomized to receive enalapril or placebo, along with background therapy that included vasodilators, digoxin, and a diuretic. At 1 year, enalapril was associated with a 40% reduction in mortality, and a 27% reduction in mortality by study end [66].

In 1991, SOLVD addressed whether treatment of HF in a heterogeneous patient population would reduce mortality. SOLVD included 2569 patients with left ventricular dysfunction (LVEF <35%). It was devised as two distinct studies that ran concurrently, a treatment study that was inclusive of patients with overt HF symptoms, and a prevention study for those with asymptomatic LV dysfunction [67]. The SOLVD treatment study demonstrated a 16% risk reduction in mortality (p = 0.0036, CI 6-28), and a 26% risk reduction in heart failure hospitalizations (p≤0.0001, CI 18-34) [67]. The SOLVD prevention study included 4228 patients with asymptomatic left ventricular dysfunction that were

randomized to enalapril (2111) or placebo (2117). In the prevention study, enalapril was associated with a 20% risk reduction of the combined end point of death and hospitalization for new HF (p = 0.001, CI 9–30) [68]. Enalapril was also associated with a 29% risk reduction in the development of HF (p≤0.001, CI 21-36).

In 1991, the second The Veterans Administration Cooperative Vasodilator Heart Failure trial (V-HEFT II) compared the effects of enalapril to those of the combination of hydralazine and isosorbide dinitrate. V-HEFT II included 804 men with heart failure and randomized them to either enalapril or the combination of hydralazine-isosorbide dinitrate. V-HEFT showed that 2-year mortality was significantly lower in the enalapril group versus the hydralazine-isosorbide dinitrate group (18% vs. 25% p = 0.016), correlating to a mortality reduction of 33.6% after 1 year, 28.2% after 2 years and 14% after 3 years [69].

Racial Differences in Response to Renin-Angiotensin-Aldosterone System Inhibition

The efficacy of RAAS inhibition in AAs has been a subject of clinical intrigue for several years. There was speculation of ACE-I inefficacy in AAs in a secondary analysis of SOLVD [31]. The analysis showed an overall mortality rate of 8.1 per 100 person years for African Americans and 5.1 per 100 person years for White Americans [31]. This difference in mortality raised speculation that there may be racial differences in the response to and benefit from ACE-I therapy [31]. The Losartan Intervention For Endpoint reduction in hypertension (LIFE) study compared an atenolol-based to a losartan-based antihypertensive regimen, and found that African Americans had a more favorable response to atenolol [70]. A meta-analysis of the 12 largest randomized clinical trials of ACE-I and beta-blockers confirmed that there has been no evidence that AAs achieve less benefit from ACE-I compared to White patients [71].

Angiotensin II Receptor Blockers

The clinical use of angiotensin receptor blockers (ARB) was established in 1995 [72]. Its vasodilatory properties made it an ideal agent in the treatment of hypertension. Its application in the management of heart failure was introduced in 2001 with the publication of the Valsartan Heart Failure Trial (VAL-HEFT). VAL-HEFT included 5010 HF patients with NYHA Class II, III, and IV symptoms. Patients were randomized to receive placebo or valsartan. VAL-HEFT showed a 13% risk reduction in the combined end point of mortality and hospitalization compared to placebo [73]. VAL-HEFT failed to show a mortality benefit when comparing valsartan to placebo [73]. The Candesartan in Heart Failure Assessment of Reduction in Mortality and morbidity (CHARM) was the first trial that showed a mortality benefit with an ARB. CHARM was a collection of three trials (CHARM-Added, CHARM-Alternative, and CHARM-Preserved). In the combined study that included 4576 patients with reduced LV function (EF < 40%), compared to placebo, the candesartan group saw a reduction in HF hospitalizations, cardiovascular mortality, and all-cause mortality [74].

The Valsartan in Myocardial Infarction (VALIANT) Trial included 4909 post-myocardial patients with systolic HF, and randomized patients to valsartan, captopril, or a combination of both captopril and valsartan [75]. In VALIANT there was no difference with regard to the primary end point of mortality. The combination of valsartan and captopril was associated with increased adverse events (hypotension, renal disturbances) that required dose reduction or complete discontinuation [75]. The ACC/AHA Guidelines for Heart Failure Management recommend that ARBs be used in patients with systolic HF with current or prior symptoms who are ACE-I intolerant, unless contraindicated, to reduce morbidity and mortality (Class I recommendation) [4].

Angiotensin-Receptor Blocker/ Neprilysin Inhibitor (ARNI)

Since the publication of the landmark studies CONSENSUS [66] and SOLVD [67], ACE-Is have been the first line treatment for HF. New compounds have recently been added to the armamentarium. Neprilysin is a neuropeptidase that degrades vasoactive elements such as bradykinin, adrenomedullin, and natriuretic peptide [76]. Early studies showed that targeting neprilysin could augment the pathophysiology of hypertension and HF [76–78]. In 2014, the Prospective Comparison of ARNI With ACEI to Determine Impact on Global Mortality and Morbidity in Heart Failure (PARADIGM-HF) was published. PARADIGM-HF randomized 9419 patients to either enalapril or the combination valsartan-sacubitril. The primary endpoint was a composite of cardiovascular death and hospitalizations. The primary outcome occurred in 21.8% in the valsartan-sacubitril group and 26.5% in the enalapril group (HR 0.80; 95% confidence interval [CI], 0.73–0.87; $p < 0.001$) [79].

Beta-Adrenergic Blockers

Activation of the sympathetic nervous system and circulating catecholamines contribute to the pathophysiology of HF. The role of beta-adrenergic blockade was first studied in small single center studies in Sweden and showed the potential of beta-blockers in the long-term management of chronic HF patients [80, 81]. The U.S. Carvedilol trial was the first large-scale beta-blocker study to demonstrate a survival benefit. The study included 1094 patients with systolic HF with an LVEF <35% [82]. Carvedilol was associated with a 65% reduction in mortality (p≤0.001), and a 27% risk reduction in hospitalizations (p≤0.001) [82]. This was followed by the Cardiac Insufficiency Bisoprolol Study II (CIBIS-II) that included 2647 NYHA Class III–IV heart failure patients with an LVEF of <35%, randomized to receive the beta-blocker bisoprolol or placebo. CBIS-II showed that bisoprolol was associated with a 32% risk reduction in all-cause mortality, and a 20% risk reduction in hospitalizations [83]. The Metoprolol CR/XL Randomized Intervention Trial in-Congestive Heart Failure (MERIT-HF) randomized 3991 HF patients with an LVEF <40%, NYHA Class II–IV to either sustained release metoprolol or to placebo. Sustained release metoprolol was associated with a 34% reduction in all-cause mortality [83].

Aldosterone Receptor Antagonist

The physiologic effects of aldosterone include sympathetic activation, sodium retention, and myocardial fibrosis formation. The Randomized Aldactone Evaluation Study (RALES) assessed whether Aldactone would reduce death from all causes in patients with severe HF [84]. RALES included 1663 NYHA Class III-IV patients with an LVEF ≤35% randomized to receive 25 mg of spironolactone or matching placebo. This study found a 30% risk reduction in all-cause mortality, a 32% risk reduction in cardiac death, and a 30% risk reduction in cardiac related hospitalizations in the spironolactone group [84, 85].

The Eplerenone in Mild Patients Hospitalized and Survival Study in Heart Failure (EMPHASIS-HF) investigated the effects of eplerenone in 2737 NYHA Class II patients. The composite endpoint of cardiovascular death or HF hospitalization was seen in 18.3% of the eplerenone group versus 25.9% of the placebo group (p≤0.001) [85, 86]. The eplerenone group saw a reduction of all-cause death and a decline in all-cause hospitalizations [86].

Heart Failure Treatment in African Americans

The mechanisms of HF in AAs remain under investigation. Studies have shown that self-described AAs have lower bioavailability of nitric oxide, and lower activation of the renin-angiotensin-aldosterone system [27, 87]. Aforementioned, V-HEFT demonstrated a survival benefit in the treatment of heart failure patients with a combination of the nitric oxide donor isosorbide dinitrate and the antioxidant hydralazine [63]. This was achieved targeting a mechanism outside of the renin-angiotensin-aldosterone system. Retrospective analysis of both V-HEFT-I and II showed a mortality benefit in AAs treated with a combination of hydralazine and isosorbide dinitrate [63]. On this basis was the AAs Heart Failure trial (A-HEFT) initiated. The investigators in A-HEFT randomized 1100 African American patients with an LVEF <35%, with NYHA Class III–IV symptoms that were on background therapy that included neurohormonal blockade to the combination of hydralazine and isosorbide dinitrate or placebo. The findings from A-HEFT showed a 43% reduction in mortality in those treated with the combination of hydralazine-isosorbide dinitrate (HR 0.57, p = 0.01) [88]. The results of A-HEFT are highly suggestive of an alternative mechanism that is independent of the renin-angiotensin-aldosterone system [88].

Devices-Implantable Cardiac Defibrillators (ICD)

Sudden cardiac death (SCD) accounts for nearly 400,000 deaths in the United States annually and patients with HF are at increased risk of life-threatening ventricular arrhythmias [89]. The Multicenter Automatic Defibrillator Implantation Trial (MADIT) investigated whether prophylactic implantation of an internal cardiac defibrillator (ICD) would improve 5-year survival in patients with ischemic HF. Eligible patients had a Q-wave or enzyme positive myocardial infarction within 3 weeks of study entry. They also had an episode of asymptomatic non-sustained ventricular tachycardia unrelated to an acute myocardial infarction. Additionally, the patient had an LVEF <35%, and inducible, sustained, non-suppressible ventricular tachyarrhythmia on electrophysiological testing [85, 90]. MADIT demonstrated that in post-MI patients with HF that were at high risk of ventricular arrhythmias, prophylactic therapy with an ICD improved survival.

The Multicenter Automatic Defibrillator Implantation Trial II (MADIT-II) was designed to evaluate the potential survival benefit of a prophylactically implanted defibrillator in the absence of electrophysiological testing to induce arrhythmias [85, 90]. MADIT-II randomized 1232 patients with prior myocardial infarctions and a LVEF ≤30% to receive an ICD or conventional medical therapy. The primary end point was death from any cause. MADIT-II showed a mortality rate of 19.8% in the conventional therapy group vs. 14.2% in the defibrillator group (hazard ratio 0.69, p = 0.016). The study confirmed the benefits of prophylactic ICD therapy that was previously reported [90].

The Sudden Cardiac Death in Heart Failure Trial (SCD-HeFT) compared amiodarone to a conservatively programmed shock-only, single lead ICD. The study assessed the risk of death from any cause in a population with mild to moderate HF and ischemic and non-ischemic HF [91]. SCD-HeFT randomized 2521 patients with LVEF ≤35%, NYHA Class II-III stable Heart failure to a single chamber ICD, amiodarone or placebo [91]. In SCD-HeFT, there were 244 deaths in the placebo group, 240 deaths in the amiodarone group, and 182 deaths in the ICD group. Amiodarone was associated with a similar risk of death compared to placebo (p = 0.53) whereas an ICD was associated with a significant decrease in the risk of death compared to placebo (p = 0.007) [85, 91].

Racial Disparities in ICD

Despite evidence supporting mortality benefit with ICD use, only about 33% of eligible patients have ICDs implanted [92, 93]. This disparity is particularly noted in women and AAs. The explanation for the disparity has not been fully charac-

terized, however, is possibly related to failure of physicians to offer implantation and patient preference. In a study of 21,059 patients eligible for ICD counseling, 4755 (22.6%) received counseling. Hispanic Americans (18%) and AAs (22.6%) were less likely to receive counseling compared to White Americans (24.3%) p = 0.01 [94]. The role of patient preference in willingness to accept cardiac procedures has been evaluated in studies. Refusal of recommended procedures was rare, but AAs and Hispanic Americans were more likely to decline recommended cardiac procedures [95]. In the Educational Videos to Reduce Racial Disparities in ICD therapy Via Innovative Designs (VIVID) study, use of a video decision aid increased patient knowledge and reduced racial differences in patient preference for ICD placement [96].

Advanced Heart Failure Therapies

Advanced HF denotes patients who have progressive heart failure that has become refractory to evidence-based medical therapies. Advanced therapies refer to surgical options such as orthotopic heart transplantation and insertion of a left ventricular assist device; and a palliative medical approach that focuses on the patient's quality of life and comfort.

Heart Transplantation

For patients who progress to end stage HF, orthotropic heart transplant is the definitive treatment. The first human heart transplant was performed on December 3, 1967, by Dr. Christian Barnard in South Africa. Dr. Barnard implanted a heart from 25-year-old Denise Darvall who was a victim of an automobile accident, into 53-year-old Louis Washkansky. The patient survived 18 days post-transplant, and died from complications related to pneumonia [97]. The first adult heart transplant in the United States was performed on January 6, 1968 by Dr. Norm Shumway. The recipient died 15 days later of multiple systemic complications [98]. In 1968, 104 heart transplants were performed with only 10 surviving the first year. The following 3 years were similar with 107 transplants performed and only 24 surviving to at least 1 year. Interest in cardiac transplant began to wane until Jean Borel's discovery of cyclosporine [99]. The use of cyclosporine as an immunosuppressant in the early 1980s improved heart transplant outcomes significantly [100]. In the United States, 2500–3000 heart transplants occur annually, with 1-year and 5-year survival being 90% and 75%, respectively [101].

Heart Transplants in African Americans and Hispanic Americans

Studies have shown that AAs and Hispanic Americans have similar transplant outcomes. These populations develop HF at younger ages and are similarly listed for transplant at younger ages compared to White Individuals [102, 103]. At the time of listing they were also found to have worse hemodynamic profiles exemplified by having a mean pulmonary capillary wedge pressure > 20 mmHg [102, 103]. AAs and Hispanic Americans were more likely to be recipients of Medicaid insurance, and to be listed for transplant at centers with lower transplant volumes [102, 103]. Hispanic Americans were found to have a 50% higher risk of dying on the waitlist or becoming too sick for transplant, and despite shorter wait times for heart transplant, Hispanic Americans were 50% more likely to have early post-transplant mortality [102]. African American's 10-year survival was found to be lower than both White and Hispanic Americans [103].

Factors that influence heart transplant outcomes can be categorized as immune and non-immune mediated. Non-immune mediated mechanisms such as metabolic risk factors (diabetes mellitus, chronic renal insufficiency, and hypertension) may contribute to accelerated graft failure and is associated with postoperative mortality [104, 105]. AAs and Hispanic Americans are more likely to possess two or more metabolic risk factors [105]. Registry studies have shown that AAs have a higher incidence of hypertension and renal insufficiency, and Hispanic Americans have a higher incidence of obesity and diabetes mellitus compared to White Americans. Other non-immune mediated processes that may contribute to worse outcomes are socioeconomic status, access to healthcare and non-compliance with immunosuppressive medications.

Studies have shown that heart transplant recipients who receive public insurance in the form of Medicare or Medicaid as compared to private insurance have experienced higher rates of mortality, hospitalizations for treated rejection, and higher rates of graft failure [106, 107].

Emani et al. in a study of 4626 heart transplant recipients dichotomized by insurance status, found that Medicaid beneficiaries bridged with a left ventricular assist device had a higher waitlist mortality (HR 1.57, p≤0.05) [108]. From a socioeconomic perspective, Hispanic Americans and AAs were less likely to have a college education, graduate degree, or possess private insurance as compared to White Americans [102, 103, 107].

Left Ventricular Assist Device (LVAD)

The genesis of mechanical circulatory support originated in 1953 with the advent of the cardiac bypass machine, which allowed for complex cardiac surgeries to be performed [109]. By 1964, the National Heart, Lung and blood Institute began funding for the "artificial heart program." [109] The long-term use of LVADs in patients with end stage heart failure was validated in the Randomized Evaluation of Mechanical Assistance for the Treatment of Congestive Heart Failure (REMATCH) study. The study included 129 patients with end stage heart failure with LVEF <25%, and NYHA Class IV symptoms; 68 patients received an LVAD, and 61 were assigned to receive optimal medical therapy. There was a 48% reduction in the risk of death from any cause (RR 0.52, CI 0.34–0.78, p = 0.001). The 1- year survival was 52% in the LVAD group versus 25%. In the medical therapy group (p = 0.002), and

2-year survival was 23% in the LVAD group and 8% in the medical therapy group (p = 0.09) [110].

The REMATCH trial demonstrated that LVADs were durable options for long-term support for patients who were not heart transplant candidates. Newer designs of LVADs involving rotary pump technology that limit pulsatility were developed. The HeartMate II trial randomized 200 patients to undergo implantation of a continuous-flow LVAD or a pulsatile-flow LVAD. The primary end point was a composite of survival at 2 years, freedom from disabling stroke, or reoperation to replace the device [111]. The primary end point was achieved in more patients in the continuous-flow arm than those assigned to pulsatile-flow devices (46% vs. 11%, HR 0.38, CI 0.27–0.54, p≤0.001) [111].

As LVAD technology has advanced, the procedure has been performed more frequently. In 2006, the early pulsatile LVAD era, 98 patients received an LVAD. This number increased significantly in the continuous-flow LVAD era to 2423 in 2014 [112]. The continuous-flow LVAD era also saw in-hospital mortality decrease from 47.2% in 2005 to 12.7% in 2011. The proportion of LVADs for destination therapy has increased from 14.7% in 2006 to 45.7% in 2014 [112].

As previously described in this chapter, AAs and Hispanic Americans have a higher risk of developing heart failure, and are diagnosed at younger ages [2]. Despite the higher rates of HF compared to White adults, historically White individuals have received approximately 75% of LVADs in the United States [113]. The factors that contribute to this disparity are complex and multifactorial. Lack of access to insurance has been implicated as a potential cause as a higher portion of racial and ethnic minorities are uninsured, and lack of insurance is a relative contraindication to LVAD implantation. Breathett et al. examined temporal changes in ventricular assist devices by race and ethnicity, in a period that corresponded to the broadening of public insurance. They found that LVAD implantation rate increased significantly among AAs but not among other racial or ethnic groups during this period [113].

Cardiomyopathies

Hypertensive Heart Disease

As discussed previously, population studies have shown that AAs have the highest risk of developing heart failure, followed by Hispanic Americans, and then White Americans (4.6, 3.4, 2.5 per 1000 person years respectively) [19]. Ethnic and racial differences exist in the pathogenesis of HF. Analysis of six landmark heart failure trials showed that AAs had a higher proportion of their HF attributed to hypertensive heart disease, whereas ischemic heart disease was the primary cause in White patients. AAs possess a threefold increased risk of developing left ventricular hypertrophy compared to age-matched White patients. The mechanisms that contribute to these racial differences are multifactorial with genetic, socioeconomic, and environmental factors playing a role. The role of nitric oxide (NO) in the pathogenesis of diseases such as hypertension, diabetes mellitus, and asthma has been an area of interest to explain these observed racial differences.

NO serves as a vascular endothelial cell-derived factor that mediates vascular smooth muscle relaxation [114–116]. NO exerts its effect by initiating signaling pathways that produce cyclic guanosine monophosphate (cGMP) in the smooth muscle cell [116]. NO-dependent vasodilation can be impaired by decreased NO production, or increased NO degradation resulting in decreased NO to exert its biologic effects [116, 117].

Cardiac Amyloidosis

Amyloidosis is a progressive systemic disease involving deposition of misfolded proteins within various organ systems. Cardiac involvement is associated with increased morbidity and mortality in patients with amyloidosis. Although several disease processes have been described to contribute to the etiology of cardiac amyloidosis, two distinct entities are responsible for the majority of the reported cases [118]. The two entities that are associated with the majority of diagnosed

Table 7.4 Cardiac amyloidosis

	AL (light-chain) [123]	ATTR [124]
Pathophysiology	Deposition of fibrils composed of monoclonal immunoglobulin light chains (associated with B cell dyscrasias)	TTR (formerly pre-albumin) is formed as a misfolded tetramer that aggregates in affected tissues
Clinical symptoms	Multi-organ involvement, b-type naturetic peptide elevated, low voltage electrocardiogram	Varies with mutation, often history of carpal tunnel 5–10 years prior
Diagnosis	Transthoracic echocardiogram with strain imaging; SPEP/UPEP/serum free light chains with abnormal light chain ratio looking for a monoclonal increase; Congo red staining	Transthoracic echocardiogram with strain imaging; technetium pyrophosphate scanning; + genetic testing to determine wild type vs. familial; consider endomyocardial biopsy
Treatment	Treat heart failure and chemotherapy to treat plasma cell dyscrasia	Tafamidis works to stabilize TTR

ATTR transthyretin amyloid, *SPEP* serum protein electrophoresis, *UPEP* urine protein electrophoresis

cases of cardiac amyloidosis are light chain amyloidosis (AL) and amyloid associated with transthyretin (ATTR) (see Table 7.4) [118]. AL cardiac amyloidosis usually occurs in the setting of plasma or B cell dyscrasias. Fibrils that are composed of monoclonal immunoglobulins are deposited within the myocardium.

TTR is a protein that is synthesized in the liver, with a role of transporting thyroid hormone and retinol-binding protein complex [119]. In its pathologic state, the tetramer dissociates and misassembles into oligomers, protofilaments, and amyloid fibrils [120]. ATTR can be caused by a mutant variant (ATTR-variant) with hereditary implications or wild type (ATTR-wt).

Several mutations have been associated with ATTR, but the Val122Ile mutation is the most common [121]. This mutation was found in 23% of AAs with ATTR, and in 3.2% of AAs without amyloidosis [121]. Penetrance of the gene is not fully understood, but it is associated with a late onset cardiomyopathy that is likely underdiagnosed because of the phenotypic resemblance to hypertensive heart disease [118].

In an autopsy study ATTR-wt was found in 25% of individuals older than 80 years of age. The exact incidence of ATTR-wt is not well known; however, its clinical manifestations are indistinguishable from ATTR-variant [118].

The clinical assessment of suspected cardiac amyloid begins with clinical suspicion of this disease entity in a patient with unexplained HF. Low voltage in the limb leads and pseudo-infarct pattern in the precordial leads of an electrocardiogram occur in 50% of patients with cardiac amyloidosis. Echocardiographic findings in late-onset disease are characterized by concentric hypertrophy, diastolic dysfunction, and biatrial enlargement. Advanced echocardiographic techniques such as the use of strain and strain rate imaging from speckle tracking can aid in the diagnosis of amyloidosis. Typically, there is greater restriction of the basal segments compared to the apical region and there may be an apical sparing pattern. Imaging modalities such as cardiac magnetic resonance imaging and radionuclide imaging have improved the detection of cardiac amyloidosis. Endomyocardial biopsy has been considered the gold standard, and its use in combination with Congo red staining and immunohistochemistry can usefully identify amyloid fibrils in up to 70% of cases.

Conclusion

HF in AAs and Hispanic Americans remains a complex and heterogeneous clinical entity. Disparities exist in risk factors, diagnosis, and treatment due to a multitude of social, economic, political, and genetic factors. Further research and investment will help to stem the tide and decrease the disparities seen with these two populations.

References

1. Ponikowski P, Anker SD, AlHabib KF, et al. Heart failure: preventing disease and death worldwide. ESC Heart Fail. 2014;1(1):4–25. https://doi.org/10.1002/ehf2.12005.

2. Benjamin EJ, Virani SS, Callaway CW, et al. Heart disease and stroke statistics—2018 update: a report from the American Heart Association. Circulation. 2018;137(12):e67–e492. https://doi.org/10.1161/CIR.0000000000000558.

3. Heidenreich PA, Albert NM, Allen LA, et al. Forecasting the impact of heart failure in the United States. Circ Heart Fail. 2013;6(3):606–19. https://doi.org/10.1161/HHF.0b013e318291329a.

4. Yancy CW, Jessup M, Bozkurt B, et al. 2 013 ACCF/AHA guideline for the Management of Heart Failure. Circulation. 2013;128(16):e240–327. https://doi.org/10.1161/CIR.0b013e31829e8776.

5. van der Meer P, Gaggin HK, Dec GW. ACC/AHA versus ESC guidelines on heart failure: JACC guideline comparison. J Am Coll Cardiol. 2019;73(21):2756–68. https://doi.org/10.1016/j.jacc.2019.03.478.

6. U.S. Census Bureau QuickFacts: United States. https://www.census.gov/quickfacts/fact/table/US/PST045218. Accessed June 13, 2019.

7. Taylor A, Wright J. Importance of race/ethnicity in clinical trials: lessons from the African-American heart failure trial (A-HeFT), the African-American study of kidney disease and hypertension (AASK), and the antihypertensive and lipid-lowering treatment to prevent heart attack trial (ALLHAT). Circulation. 2005;112(23):3654–60. https://doi.org/10.1161/CIRCULATIONAHA.105.540443.

8. Weinick RM, Jacobs EA, Stone LC, Ortega AN, Burstin H. Hispanic healthcare disparities: challenging the myth of a monolithic Hispanic population. Med Care. 2004;42(4):313. https://doi.org/10.1097/01.mlr.0000118705.27241.7c.

9. Novello AC, Wise PH, Kleinman DV. Hispanic health: time for data, time for action. JAMA. 1991;265(2):253–5. https://doi.org/10.1001/jama.1991.03460020107038.

10. Vivo RP, Krim SR, Cevik C, Witteles RM. Heart failure in Hispanics. J Am Coll Cardiol. 2009;53(14):1167–75. https://doi.org/10.1016/j.jacc.2008.12.037.

11. LaVeist TA. Beyond dummy variables and sample selection: what health services researchers ought to know about race as a variable. Health Serv Res. 1994;29(1):1–16.

12. Williams DR, Jackson JS. Race/ethnicity and the 2000 census: recommendations for African American and other black populations in the United States. Am J Public Health. 2000;90(11):1728–30. https://doi.org/10.2105/ajph.90.11.1728.

13. Agyemang C, Bhopal R, Bruijnzeels M. Negro, Black, Black African, African Caribbean, African American or what? Labelling African origin populations in the health arena in the 21st century. J Epidemiol Community Health. 2005;59(12):1014–8. https://doi.org/10.1136/jech.2005.035964.

14. Black/African American – The Office of Minority Health. https://www.minorityhealth.hhs.gov/omh/browse.aspx?lvl=3&lvlid=61. Accessed June 14, 2019.

15. Levy D, Kenchaiah S, Larson MG, et al. Long-term trends in the incidence of and survival with heart failure. N Engl J Med. 2002;347(18):1397–402. https://doi.org/10.1056/NEJMoa020265.

16. Barker WH, Mullooly JP. Getchell William. Changing incidence and survival for heart failure in a well-defined older population, 1970–1974 and 1990–1994. Circulation. 2006;113(6):799–805. https://doi.org/10.1161/CIRCULATIONAHA.104.492033.

17. Huffman MD, Berry JD, Ning H, et al. Lifetime risk for heart failure among White and Black Americans: cardiovascular lifetime risk pooling project. J Am Coll Cardiol. 2013;61(14):1510–7. https://doi.org/10.1016/j.jacc.2013.01.022.

18. Gerber Y, Weston SA, Redfield MM, et al. A contemporary appraisal of the heart failure epidemic in Olmsted County, Minnesota, 2000 to 2010. JAMA Intern Med. 2015;175(6):996–1004. https://doi.org/10.1001/jamainternmed.2015.0924.

19. Bahrami H, Kronmal R, Bluemke DA, et al. Differences in the incidence of congestive heart failure by ethnicity: the multi-ethnic study of atherosclerosis. Arch Intern Med. 2008;168(19):2138–45. https://doi.org/10.1001/archinte.168.19.2138.

20. Chang PP, Chambless LE, Shahar E, et al. Incidence and survival of hospitalized acute decompensated heart failure in four US communities (from the atherosclerosis risk in communities study). Am J Cardiol. 2014;113(3):504–10. https://doi.org/10.1016/j.amjcard.2013.10.032.

21. Lloyd-Jones Donald M, Yuling H, Darwin L, et al. Defining and setting National Goals for cardiovascular health promotion and disease reduction. Circulation. 2010;121(4):586–613. https://doi.org/10.1161/CIRCULATIONAHA.109.192703.

22. Loehr LR, Rosamond WD, Chang PP, Folsom AR, Chambless LE. Heart failure incidence and survival (from the atherosclerosis risk in communities study). Am J Cardiol. 2008;101(7):1016–22. https://doi.org/10.1016/j.amjcard.2007.11.061.

23. Pandey DK, Labarthe DR, Goff DC, Chan W, Nichaman MZ. Community-wide coronary heart disease mortality in Mexican Americans equals or exceeds that in non-Hispanic whites: the Corpus Christi heart project. Am J Med. 2001;110(2):81–7. https://doi.org/10.1016/S0002-9343(00)00667-7.

24. Hunt KJ, Resendez RG, Williams K, Haffner SM, Stern MP, Hazuda HP. All-cause and cardiovascular

mortality among Mexican-American and non-Hispanic White older participants in the San Antonio heart study— evidence against the "Hispanic paradox.". Am J Epidemiol. 2003;158(11):1048–57. https://doi.org/10.1093/aje/kwg249.

25. Dunlay SM, Weston SA, Jacobsen SJ, Roger VL. Risk factors for heart failure: a population-based case-control study. Am J Med. 2009;122(11):1023–8. https://doi.org/10.1016/j.amjmed.2009.04.022.

26. Kalogeropoulos A, Georgiopoulou V, Kritchevsky SB, et al. Epidemiology of incident heart failure in a contemporary elderly cohort: the health, aging, and body composition study. Arch Intern Med. 2009;169(7):708–15. https://doi.org/10.1001/archinternmed.2009.40.

27. Yancy CW. Heart failure in African Americans: a cardiovascular enigma. J Card Fail. 2000;6(3):183–6. https://doi.org/10.1054/jcaf.2000.17610.

28. Centers for Disease Control and Prevention (CDC). Prevalence of diabetes among Hispanics–selected areas, 1998-2002. MMWR Morb Mortal Wkly Rep. 2004;53(40):941–4.

29. War d BW. Early Release of Selected Estimates Based on Data From the 2015 National Health Interview Survey (05/2016). 2015:120.

30. Trends in Obesity Among Adults in the United States, 2005 to 2014 | Obesity | JAMA | JAMA Network. https://jamanetwork-com.ezproxy.galter.northwestern.edu/journals/jama/fullarticle/2526639. Accessed June 17, 2019.

31. Dries DL, Exner DV, Gersh BJ, Cooper HA, Carson PE, Domanski MJ. Racial differences in the outcome of left ventricular dysfunction. N Engl J Med. 1999;340(8):609–16. https://doi.org/10.1056/NEJM199902253400804.

32. Willett WC, Sacks F, Trichopoulou A, et al. Mediterranean diet pyramid: a cultural model for healthy eating. Am J Clin Nutr. 1995;61(6):1402S–6S. https://doi.org/10.1093/ajcn/61.6.1402S.

33. Dietary Sodium and the Dietary Approaches to Stop Hypertension (DASH) Diet | NEJM. New England Journal of Medicine. https://www-nejm-org.ezproxy.galter.northwestern.edu/doi/10.1056/NEJM200101043440101?url_ver=Z39.88-2003&rfr_id=ori%3Arid%3Acrossref.org&rfr_dat=cr_pub%3Dwww-ncbi-nlm-nih-gov.ezproxy.galter.northwestern.edu. Accessed June 13, 2019.

34. Sanches Machado d'Almeida K, Ronchi Spillere S, Zuchinali P, Corrêa Souza G. Mediterranean diet and other dietary patterns in primary prevention of heart failure and changes in cardiac function markers: a systematic review. Nutrients. 2018;10(1) https://doi.org/10.3390/nu10010058.

35. Levitan EB, Wolk A, Mittleman MA. Consistency with the DASH diet and incidence of heart failure. Arch Intern Med. 2009;169(9):851–7. https://doi.org/10.1001/archinternmed.2009.56.

36. Levitan EB, Wolk A, Mittleman MA. Relation of consistency with the dietary approaches to stop hypertension diet and incidence of heart fail-

ure in men aged 45 to 79 years. Am J Cardiol. 2009;104(10):1416–20. https://doi.org/10.1016/j.amjcard.2009.06.061.

37. Lara KM, Levitan EB, Gutierrez OM, et al. Dietary patterns and incident heart failure in U.S. adults without known coronary disease. J Am Coll Cardiol. 2019;73(16):2036–45. https://doi.org/10.1016/j.jacc.2019.01.067.

38. Contribution of Major Diseases to Disparities in Mortality | NEJM. New England Journal of Medicine. https://www-nejm-org.ezproxy.galter.northwestern.edu/doi/10.1056/NEJMsa012979?url_ver=Z39.88-2003&rfr_id=ori%3Arid%3Acrossref.org&rfr_dat=cr_pub%3Dwww-ncbi-nlm-nih-gov.ezproxy.galter.northwestern.edu. Accessed June 13, 2019.

39. Chen L, Simonsen N, Liu L. Racial differences of Pediatric hypertension in relation to birth weight and body size in the United States. PLoS One. 2015;10(7):e0132606. https://doi.org/10.1371/journal.pone.0132606.

40. Carson AP, Howard G, Burke GL, Shea S, Levitan EB, Muntner P. Ethnic differences in hypertension incidence among middle-aged and older adults: the multi-ethnic study of atherosclerosis. Hypertension. 2011;57(6):1101–7. https://doi.org/10.1161/HYPERTENSIONAHA.110.168005.

41. Howard G, Safford MM, Moy CS, et al. Racial differences in the incidence of cardiovascular risk factors in older Black and White adults. J Am Geriatr Soc. 2017;65(1):83–90. https://doi.org/10.1111/jgs.14472.

42. Fuchs FD. Why do black Americans have higher prevalence of hypertension?: an enigma still unsolved. Hypertension. 2011;57(3):379–80. https://doi.org/10.1161/HYPERTENSIONAHA.110.163196.

43. Howard G, Cushman M, Moy CS, et al. Association of Clinical and Social Factors with Excess Hypertension Risk in Black compared with White US adults. JAMA. 2018;320(13):1338–48. https://doi.org/10.1001/jama.2018.13467.

44. My Life Check - Life's Simple 7. http://www.heart.org/HEARTORG/Conditions/My-Life-Check%E2%80%94Lifes-Simple-7_UCM_471453_Article.jsp#.XQFLWNNKgUt. Accessed June 12, 2019.

45. Aferdita S, Sameera T, Adolfo C, et al. Ideal cardiovascular health, cardiovascular Remodeling, and heart failure in blacks. Circ Heart Fail. 2017;10(2):e003682. https://doi.org/10.1161/CIRCHEARTFAILURE.116.003682.

46. Casagrande SS, Aviles-Santa L, Corsino L, et al. Hemoglobin A1c, blood pressure, and LDL-cholesterol control among Hispanic/Latino adults with diabetes: results from the Hispanic community health study/study of Latinos (HCHS/SOL). Endocr Pract. 2017;23(10):1232–53. https://doi.org/10.4158/EP171765.OR.

47. Yancy CW, Jessup M, Bozkurt B, et al. 2013 ACCF/AHA guideline for the Management of Heart

Failure: executive summary: a report of the American College of Cardiology Foundation/American Heart Association task force on practice guidelines. J Am Coll Cardiol. 2013;62(16):1495–539. https://doi.org/10.1016/j.jacc.2013.05.020.

48. Pandey A, Omar W, Ayers C, et al. Sex and race differences in lifetime risk of heart failure with preserved ejection fraction and heart failure with reduced ejection fraction. Circulation. 2018;137(17):1814–23. https://doi.org/10.1161/CIRCULATIONAHA.117.031622.

49. Joseph Y, Rodriguez CJ, Brandon S, et al. Prognosis of individuals with asymptomatic left ventricular systolic dysfunction in the multi-ethnic study of atherosclerosis (MESA). Circulation. 2012;126(23):2713–9. https://doi.org/10.1161/CIRCULATIONAHA.112.112201.

50. Friedman GD, Cutter GR, Donahue RP, et al. Cardia: study design, recruitment, and some characteristics of the examined subjects. J Clin Epidemiol. 1988;41(11):1105–16. https://doi.org/10.1016/0895-4356(88)90080-7.

51. Bibbins-Domingo K, Pletcher MJ, Lin F, et al. Racial differences in incident heart failure among Young adults. N Engl J Med. 2009;360(12):1179–90. https://doi.org/10.1056/NEJMoa0807265.

52. Glynn P, Lloyd-Jones DM, Feinstein MJ, Carnethon M, Khan SS. Disparities in cardiovascular mortality related to heart failure in the United States. J Am Coll Cardiol. 2019;73(18):2354–5. https://doi.org/10.1016/j.jacc.2019.02.042.

53. Vivo RP, Krim SR, Krim NR, et al. Care and outcomes of Hispanic patients admitted with heart failure with preserved or reduced ejection fraction. Circ Heart Fail. 2012;5(2):167–75. https://doi.org/10.1161/CIRCHEARTFAILURE.111.963546.

54. Goyal P, Paul T, Almarzooq ZI, et al. Sex- and race-related differences in characteristics and outcomes of hospitalizations for heart failure with preserved ejection fraction. J Am Heart Assoc. 2017;6(4) https://doi.org/10.1161/JAHA.116.003330.

55. Setoguchi S, Stevenson LW, Schneeweiss S. Repeated hospitalizations predict mortality in the community population with heart failure. Am Heart J. 2007;154(2):260–6. https://doi.org/10.1016/j.ahj.2007.01.041.

56. Reis SE, Holubkov R, Edmundowicz D, et al. Treatment of patients admitted to the hospital with congestive heart failure: specialty-related disparities in practice patterns and outcomes. J Am Coll Cardiol. 1997;30(3):733–8. https://doi.org/10.1016/S0735-1097(97)00214-3.

57. Harjai KJ, Boulos LM, Smart FW, et al. Effects of caregiver specialty on cost and clinical outcomes following hospitalization for heart failure. Am J Cardiol. 1998;82(1):82–5.

58. Auerbach AD, Hamel MB, Califf RM, et al. Patient characteristics associated with care by a cardiologist among adults hospitalized with severe congestive heart failure. J Am Coll Cardiol.

2000;36(7):2119–25. https://doi.org/10.1016/S0735-1097(00)01005-6.

59. Breathett K, Liu WG, Allen LA, et al. African Americans are less likely to receive care by a cardiologist during an intensive care unit admission for heart failure. JACC Heart Failure. 2018;6(5):413–20. https://doi.org/10.1016/j.jchf.2018.02.015.

60. Joynt KE, Orav EJ, Jha AK. Thirty-day readmission rates for Medicare beneficiaries by race and site of care. JAMA. 2011;305(7):675–81. https://doi.org/10.1001/jama.2011.123.

61. Burch GE, Walsh JJ, Black WC. Value of prolonged bed rest in Management of Cardiomegaly. JAMA. 1963;183(2):81–7. https://doi.org/10.1001/jama.1963.03700020031008.

62. Guiha NH, Cohn JN, Mikulic E, Franciosa JA, Limas CJ. Treatment of refractory heart failure with infusion of nitroprusside. N Engl J Med. 1974;291(12):587–92. https://doi.org/10.1056/nejm197409192911201.

63. Cohn JN, Archibald DG, Ziesche S, et al. Effect of vasodilator therapy on mortality in chronic congestive heart failure. N Engl J Med. 1986;314(24):1547–52. https://doi.org/10.1056/nejm198606123142404.

64. Ferreira SH. Angiotensin converting enzyme: history and relevance. Semin Perinatol. 2000;24(1):7–10. https://doi.org/10.1016/S0146-0005(00)80046-4.

65. Lipkin DP, Poole-Wilson PA. Treatment of chronic heart failure: a review of recent drug trials. Br Med J (Clin Res Ed). 1985;291(6501):993–6. https://doi.org/10.1136/bmj.291.6501.993.

66. The Consensus Trial Study Group. Effects of Enalapril on mortality in severe congestive heart failure. N Engl J Med. 1987;316(23):1429–35. https://doi.org/10.1056/nejm198706043162301.

67. The Consensus Trial Study Group. Effect of Enalapril on survival in patients with reduced left ventricular ejection fractions and congestive heart failure. N Engl J Med. 1991;325(5):293–302. https://doi.org/10.1056/nejm199108013250501.

68. The Consensus Trial Study Group. Effect of Enalapril on mortality and the development of heart failure in asymptomatic patients with reduced left ventricular ejection fractions. N Engl J Med. 1992;327(10):685–91. https://doi.org/10.1056/nejm199209033271003.

69. Cohn JN, Johnson G, Ziesche S, et al. A comparison of Enalapril with hydralazine–isosorbide Dinitrate in the treatment of chronic congestive heart failure. N Engl J Med. 1991;325(5):303–10. https://doi.org/10.1056/nejm199108013250502.

70. Julius S, Alderman MH, Beevers G, et al. Cardiovascular risk reduction in hypertensive black patients with left ventricular hypertrophy: the life study. J Am Coll Cardiol. 2004;43(6):1047–55. https://doi.org/10.1016/j.jacc.2003.11.029.

71. Shekelle PG, Rich MW, Morton SC, et al. Efficacy of angiotensin-converting enzyme inhibitors and beta-blockers in the management of left ventricular systolic dysfunction according to race, gender, and diabetic status: a meta-analysis of major clinical

trials. J Am Coll Cardiol. 2003;41(9):1529–38. https://doi.org/10.1016/S0735-1097(03)00262-6.

72. Abraham HMA, White CM, White WB. The comparative efficacy and safety of the angiotensin receptor blockers in the management of hypertension and other cardiovascular diseases. Drug Saf. 2015;38(1):33–54. https://doi.org/10.1007/s40264-014-0239-7.

73. Cohn JN, Tognoni G. A randomized trial of the angiotensin-receptor blocker valsartan in chronic heart failure. N Engl J Med. 2001;345(23):1667–75. https://doi.org/10.1056/NEJMoa010713.

74. Young JB, Dunlap ME, Pfeffer MA, et al. Mortality and morbidity reduction with candesartan in patients with chronic heart failure and left ventricular systolic dysfunction. Circulation. 2004;110(17):2618–26. https://doi.org/10.1161/01.CIR.0000146819.43235.A9.

75. Pfeffer MA, McMurray JJV, Velazquez EJ, et al. Valsartan, captopril, or both in myocardial infarction complicated by heart failure, left ventricular dysfunction, or both. N Engl J Med. 2003;349(20):1893–906. https://doi.org/10.1056/NEJMoa032292.

76. Cruden NLM, Fox KAA, Ludlam CA, Johnston NR, Newby DE. Neutral endopeptidase inhibition augments vascular actions of bradykinin in patients treated with angiotensin-converting enzyme inhibition. Hypertension. 2004;44(6):913–8. https://doi.org/10.1161/01.HYP.0000146483.78994.56.

77. Wilkinson IB, McEniery CM, Bongaerts KH, MacCallum H, Webb DJ, Cockcroft JR. Adrenomedullin (ADM) in the human forearm vascular bed: effect of neutral endopeptidase inhibition and comparison with proadrenomedullin NH2-terminal 20 peptide (PAMP). Br J Clin Pharmacol. 2001;52(2):159–64. https://doi.org/10.1046/j.0306-5251.2001.1420.x.

78. Rademaker MT, Charles CJ, Espiner EA, Nicholls MG, Richards AM, Kosoglou T. Neutral endopeptidase inhibition: augmented atrial and brain natriuretic peptide, haemodynamic and natriuretic responses in ovine heart failure. Clin Sci. 1996;91(3):283–91. https://doi.org/10.1042/cs0910283.

79. McMurray JJV, Packer M, Desai AS, et al. Angiotensin–Neprilysin inhibition versus Enalapril in heart failure. N Engl J Med. 2014;371(11):993–1004. https://doi.org/10.1056/NEJMoa1409077.

80. Waagstein F, Hjalmarson A, Varnauskas E, Wallentin I. Effect of chronic beta-adrenergic receptor blockade in congestive cardiomyopathy. Br Heart J. 1975;37(10):1022–36. https://doi.org/10.1136/hrt.37.10.1022.

81. Funck-Brentano C. Beta-blockade in CHF: from contraindication to indication. Eur Heart J Suppl. 2006;8(suppl_C):C19–27. https://doi.org/10.1093/eurheartj/sul010.

82. Packer M, Bristow MR, Cohn JN, et al. The effect of carvedilol on morbidity and mortality in patients with chronic heart failure. N Engl J Med. 1996;334(21):1349–55. https://doi.org/10.1056/nejm199605233342101.

83. Drummond GA, Squire IB. The cardiac insufficiency Bisoprolol study II (CIBIS-II): a randomised trial. Lancet (London, England). 1999;353(9146):9–13.

84. Pitt B, Zannad F, Remme WJ, et al. The effect of spironolactone on morbidity and mortality in patients with severe heart failure. N Engl J Med. 1999;341(10):709–17. https://doi.org/10.1056/nejm199909023411001.

85. Okwuosa IS, Princewill O, Nwabueze C, et al. The ABCs of managing systolic heart failure: past, present, and future. Cleve Clin J Med. 2016;83(10):753–65. https://doi.org/10.3949/ccjm.83a.16006.

86. Zannad F, McMurray JJV, Krum H, et al. Eplerenone in patients with systolic heart failure and mild symptoms. N Engl J Med. 2011;364(1):11–21. https://doi.org/10.1056/NEJMoa1009492.

87. Gillum RF. Pathophysiology of hypertension in blacks and whites. A review of the basis of racial blood pressure differences. Hypertension (Dallas, Tex: 1979). 1979;1(5):468–75.

88. Taylor AL, Ziesche S, Yancy C, et al. Combination of isosorbide Dinitrate and hydralazine in blacks with heart failure. N Engl J Med. 2004;351(20):2049–57. https://doi.org/10.1056/NEJMoa042934.

89. Saour B, Smith B, Yancy CW. Heart failure and sudden cardiac death. Cardiac Electrophysiol Clin. 2017;9(4):709–23. https://doi.org/10.1016/j.ccep.2017.07.010.

90. Moss AJ, Zareba W, Hall WJ, et al. Prophylactic implantation of a defibrillator in patients with myocardial infarction and reduced ejection fraction. N Engl J Med. 2002;346(12):877–83. https://doi.org/10.1056/NEJMoa013474.

91. Bardy GH, Lee KL, Mark DB, et al. Amiodarone or an implantable cardioverter–defibrillator for congestive heart failure. N Engl J Med. 2005;352(3):225–37. https://doi.org/10.1056/NEJMoa043399.

92. Hernandez AF, Fonarow GC, Liang L, et al. Sex and racial differences in the use of implantable cardioverter-defibrillators among patients hospitalized with heart failure. JAMA. 2007;298(13):1525–32. https://doi.org/10.1001/jama.298.13.1525.

93. Al-Khatib SM, Hellkamp AS, Hernandez AF, et al. Trends in use of implantable cardioverter-defibrillator therapy among patients hospitalized for heart failure: have the previously observed sex and racial disparities changed over time? Circulation. 2012;125(9):1094–101. https://doi.org/10.1161/CIRCULATIONAHA.111.066605.

94. Hess PL, Hernandez AF, Bhatt DL, et al. Sex and race/ethnicity differences in implantable cardioverter-defibrillator Counseling and use among patients hospitalized with heart failure: findings from the get with the guidelines-heart failure program. Circulation. 2016;134(7):517–26. https://doi.org/10.1161/CIRCULATIONAHA.115.021048.

95. Gordon HS, Paterniti DA, Wray NP. Race and patient refusal of invasive cardiac procedures. J Gen Intern Med. 2004;19(9):962–6. https://doi.org/10.1111/j.1525-1497.2004.30131.x.

96. Thomas KL, Zimmer LO, Dai D, Al-Khatib SM, Allen LaPointe NM, Peterson ED. Educational videos to reduce racial disparities in ICD therapy via innovative designs (VIVID): a randomized clinical trial. Am Heart J. 2013;166(1):157–63. https://doi.org/10.1016/j.ahj.2013.03.031.

97. Alivizatos PA. Fiftieth anniversary of the first heart transplant: the progress of American medical research, the ethical dilemmas, and Christiaan Barnard. Proc (Bayl Univ Med Cent). 2017;30(4):475–7. https://doi.org/10.1080/08998280.2017.11930236.

98. Silbergleit A, Norman E. Shumway and the early heart transplants. Tex Heart Inst J. 2006;33(2):274–5.

99. Borel JF, Kis ZL, Beveridge T. The history of the discovery and development of cyclosporine (Sandimmune®). In: Merluzzi VJ, Adams J, editors. The search for anti-inflammatory drugs: case histories from concept to clinic. Boston: Birkhäuser Boston; 1995. p. 27–63. https://doi.org/10.1007/978-1-4615-9846-6_2.

100. Sivathasan C. Experience with cyclosporine in heart transplantation. Transplant Proc. 2004;36(2, Supplement):S346–8. https://doi.org/10.1016/j.transproceed.2004.01.072.

101. Alraies MC, Eckman P. Adult heart transplant: indications and outcomes. J Thorac Dis. 2014;6(8):1120–8. https://doi.org/10.3978/j.issn.2072-1439.2014.06.44.

102. Singh Tajinder P, Almond Christopher S, Taylor David O, Milliren Carly E, Graham DA. Racial and ethnic differences in wait-list outcomes in patients listed for heart transplantation in the United States. Circulation. 2012;125(24):3022–30. https://doi.org/10.1161/CIRCULATIONAHA.112.092643.

103. Allen JG, Weiss ES, Arnaoutakis GJ, et al. The impact of race on survival after heart transplantation: an analysis of more than 20,000 patients. Ann Thorac Surg. 2010;89(6):1956–64. https://doi.org/10.1016/j.athoracsur.2010.02.093.

104. Suryanarayana PG, Copeland H, Friedman M, Copeland JG. Cardiac transplantation in African Americans: a single-Center experience. Clin Cardiol. 2014;37(6):331–6. https://doi.org/10.1002/clc.22275.

105. Kilic A, Conte JV, Shah AS, Yuh DD. Orthotopic heart transplantation in patients with metabolic risk factors. Ann Thorac Surg. 2012;93(3):718–24. https://doi.org/10.1016/j.athoracsur.2011.11.054.

106. Kilic A, Higgins Robert SD, Whitson Bryan A, Kilic A. Racial disparities in outcomes of adult heart transplantation. Circulation. 2015;131(10):882–9. https://doi.org/10.1161/CIRCULATIONAHA.114.011676.

107. DuBay DA, MacLennan PA, Reed RD, et al. Insurance type and solid organ transplantation outcomes: a historical perspective on how Medicaid expansion might impact transplantation outcomes. J Am Coll Surg. 2016;223(4):611–620.e4. https://doi.org/10.1016/j.jamcollsurg.2016.07.004.

108. Emani S, Tumin D, Foraker RE, Hayes D Jr, Smith SA. Impact of insurance status on heart transplant wait-list mortality for patients with left ventricular assist devices. Clin Transplant. 2017;31(2) https://doi.org/10.1111/ctr.12875.

109. Prinzing A, Herold U, Berkefeld A, Krane M, Lange R, Voss B. Left ventricular assist devices-current state and perspectives. J Thorac Dis. 2016;8(8):E660–6. https://doi.org/10.21037/jtd.2016.07.13.

110. Rose EA, Gelijns AC, Moskowitz AJ, et al. Long-term use of a left ventricular assist device for end-stage heart failure. N Engl J Med. 2001;345(20):1435–43. https://doi.org/10.1056/NEJMoa012175.

111. Slaughter MS, Rogers JG, Milano CA, et al. Advanced heart failure treated with continuous-flow left ventricular assist device. N Engl J Med. 2009;361(23):2241–51. https://doi.org/10.1056/NEJMoa0909938.

112. Kirklin JK, Naftel DC, Pagani FD, et al. Seventh INTERMACS annual report: 15,000 patients and counting. J Heart Lung Transplant. 2015;34(12):1495–504. https://doi.org/10.1016/j.healun.2015.10.003.

113. Breathett K, Allen Larry A, Helmkamp L, et al. Temporal trends in contemporary use of ventricular assist devices by race and ethnicity. Circ Heart Fail. 2018;11(8):e005008. https://doi.org/10.1161/CIRCHEARTFAILURE.118.005008.

114. Furchgott RF, Zawadzki JV. The obligatory role of endothelial cells in the relaxation of arterial smooth muscle by acetylcholine. Nature. 1980;288(5789):373–6.

115. Stuart-Smith K. Demystified. Nitric oxide. Mol Pathol. 2002;55(6):360–6. https://doi.org/10.1136/mp.55.6.360.

116. Ignarro LJ, Buga GM, Wood KS, Byrns RE, Chaudhuri G. Endothelium-derived relaxing factor produced and released from artery and vein is nitric oxide. Proc Natl Acad Sci U S A. 1987;84(24):9265–9. https://doi.org/10.1073/pnas.84.24.9265.

117. Mata-Greenwood E, Chen D-B. Racial differences in nitric oxide-dependent vasorelaxation. Reprod Sci. 2008;15(1):9–25. https://doi.org/10.1177/1933719107312160.

118. Banypersad SM, Moon JC, Whelan C, Hawkins PN, Wechalekar AD. Updates in cardiac amyloidosis: a review. J Am Heart Assoc. 1(2):e000364. https://doi.org/10.1161/JAHA.111.000364.

119. Vieira M, Saraiva MJ. Transthyretin: a multifaceted protein. BMC. 2014;5(1):45. https://doi.org/10.1515/bmc-2013-0038.

120. Colon W, Kelly JW. Partial denaturation of transthyretin is sufficient for amyloid fibril formation in vitro. Biochemistry. 1992;31(36):8654–60. https://doi.org/10.1021/bi00151a036.

121. Jacobson DR, Pastore RD, Yaghoubian R, et al. Variant-sequence transthyretin (isoleucine 122) in late-onset cardiac amyloidosis in Black Americans. N Engl J Med. 1997;336(7):466–73. https://doi.org/10.1056/nejm199702133360703.

122. Yancy CW, et al. 2017 ACC/AHA/HFSA Focused Update of the 2013 ACCF/AHA Guideline for the Management of Heart Failure: A Report of the American College of Cardiology/American Heart Association Task Force on Clinical Practice Guidelines and the Heart Failure Society of America. J Am Coll Cardiol. 2017;70(6):776–803.

123. Falk RH, Alexander KM, Liao R, Dorbala S. AL (Light-Chain) cardiac amyloidosis: a review of diagnosis and therapy. J Am Coll Cardiol. 2016;68(12):1323–41.

124. Ruberg FL, et al. Transthyretin amyloid cardiomyopathy: JACC state-of-the-art review. J Am Coll Cardiol. 2019;73(22):2872–91.

Heterogeneity, Nativity, and Disaggregation of Cardiovascular Risk and Outcomes in Hispanic Americans

8

Vanessa Blumer and Fatima Rodriguez

Introduction

Cardiovascular disease (CVD) is the leading cause of death among Hispanic Americans, who currently comprise the largest and one of the fastest growing minority groups in the United States [1]. The rapid growth of this population has led to an increased interest in better understanding their risk factors and CVD outcomes. Hispanic individuals appear to have decreased cardiovascular risk when compared to non-Hispanic individuals with similar risk factor burden [2], and growing evidence suggests that cardiovascular risk and disease rates may vary among the highly heterogenous Hispanic subgroups [3]. This chapter reviews the importance of unpacking Hispanic heterogeneity through understanding of Hispanic immigration patterns and disaggregation of cardiovascular risk and outcomes.

Who Is Hispanic? US Census History

Hispanics/Latinos are a heterogeneous group of individuals of any race, ancestry, ethnicity, or combination, who have origins in South America, Central America, Mexico, the Caribbean, or any other Spanish-speaking country or culture [4]. The terms *Hispanic* and *Latino* are often used as synonyms and interchangeably, yet for the purpose of this book chapter, the term Hispanic will be preferentially used.

Despite the long history of Hispanic immigration in the United States, there was no attempt to count this group separately in the US Census until the late twentieth century. Behind the current Hispanic definition of the US Census Bureau, there are multiple decades of revised question wording on census forms and shifting answer categories—all of which serve as a testament of the challenges to define this fast-growing population and reflect evolving cultural norms about what it means to be Hispanic in the United States today.

The first attempt to count Hispanic Americans appeared in the 1930 Census which had a one-time inclusion for "Mexican" as a category in the race question. Thereafter, the initial major attempt to estimate the size of the Hispanic population for the entire nation was in the 1970 Census. In the 1970 Census, forms were completed by residents themselves and a "person's origin or descent" was inquired; the categories in the 1970 Census included "Mexican, Puerto

V. Blumer
Division of Cardiology, Duke University Medical Center, Durham, NC, USA
e-mail: vanessa.blumer@duke.edu

F. Rodriguez (✉)
Division of Cardiovascular Medicine, Stanford University, Stanford, CA, USA
e-mail: frodrigu@stanford.edu

K. C. Ferdinand et al. (eds.), *Cardiovascular Disease in Racial and Ethnic Minority Populations*, Contemporary Cardiology, https://doi.org/10.1007/978-3-030-81034-4_8

Rican, Cuban, Central or South American, and other Spanish." This question did not appear to work very well, leading to an undercount of about one million Hispanic individuals. One reason for this was that many second-generation Hispanic Americans did not select one of the Hispanic groups because the question did not include terms like "Mexican American." The wording also resulted in hundreds of thousands of people living in the south or central regions of the United States to be mistakenly included in the "Central or South American" category. In 1980, the question was modified to further specify that it pertained to Hispanics: "Is this person of Spanish/Hispanic origin or descent?" Furthermore, the categories were broadened to include "Mexican, Mexican-Amer., Chicano, Puerto Rican, Cuban, or other Spanish/Hispanic." In 2000, the term "Latino" was added to make the question read, "Is this person Spanish, Hispanic, or Latino?" Additionally, the response category was reworded to "Yes, another Hispanic, Latino, or Spanish origin," and a list of examples was provided ("Argentinean, Colombian, Dominican, Nicaraguan, Salvadoran, Spaniard, etc.") in an attempt to elicit a specific response [5, 6]. In more recent years, the US Census Bureau has studied an alternative approach to counting Hispanic Americans that combines questions that ask about Hispanic origin and race. However, this change will not appear in the 2020 census. The 2020 US Census will continue to ask, "Is this person of Hispanic, Latino, or Spanish origin?," and the possible answers are similar to those reported in the 2000 US Census [6].

Hispanic Immigration in the United States

Hispanic Americans are the fastest growing minority group in the United States, currently comprising 18% of the population (Fig. 8.1). According to the US Census Bureau [7], that population is expected to increase from 55 million in 2014 to 119 million by 2060; by that time, Hispanic individuals will represent nearly one-third of the US population (29% of the total US

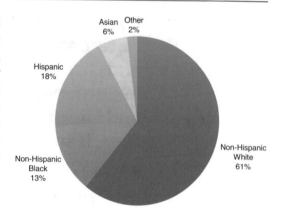

Fig. 8.1 US population by self-reported race and ethnicity. Racial groups include only non-Hispanics. Hispanic individuals may be of any race. Figure based on data from Tabulations of US Census Bureau Statistics; 2018 population estimates. https://www.census.gov/quickfacts/fact/table/US/RHI725217

population). The growing US Hispanic population is drawn from an increasingly diverse mix of countries. Traditionally, the three largest subgroups in the United States, as defined in the US Census, have been those of Mexican, Puerto Rican, and Cuban origin. Over the past years, Mexicans in the United States increased by 54%, Puerto Ricans grew by 36%, whereas the Cuban population increased by 44% [7, 8]. However, the landscape of the Hispanic population in the United States is dynamic, with a greater diversity of nationalities adding their numbers to the already established subgroups. Five other Hispanic origin groups have populations that exceed or are very close to one million people— Salvadorans, Dominicans, Guatemalans, Colombians, and Hondurans—and each of these groups has also seen their population increase over the past decade [9]. Moreover, the geographic distribution of the US Hispanic population has also dramatically changed (Fig. 8.2). According to 2017 US Census data, the states with a population of one million or more Hispanic residents has extended to Arizona, California, Colorado, Florida, Georgia, Illinois, New Jersey, New York, and Texas [10]. This demographic shift underscores the potential impact that Hispanic health may have in shaping the health profile of the United States. Hence,

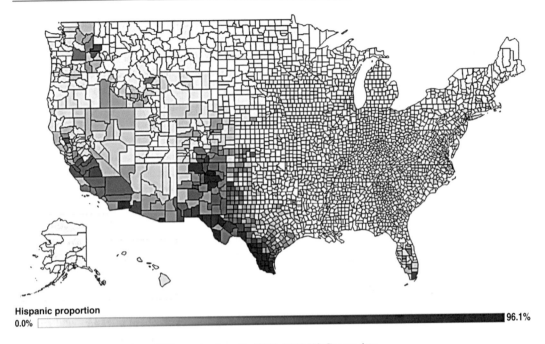

Hispanic proportion
0.0%   96.1%

Fig. 8.2 Hispanic proportion of US counties from the 2000–2010 US Census data

understanding the fundamental determinants of Hispanic health is crucial for all populations.

A thorough understanding of the cardiovascular risk and outcomes in Hispanic Americans has been hindered by the paucity of data acknowledging the profound heterogeneity of this ethnic and multiracial group. Although Hispanic Americans share the same language, they have very diverse backgrounds, and their migration history and patterns of settlement in the United States vary. Hispanic individuals are a diverse population with different genetic profiles, sociocultural practices, and socioeconomic status [11, 12]. In this regard, the Hispanic population should not be considered as a single group and their distinct individual characteristics should be considered when analyzing their potential risk factors and specific CVD outcomes.

Hispanic counterparts despite their tendency of having lower levels of income, education, worse healthcare access, and greater adverse baseline CVD risk profiles [13].

Although CVD is the leading cause of death in the Hispanic population, when studied in aggregate, Hispanic Americans experience better outcomes than non-Hispanic individuals. The rationale for this observation has been supported by several theories that include, but are not limited to, a healthy Hispanic immigrant effect, duration of residence in the United States and acculturation, socioeconomic status (SES), as well as health behaviors and genetic, geographic, and psychosocial baseline characteristics (Fig. 8.3). However, the exact underlying mechanism to explain this phenomenon remains uncertain.

The Hispanic Paradox

Over 30 years ago, Kyriakos Markides coined the term "Hispanic paradox" to describe the epidemiological finding that Hispanic individuals in the United States live longer than their non-

Healthy Migrant and Statistical Immortality

The healthy migrant theory postulates that Hispanic individuals who emigrate are more likely to be younger and healthier individuals

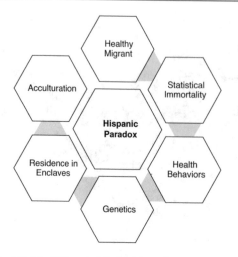

Fig. 8.3 The "Hispanic Paradox" describes the epidemiological mystery of why Hispanics in the US live longer than their white counterparts despite generally lower socioeconomic status and health care access. Many theories have been proposed to support or refute the Hispanic Paradox

than those who do not migrate, positioning the immigrant population at an advantage when compared to the US host population. The statistical immortality theory, also known as salmon bias theory, proposes that migrants return to their native country to die, in that way underestimating mortality rates in the United States.

These theories have been challenged by more recent studies. Using a decade of national data, a recent study found that foreign-born Cubans, Mexicans, and Puerto Ricans experienced higher age-adjusted CVD mortality than their US-born counterparts [3]. This analysis supports the Hispanic paradox by showing that both foreign- and US-born Hispanic adults have lower CVD mortality than non-Hispanic White (NHW) adults, but contradicts the healthy immigrant effect by means of showing that foreign-born Hispanic adults have higher mortality rates than US-born Hispanic adults. Prior studies suggesting the feasibility of the healthy migrant effect and salmon bias theory have focused primarily on Mexicans [14], the aforementioned analysis included a heterogeneous population of Hispanic subgroups potentially explaining the contrasting findings.

Genetics and Healthier Behaviors

It has been speculated that Hispanic individuals have diverse genetic backgrounds and also acquired healthier behaviors that could result in better health outcomes, potentially protecting Hispanic patients against the effects of lower socioeconomic status compared with other race/ethnic groups in the United States.

Hispanic Americans are very genetically diverse as a result of extensive geographic origins within the Americas, as well as having assorted patterns of immigration from other continents. Moreover, Hispanic individuals have admixed genomes consisting of three predominant continental ancestries and racial influences: indigenous American (primarily of South and Central America, Mexico, and the Caribbean islands), European as a result of colonization, and African as a result of slave transport from West Africa [12]. Accounting for this genetic heterogeneity is crucial, as there might be a genetic basis to the well-described distinct phenotypic variation among Hispanic Americans in the United States.

There are also data identifying specific health behaviors that could modify the impact of CVD in this population. As an example, data from the Hispanic Health and Nutrition Examination Survey (HHANES) examined several health risk behaviors (cigarette smoking, alcohol use, dietary practices, and recency of health screening) of Mexican American, Cuban American, and Puerto Rican adults [15]. According to this analysis, a greater percentage of men when compared to women smoked cigarettes and used alcohol. Heavy smoking was most prevalent for Cuban American males, and heavy drinking was most prevalent in Mexican American and Puerto Rican men. Furthermore, greater acculturation was associated with increased alcohol use (particularly for females). The Puerto Rican diet was less balanced than that of the other two groups. Concerningly, screening (including Pap smear in women) was lower for those who smoked cigarettes and for those with poor dietary practices, indicating that there are disparities in healthcare in distinct Hispanic populations.

Residence in Ethnic Enclaves

Residential segregation has been implicated as a key contributor to ethnic health disparities. Most of the understanding of the segregation-health relationship is derived from studies that examined Black-White segregation and its impacts on Black Americans [16–21]. According to these studies, Black residential segregation has been associated with worse health risks and disease profiles. Given that Hispanic Americans are also disproportionately exposed to neighborhood disadvantage, it has been hypothesized that Hispanic enclaves may also negatively influence health consequences for Hispanic individuals. Conversely, some have proposed that residence in enclaves or increasing neighborhood ethnic density may be protective for Hispanic individuals by providing an environment with more salubrious cultural habits (i.e., improved nutrition and lower smoking rates) and added social cohesion and support [22]. Hence, the evidence is conflicting, and it is unclear whether segregation in Hispanic Americans should be considered protective or even has deleterious effects on health outcomes [23–25].

Most recently, using a decade of national data, Rodriguez et al. [26] found that Hispanic ethnic density is positively correlated with CVD mortality among both Hispanic Americans and NHWs. However, this finding persisted for Hispanic Americans after adjusting for county-level socioeconomic, demographic, and healthcare factors. The finding that Hispanic ethnic density is associated with increased CVD mortality challenges existing concepts about the protective effect of cultural enclaves among Hispanic individuals, and suggests that residence in Hispanic ethnic enclaves is unlikely to explain the Hispanic paradox in CVD mortality.

Acculturation

Acculturation refers to the process through which foreigners adapt to the customs, values, and traditions of a host country [3]. The acculturation hypothesis suggests that Hispanic cultural inclination may result in healthier behaviors that lead to better health outcomes; consequently, foreign-born Hispanics have better cardiovascular health than their US-born counterparts. However, this health advantage among foreign-born Hispanics seems to fade in time, likely influenced by an increased exposure to different sociocultural and environmental factors (increased *acculturation*) that lead to adverse changes in dietary practices, physical activity levels, and weight [17]. Compared with foreign-born Hispanics, US-born Hispanics tend to have a higher prevalence of the major CVD risk factors such as obesity, smoking, and hypertension [27]. Although a standard acculturation metric is not fully agreed upon [28], frequently studied measures of acculturation include English language proficiency, nativity (US-born or foreign-born), years of residence in the United States, and citizenship status.

A recent analysis using data from the Hispanic Community Health Study/Study of Latinos (HCHS/SOL) assessed the relationship of nativity and length of residence in the United States (a commonly used proxy for acculturation), with low CV risk prevalence in a diverse group of Hispanics. The study showed that women who had lived in the United States for less than 10 years were significantly more likely to have low CV risk than those born in the United States after adjusting for sociodemographic characteristics, diet, physical activity, and ethnic discrimination. Among men, there was no association between length of residence and low CV risk in any group except among Dominicans, where low CV risk prevalence was highest for those who had lived in the United States ≥10 years [17].

Regrettably, the majority of studies exploring the association between acculturation and CVD have predominantly studied a single Hispanic subgroup (mostly Mexican populations). The acculturation process experienced by Hispanic Americans with increasing time spent in the United States or across generations may vary by country of origin. A 10-year national study showed that foreign-born Hispanic adults experienced higher age-adjusted mortality rates from CVD compared with US-born Hispanic adults, yet this difference was particular pronounced among Cubans and Puerto Ricans [3]. These results serve to emphasize the importance of data disaggregation by Hispanic subgroup and suggest that granulizing data even further by nativity status demonstrates further heterogeneity in outcomes.

Socioeconomic Status

Low socioeconomic status (SES) has been shown to consistently result in adverse health outcomes across race/ethnic groups. Some studies have proposed that the higher burden of metabolic risk factors among Hispanic Americans can be partially explained by their lower SES, because patients with lower SES tend to have lower health literacy and below average access to preventive care [1]. Research exploring this association has been limited to lower SES Hispanic populations studied cross-sectionally [8] and has failed to account for the cultural diversity in Hispanic Americans [29].

Among the frequently used metrics for SES, education ranks among the strongest and most consistent in its association with health risk factors [30]. A recently published retrospective cohort analysis of participants from the Cooper Center Longitudinal Study, documented persistent health disparities in cardiovascular risk factors for well-educated Hispanics compared with NHW individuals. In this analysis, Hispanics had a higher prevalence of metabolic syndrome, diabetes, and lower fitness than NHW individuals. However, there was no evidence of a Hispanic paradox, with no significant ethnic differences in estimated ASCVD risk, subclinical coronary atherosclerosis (as measured by CAC score), and all-cause mortality [31]. Interestingly, the cohort analyzed included participants who were highly acculturated, and increased acculturation has been linked to higher rates of obesity, hypertension, diabetes, and risk of cardiovascular disease [32, 33]. This study challenges the well-described epidemiologic association between high SES and improved health outcomes [30, 34–36], and suggests that the Hispanic Paradox might be influenced by a multitude of factors.

Many theories have been proposed to support or refute the Hispanic Paradox; however, most of the proposed theories have failed to account for the increasing heterogeneity of the Hispanic population. A better understanding of the disaggregated risk affecting the Hispanic population and its subgroups is fundamental to improve cardiovascular health of Hispanic Americans residing in the United States. While the existence of a Hispanic paradox remains controversial across all groups, identifying potential protective factors that may result in improved outcomes may offer potential targets for interventions.

Heterogeneity and Disaggregation of Cardiovascular Risk in Hispanic Americans

By 2060, 1 in 3 individuals in the United States will be of Hispanic origin [7] and cardiovascular disease is the leading cause of death among Hispanic Americans [8]. Despite this remarkable projected growth, there remains paucity of data on this diverse group. Efforts to provide a detailed and comprehensive description of cardiovascular risk factors, risk assessment, and disease-related outcomes in Hispanic Americans have been challenged by a variety of factors, including the understudied heterogeneity of Hispanics living in the United States and the lack of disaggregation of their cardiovascular risk.

Hispanic individuals living in the United States represent an increasing population of diverse nationalities with rapidly evolving new Hispanic groups adding their numbers to the well-established population of Mexican, Puerto Rican, and Cuban origin, traditionally known to be the largest Hispanic subgroups in the United States. Within each of these ethnic groups, even more heterogeneity exists given the diverse racial subgroups, with varying Native American, European, and African ancestry [12]. As previously mentioned, available information suggests that the health status, risk factors, and outcomes in Hispanics residing in the United States differ depending on their nativity, generational status, degree of acculturation, genetics and individual health behaviors, among others. Moreover, there is still a relative lack of disaggregated epidemiological data in the study of cardiovascular disease, which likely leads to misinterpretations with respect to true associations between CVD risk factors and incident illness.

In 2014, the American Heart Association (AHA) issued a scientific advisory statement highlighting the public health burden of CVD in Hispanic Americans and calling for the development of culturally tailored interventions and highlighting the need of acknowledging Hispanic individuals in the nation's heart health improvement goals [8, 12]. Cardiovascular research has relied heavily on national surveys of US Hispanics such as the National Health and Nutrition Examination Surveys (NHANES) [37], the National Health Interview Survey (NHIS) [38], and the Behavioral Risk Factor Surveillance System (BRFSS) [8, 38, 39]. However, these surveys have studied Hispanic Americans as an aggregated group without systematically identifying their background of origin and unique factors. In 2007, NHANES set forward efforts to include not only Mexican Americans, but to oversample all Hispanic Americans. Although Mexicans have been traditionally the largest Hispanic group in the United States and thus the most vastly studied, failure to consider other Hispanic subgroups leads to an incomplete understanding of the true burden of CVD risk factors and disease across all Hispanics living in the United States.

In recognition of the limited and scant data on Hispanic health and disease, the National Heart, Lung, and Blood Institute has funded a large prospective cohort, the Hispanic Community Health Study/Study of Latinos (HCHS/SOL) [40], that explicitly seeks to examine heterogeneity among the Hispanics. HCHS/SOL has enrolled over 16,000 people of Hispanic origin; specifically, individuals from Cuba, Puerto Rico, Dominican Republic, Mexico, and Central/South America were recruited through four field centers in Miami, San Diego, Chicago, and the Bronx area of New York. Of these, approximately 13,000 consenting HCHS/SOL participants were extensively genotyped. Hence, the HCHS/SOL study

has the potential to explore the heterogeneity in CVD risk, course, and outcomes between Hispanic individuals of different origins and backgrounds and disentangle the mechanisms behind these differences.

Risk Factors

Data from the HCHS/SOL have yielded several important findings in regard to CVD risk factors in Hispanic Americans and specific Hispanic subgroups. Among them, it is important to highlight that while Hispanics have historically been considered to have particularly high risk of diabetes mellitus and obesity (and indeed, data from HCHS/SOL demonstrate that rates of these risk factors are higher than those reported for NHWs in national surveys), a contemporary analysis performed by Daviglus et al. based on HCHS/SOL data shows that the risk factors most highly prevalent among US Hispanics are, in descending order, hypercholesterolemia, obesity, smoking, and HTN for men, and obesity, hypercholesterolemia, and HTN for women [42]. This analysis demonstrated that an alarmingly large proportion of men and women (80% and 71%, respectively) had at least one major CVD risk factor; furthermore, the prevalence of three or more adverse CVD risk factors was highest among men and women of Puerto Rican background, and was significantly higher among participants with lower educational attainment.

Baseline findings from contemporary HCHS/SOL study have provided a new standard and demonstrate that significant burdens in CVD risk exist among all major Hispanic background groups in the United States [1]. However, there are marked variations in rates of individual risk factors by Hispanic background group, with some groups experiencing much lower rates of some risk factors than previously reported for Hispanic individuals and others experiencing higher burdens.

than all other race/ethnic groups. A detailed summary of these findings by Hispanic group and sex can be found in Fig. 8.4.

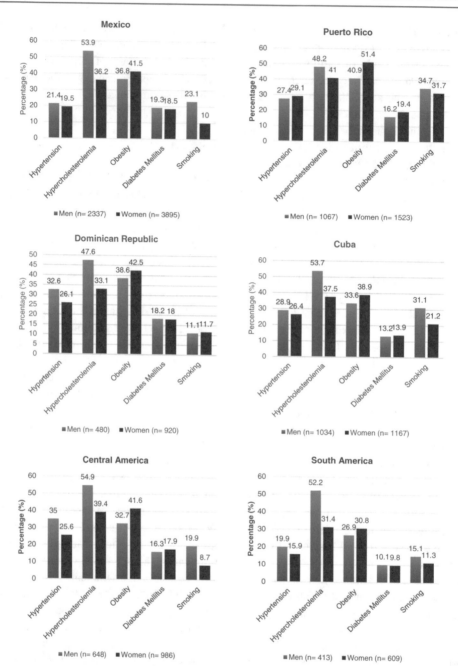

Fig. 8.4 Age-standardized prevalence of cardiovascular disease risk factors for HCHS/SOL participants by Hispanic group and sex. This figure based on data from Daviglus et al. [41]. All values were weighted for survey design and non-response and age-standardized to Census 2010 US population. (Cardiovascular disease risk factors were defined as follows based on current national guidelines: hypercholesterolemia, total cholesterol >240 mg/dL, LDL cholesterol >160 mg/dL, HDL cholesterol <40 mg/dL, or receiving cholesterol-lowering medication; hypertension, systolic blood pressure > 140 mm Hg, diastolic blood pressure > 90 mm Hg, or receiving antihypertensive medication; obesity, body mass index >30.0 kg/m^2; diabetes mellitus, fasting plasma glucose >126 mg/dL, 2-h-postload plasma glucose >200 mg/dL, an HbA1c >6.5%, or use of anti-hyperglycemic medications; smoking, currently smoking cigarettes). Figure reproduced by permission from Rodriguez et al. [26]. Copyright © 2018 Published on behalf of the American Heart Association, Inc., by Wiley Blackwell

Risk Assessment

One of the first studies to examine CV risk factors and subclinical CVD in disaggregated Hispanic groups was published by Rodriguez et al. in 2005 [43]. According to their report, there is a differential prevalence of hypertension, left ventricular hypertrophy (LVH) and abnormal left ventricular remodeling across Hispanic subgroups, clearly illustrating the heterogeneity of the Hispanic population. Specifically, Caribbean-origin Hispanic individuals had a twofold increased odds of LVH compared to non-Hispanic White individuals which was explained, in part due to an elevated prevalence of hypertension. Mexican-origin Hispanic subjects had a similar twofold increased odds of LVH compared to non-Hispanic White subjects despite no increase in the prevalence of hypertension. All Hispanic subgroups had a significantly higher prevalence of concentric and eccentric hypertrophy compared to non-Hispanic White groups.

Although CVD is the leading cause of death for Hispanic Americans and prior work has clearly acknowledged a marked heterogeneity in CVD risk and mortality patterns in this population, studies exploring racial/ethnic disparities in CVD are limited. Specifically, assessment of atherosclerotic cardiovascular disease (ASCVD) has mainly focused on differences between Black individuals and NHW individuals, yet the ASCVD burden in Hispanic Americans has been understudied and is not fully understood [44–47]. As an example, the recent 2018 update to the 2013 prevention guidelines released by the American Heart Association (AHA) and the American College of Cardiology (ACC) relies on pooled cohort equations (PCE) to guide recommendations for risk stratification and lipid therapy decisions [48, 49]. The ACC/AHA Work Group, which developed the risk estimator algorithm, acknowledges that it was designed for use only in men and women of NHW or African American descent, and that the risk estimator may not accurately predict risk in other racial/ethnic groups, such as Hispanic individuals [50]. Despite increasing diversity in the United States, the PCE have not been validated in aggregated or disaggregated representative Hispanic populations, who are known to have heterogenous cardiovascular risk and outcomes, and uncertainty remains regarding the predictive value of cardiovascular risk prediction tools in specific populations, such as Hispanic individuals [51–53].

A recent study by Rodriguez et al. in 2019 tested the accuracy of the PCE for disaggregated Asian and Hispanic subgroups [54]. Their cohort consisted of electronic health record (EHR) data from a community-based, outpatient healthcare system in Northern California, and included 231,622 eligible adults between 40 and 79 years of age. The authors found that the PCE generally overestimate ASCVD risk across diverse populations by 20–60%. However, there was marked heterogeneity by disaggregated Asian and Hispanic subgroups. The extent of overestimation of ASCVD risk varied by disaggregated racial/ethnic subgroups, with a predicted-to-observed ratio of ASCVD events ranging from 1.1 for Puerto Rican patients to 1.9 for Chinese patients. These findings are immensely relevant when attempting to estimate CVD risk in Hispanic individuals, and have important implications for the use of the EHR-based variables in ASCVD risk prediction across diverse populations.

CVD Outcomes

Much of the original data regarding the statistical tabulations for CVDs is derived from the *Heart Disease and Stroke Statistics* published by the AHA [55]. The 2019 report indicates that approximately 121.5 million or almost 1 in 2 adults in the United States (48%) have at least one type of CVD. CVD is an umbrella term referring to the cluster of conditions affecting the heart and circulatory system. Generally, the term CVD includes, but is not limited to, coronary artery disease (CAD), peripheral vascular disease (PVD) (including carotid artery disease, aortic aneurysms, and intermittent claudication), and other cardiac-related conditions (such as stroke, congenital heart disease, arrhythmias, and congestive heart failure). CVD as an aggregate constitutes the leading cause of death among Hispanic Americans, as it is among the rest of the US population [8].

Knowledge regarding CVD outcomes in Hispanic Americans has been hindered by paucity of studies analyzing the impact of CVD in a disaggregated manner. As such, most of the evidence is limited to prevalence and incidence of CVD in primarily Mexican Americans given their historically larger numerical presence within the United States. Using a decade of national data, Rodriguez et al. [56] found marked heterogeneity in CVD mortality patterns among the three largest Hispanic subgroups. According to their analysis, Mexicans experience higher cerebrovascular disease mortality rates compared with other Hispanic subgroups, but still lower rates compared with NHWs. Puerto Ricans and Mexicans are younger at the time of CVD death than Cubans and NHWs. After adjustment for age, Puerto Ricans and Cubans experience CVD mortality rates comparable to those of NHWs but have overall higher rates of ischemic and hypertensive heart disease. This landmark study once again highlights the importance of disaggregating data when analyzing CVD related risks and outcomes in Hispanic Americans. Furthermore, findings from this study challenge the previously discussed Hispanic mortality paradox; whether this paradox is true in all Hispanic subgroups and across different types of CVD remains a matter of controversy.

Emerging Concepts and Future Directions

The growing focus on precision medicine has the potential to improve our understanding of cardiovascular health and disease among Hispanic individuals. For example, polygenic risk scores (PRS) based on an individual's genome sequence are emerging as potentially powerful biomarkers to predict the risk to develop CAD and could pave the way toward more targeted strategies prevent CAD-related adverse events [57].

The goal of PRSs is to stratify patients into risk categories considering their genetic mutations.

PRSs are typically constructed based on published results from Genome-Wide Association Studies (GWASs), the majority of which have been performed in large populations of European ancestry individuals [58, 59]. However, the major ethical and scientific challenge surrounding clinical implementation of PRS is that those available today are several times more accurate in individuals of European ancestry than other ancestries, including non-Hispanic Black and Hispanic individuals. Hispanic Americans in disaggregation have a high level of genetic diversity and there is an important need for genetic-analysis tools suited to the multi-way admixture and high diversity of Hispanic populations [12]. Hence, further initiatives for participant recruitment and data collection in Hispanic studies are clearly required to fill this gap. The HCHS/SOL provides data from 12,803 individuals that consented to genetic studies and were successfully genotyped on a genome-wide SNP array, genetic analyses arising from this subpopulation can have a tremendous impact in this field and lead to relevant contributions. Including a categorical variable for ethnic group, such as Hispanic background, might have several useful applications in GWASs, as it can increase precision by controlling for complex cultural and environmental differences, it can help to control confounding by ancestry, and it can serve to aid detection of group-specific genetic effects [12].

Because racial and ethnic minority groups will constitute an increasingly larger proportion of the US population in coming years, improving the cardiovascular health of these groups is of paramount importance. Hispanic Americans are the largest ethnic minority in the United States, and this is not expected to change within the next 20–40 years. Hence, they are uniquely important to public health nationwide. The current aggregate classification of Hispanic individuals masks the heterogeneity in this population, leading to an incomplete understanding of CVD risks and outcomes among Hispanic subgroups. It is crucial to expand our data collection in existent databases to include more granular data that could better disaggregate CVD profiles, and thus better target patient-specific interventions.

Conclusion

The Hispanic population in the United States has increased dramatically, now comprising the nation's largest minority group. CVD is the leading cause of death among Hispanic individuals in the United States, yet there are notable variations in risk, prevalence, and outcomes across groups and subgroups of Hispanics living in the United States. Largely driven by improvements of data collection and the HCHS/SOL, recent years have seen an increase in literature examining differences among Hispanic Americans. Unpacking the diversity within Hispanic Americans and disaggregating their risk is important to develop targeted CVD preventive efforts and therapies.

References

1. Daviglus ML, Pirzada A, Talavera GA. Cardiovascular disease risk factors in the Hispanic/Latino population: lessons from the Hispanic community health study/study of Latinos (HCHS/SOL). Prog Cardiovasc Dis. 2014;57(3):230–6.
2. Lopez-Jimenez F, Lavie CJ. Hispanics and cardiovascular health and the "Hispanic paradox": what is known and what needs to be discovered? Prog Cardiovasc Dis. 2014;57(3):227–9.
3. Rodriguez F, Hastings KG, Hu J, Lopez L, Cullen M, Harrington RA, et al. Nativity status and cardiovascular disease mortality among Hispanic adults. J Am Heart Assoc. 2017;6(12):e007207.
4. Bureau USC. Hispanic Origin 2018. Available from: https://www.census.gov/topics/population/hispanic-origin/about.html
5. Cohn DV. Census History: Counting Hispanics 2010. Available from: https://www.pewsocialtrends.org/2010/03/03/census-history-counting-hispanics-2/
6. M Lopez JK, JS Passel. Who is Hispanic? 2019. Available from: https://www.pewresearch.org/fact-tank/2019/11/11/who-is-hispanic/
7. Bureau USC. Quick Facts, Hispanic or Latino 2018. Available from: https://www.census.gov/quickfacts/fact/table/US/RHI725217
8. Rodriguez CJ, Allison M, Daviglus ML, Isasi CR, Keller C, Leira EC, et al. Status of cardiovascular disease and stroke in Hispanics/Latinos in the United States: a science advisory from the American Heart Association. Circulation. 2014;130(7):593–625.
9. Statista. Hispanic population groups in the United States, by country of origin 2017 2018. Updated Apr 29 2019. Available from: https://www.statista.com/statistics/234852/us-hispanic-population/
10. Bureau UC. Hispanic Heritage Month 2018 2018. Updated Sept 13 2019. Available from: https://www.census.gov/newsroom/facts-for-features/2018/hispanic-heritage-month.html
11. Morales LS, Lara M, Kington RS, Valdez RO, Escarce JJ. Socioeconomic, cultural, and behavioral factors affecting Hispanic health outcomes. J Health Care Poor Underserved. 2002;13(4):477–503.
12. Conomos MP, Laurie CA, Stilp AM, Gogarten SM, McHugh CP, Nelson SC, et al. Genetic diversity and association studies in US Hispanic/Latino populations: applications in the Hispanic community health study/study of Latinos. Am J Hum Genet. 2016;98(1):165–84.
13. Markides KS, Coreil J. The health of Hispanics in the southwestern United States: an epidemiologic paradox. Public Health Rep (Washington, DC: 1974). 1986;101(3):253–65.
14. Hunt KJ, Williams K, Resendez RG, Hazuda HP, Haffner SM, Stern MP. All-cause and cardiovascular mortality among diabetic participants in the San Antonio heart study: evidence against the "Hispanic paradox". Diabetes Care. 2002;25(9):1557–63.
15. Marks G, Garcia M, Solis JM. Health risk behaviors of Hispanics in the United States: findings from HHANES, 1982-84. Am J Public Health. 1990;80(Suppl):20–6.
16. Greer S, Kramer MR, Cook-Smith JN, Casper ML. Metropolitan racial residential segregation and cardiovascular mortality: exploring pathways. J Urban Health Bull N Y Acad Med. 2014;91(3):499–509.
17. Kershaw KN, Diez Roux AV, Burgard SA, Lisabeth LD, Mujahid MS, Schulz AJ. Metropolitan-level racial residential segregation and black-white disparities in hypertension. Am J Epidemiol. 2011;174(5):537–45.
18. Do DP, Frank R, Zheng C, Iceland J. Hispanic segregation and poor health: it's not just black and white. Am J Epidemiol. 2017;186(8):990–9.
19. Subramanian SV, Acevedo-Garcia D, Osypuk TL. Racial residential segregation and geographic heterogeneity in black/white disparity in poor self-rated health in the US: a multilevel statistical analysis. Soc Sci Med. 2005;60(8):1667–79.
20. Jackson SA, Anderson RT, Johnson NJ, Sorlie PD. The relation of residential segregation to all-cause mortality: a study in black and white. Am J Public Health. 2000;90(4):615–7.
21. Kramer MR, Hogue CR. Place matters: variation in the black/white very preterm birth rate across U.S. metropolitan areas, 2002-2004. Public Health Rep (Washington, DC: 1974). 2008;123(5):576–85.
22. Osypuk TL, Diez Roux AV, Hadley C, Kandula NR. Are immigrant enclaves healthy places to live?

The multi-ethnic study of atherosclerosis. Soc Sci Med. 2009;69(1):110–20.

23. Kershaw KN, Osypuk TL, Do DP, De Chavez PJ, Diez Roux AV. Neighborhood-level racial/ethnic residential segregation and incident cardiovascular disease: the multi-ethnic study of atherosclerosis. Circulation. 2015;131(2):141–8.

24. Li K, Wen M, Henry KA. Ethnic density, immigrant enclaves, and Latino health risks: a propensity score matching approach. Soc Sci Med. 2017;189:44–52.

25. Eschbach K, Ostir GV, Patel KV, Markides KS, Goodwin JS. Neighborhood context and mortality among older Mexican Americans: is there a barrio advantage? Am J Public Health. 2004;94(10):1807–12.

26. Rodriguez F, Hu J, Kershaw K, Hastings KG, Lopez L, Cullen MR, et al. County-level Hispanic ethnic density and cardiovascular disease mortality. J Am Heart Assoc. 2018;7(19):e009107.

27. Dominguez K, Penman-Aguilar A, Chang MH, Moonesinghe R, Castellanos T, Rodriguez-Lainz A, et al. Vital signs: leading causes of death, prevalence of diseases and risk factors, and use of health services among Hispanics in the United States - 2009-2013. MMWR Morb Mortal Wkly Rep. 2015;64(17):469–78.

28. Alegria M. The challenge of acculturation measures: what are we missing? A commentary on Thomson & Hoffman-Goetz. Soc Sci Med. 2009;69(7):996–8.

29. Shaw PM, Chandra V, Escobar GA, Robbins N, Rowe V, Macsata R. Controversies and evidence for cardiovascular disease in the diverse Hispanic population. J Vasc Surg. 2018;67(3):960–9.

30. Winkleby MA, Jatulis DE, Frank E, Fortmann SP. Socioeconomic status and health: how education, income, and occupation contribute to risk factors for cardiovascular disease. Am J Public Health. 1992;82(6):816–20.

31. Rodriguez F, Leonard D, DeFina L, Barlow CE, Willis BL, Haskell WL, et al. Association of educational attainment and cardiovascular risk in Hispanic individuals: findings from the Cooper Center longitudinal study. JAMA Cardiol. 2019;4(1):43–50.

32. Lutsey PL, Diez Roux AV, Jacobs DR Jr, Burke GL, Harman J, Shea S, et al. Associations of acculturation and socioeconomic status with subclinical cardiovascular disease in the multi-ethnic study of atherosclerosis. Am J Public Health. 2008;98(11):1963–70.

33. Koya DL, Egede LE. Association between length of residence and cardiovascular disease risk factors among an ethnically diverse group of United States immigrants. J Gen Intern Med. 2007;22(6):841–6.

34. Adler NE, Ostrove JM. Socioeconomic status and health: what we know and what we don't. Ann N Y Acad Sci. 1999;896:3–15.

35. Kimbro RT, Bzostek S, Goldman N, Rodriguez G. Race, ethnicity, and the education gradient in health. Health Affairs (Project Hope). 2008;27(2):361–72.

36. Sorlie PD, Backlund E, Keller JB. US mortality by economic, demographic, and social characteristics: the National Longitudinal Mortality Study. Am J Public Health. 1995;85(7):949–56.

37. Prevention CfDCa. National Health and Nutrition Examination Survey (NHANES) 2019 [updated May 8 2019; cited 2019 2019]. Available from: https://www.cdc.gov/nchs/nhanes/index.htm

38. Prevention CfDCa. Behavioral Risk Factor Surveillance System (BRFSS) 2019. Updated April 17, 2019. Available from: https://www.cdc.gov/nchs/nhis/index.htm

39. Balfour PC Jr, Ruiz JM, Talavera GA, Allison MA, Rodriguez CJ. Cardiovascular disease in Hispanics/Latinos in the United States. J Lat Psychol. 2016;4(2):98–113.

40. Study HCH. Hispanic Community Health Study/Study of Latinos, Study Overview. Available from: https://sites.cscc.unc.edu/hchs/StudyOverview

41. Daviglus ML, Talavera GA, Aviles-Santa ML, Allison M, Cai J, Criqui MH, et al. Prevalence of major cardiovascular risk factors and cardiovascular diseases among Hispanic/Latino individuals of diverse backgrounds in the United States. JAMA. 2012;308(17):1775–84.

42. Rodriguez CJ, Diez-Roux AV, Moran A, Jin Z, Kronmal RA, Lima J, et al. Left ventricular mass and ventricular remodeling among Hispanic subgroups compared with non-Hispanic blacks and whites: MESA (Multi-ethnic study of atherosclerosis). J Am Coll Cardiol. 2010;55(3):234–42.

43. Mainous AG 3rd, Majeed A, Koopman RJ, Baker R, Everett CJ, Tilley BC, et al. Acculturation and diabetes among Hispanics: evidence from the 1999-2002 National Health and nutrition examination survey. Public Health Rep (Washington, DC: 1974). 2006;121(1):60–6.

44. Davidson JA, Kannel WB, Lopez-Candales A, Morales L, Moreno PR, Ovalle F, et al. Avoiding the looming Latino/Hispanic cardiovascular health crisis: a call to action. Ethn Dis. 2007;17(3):568–73.

45. Lara M, Gamboa C, Kahramanian MI, Morales LS, Bautista DEH. Acculturation and Latino health in the United States: a review of the literature and its sociopolitical context. Annu Rev Public Health. 2005;26(1):367–97.

46. Derby CA, Wildman RP, McGinn AP, Green RR, Polotsky AJ, Ram KT, et al. Cardiovascular risk factor variation within a Hispanic cohort: SWAN, the Study of Women's Health Across the Nation. Ethn Dis. 2010;20(4):396–402.

47. Stone Neil J, Robinson Jennifer G, Lichtenstein Alice H, Bairey Merz CN, Blum Conrad B, Eckel Robert H, et al. 2013 ACC/AHA guideline on the treatment of blood cholesterol to reduce atherosclerotic cardiovascular risk in adults. Circulation. 2014;129(25_suppl_2):S1–S45.

48. Grundy Scott M, Stone Neil J, Bailey Alison L, Beam C, Birtcher Kim K, Blumenthal Roger S, et al. 2018 AHA/ACC/AACVPR/AAPA/ABC/ACPM/ADA/AGS/APhA/ASPC/NLA/PCNA guideline on the

Management of Blood Cholesterol: a report of the American College of Cardiology/American Heart Association task force on clinical practice guidelines. Circulation. 2019;139(25):e1082–e143.

49. Goff David C, Lloyd-Jones Donald M, Bennett G, Coady S, D'Agostino Ralph B, Gibbons R, et al. 2013 ACC/AHA guideline on the assessment of cardiovascular risk. Circulation. 2014;129(25_suppl_2):S49–73.

50. DeFilippis AP, Young R, Carrubba CJ, McEvoy JW, Budoff MJ, Blumenthal RS, et al. An analysis of calibration and discrimination among multiple cardiovascular risk scores in a modern multiethnic cohort. Ann Intern Med. 2015;162(4):266–75.

51. Karmali KN, Goff DC Jr, Ning H, Lloyd-Jones DM. A systematic examination of the 2013 ACC/AHA pooled cohort risk assessment tool for atherosclerotic cardiovascular disease. J Am Coll Cardiol. 2014;64(10):959–68.

52. Muntner P, Colantonio LD, Cushman M, Goff DC Jr, Howard G, Howard VJ, et al. Validation of the atherosclerotic cardiovascular disease pooled cohort risk equations. JAMA. 2014;311(14):1406–15.

53. Rodriguez FCS, Blum MR, Coulet A, Basu S, Palaniappan LP. Atherosclerotic cardiovascular disease risk prediction in disaggregated Asian and Hispanic subgroups using electronic health records. J Am Heart Assoc. 2019;8(14):e011874.

54. Benjamin Emelia J, Muntner P, Alonso A, Bittencourt Marcio S, Callaway Clifton W, Carson April P, et al. Heart disease and stroke statistics—2019 update: a report from the American Heart Association. Circulation. 2019;139(10):e56–e528.

55. Rodriguez F, Hastings KG, Boothroyd DB, Echeverria S, Lopez L, Cullen M, et al. Disaggregation of cause-specific cardiovascular disease mortality among Hispanic subgroups. JAMA Cardiol. 2017;2(3):240–7.

56. Wunnemann F, Sin Lo K, Langford-Avelar A, Busseuil D, Dube MP, Tardif JC, et al. Validation of genome-wide polygenic risk scores for coronary artery disease in French Canadians. Circulation Genomic Precision Med. 2019;12(6):e002481.

57. Martin AR, Kanai M, Kamatani Y, Okada Y, Neale BM, Daly MJ. Clinical use of current polygenic risk scores may exacerbate health disparities. Nat Genet. 2019;51(4):584–91.

58. Grinde KE, Qi Q, Thornton TA, Liu S, Shadyab AH, Chan KHK, et al. Generalizing polygenic risk scores from Europeans to Hispanics/Latinos. Genet Epidemiol. 2019;43(1):50–62.

59. Manichaikul A, Palmas W, Rodriguez CJ, Peralta CA, Divers J, Guo X, et al. Population structure of Hispanics in the United States: the multi-ethnic study of atherosclerosis. PLoS Genet. 2012;8(4):e1002640-e.

Cardiovascular Epidemiology in Hispanics/Latinos: Lessons Learned from HCHS/SOL

César J. Herrera, Manuel Hache-Marliere, and Carlos J. Rodriguez

The Hispanic/Latino Horizon

The United States census classifies Hispanic/Latino (from now on referred here as Hispanics) as self-identified individuals of Mexican, Cuban, Puerto Rican, Central or South American, and any other Spanish culture origin. Note that this definition is not race but rather ethnic-based, an important characterization given the heterogeneity of this population where European, African, and indigenous/native ancestries vary from nation to nation. Of the more than 319 million people living in the United States (US) in 2014, Hispanics constitute the largest minority ethnic group with over 57 million that represent 17.4% of the total population; projections indicate that this figure will reach 119 million in 2060, meaning that in less than four decades more than one in four Americans will be of Hispanic origin. It is also important to recognize that up to 40% of Hispanics residing in the US are foreign-born, a factor to consider when analyzing and establishing conclusions from epidemiological data [1].

Inherently, Hispanics are a complex heterogeneous group whose members come from several different countries each with mixed genetic backgrounds (mostly Caucasian in South America, Amerindian in Central America, and African in the Caribbean); carry the different historical burden, societal structures, and practices; and yet, they hold a common identity in the United States that somehow blurs the race vs. ethnic divide. It must be acknowledged that understanding this diverse but closely related substrate is paramount in the process of beginning to grasp the various behaviors—deleterious and protective—the relevant cardiovascular (CV) risk factors, and the morbidities affecting this unique community.

Furthermore, to consider geographical proximity as a common link among Hispanics would be oblivious of the rich history of origins of each region where ethnic enclaves may simultaneously share Mesoamerican roots, admixtures of multi-European colonialism, or post-Columbian Afro-Caribbean heritage haplogroups. The relatively young and recent migrant waves of Hispanics to the United States by itself carry a weight onto potential epigenetic changes related to the new and unfamiliar environment, let alone

C. J. Herrera
Montefiore Center for Heart and Vascular Care, New York City, NY, USA

CEDIMAT Cardiovascular Center, Santo Domingo, Dominican Republic
e-mail: cjherrera@cedimat.net

M. Hache-Marliere
Internal Medicine, Jacobi Medical Center, New York City, NY, USA

C. J. Rodriguez (✉)
Montefiore Center for Heart and Vascular Care, New York City, NY, USA

Division of Cardiovascular Medicine, Albert Einstein College of Medicine, New York City, NY, USA
e-mail: carlos.rodriguez@einsteinmed.org

© Springer Nature Switzerland AG 2021
K. C. Ferdinand et al. (eds.), *Cardiovascular Disease in Racial and Ethnic Minority Populations*, Contemporary Cardiology, https://doi.org/10.1007/978-3-030-81034-4_9

the complexities of acculturation and adaptation of new habits, values, and behaviors.

To date, it is unequivocally agreed that CV disease is the leading cause of death among Hispanics in the US, a fact that unfortunately is only worsened by the existence of a larger, over-reaching, and complex underlying problem of major proportions given the relative youth of this ethnic group: the prevailing high rates of CV risk factors across most ages and subgroups of Hispanics that have made this country home.

Despite accounting for a large sector of the US population, Hispanics, as a minority, until recently were unaccounted for in clinical guidelines; large-scale epidemiological studies capable of providing an evidence-based foundation for risk assessment and management recommendations were lacking, and therefore, public health policies were significantly hampered.

Furthermore, national surveys such as NHANES (the National Health and Nutrition Examination), NHIS (the National Heath Interview), and BRFSS (the Behavioral Risk Factor Surveillance System) at least until 2010 reported data on Hispanics as a single ethnic group of predominantly Mexican descent not taking into account the already mentioned diversity that defines them [2–5].

The first major survey that looked at Hispanics as a multifaceted group was the Hispanic Health and Nutrition Examination Study (HHANES) conducted between 1982 and 1984; it examined subjects in a one-time cross-sectional pattern similar to NHANES and included a sample of 11,653 individuals of Mexican, Puerto Rican, and Cuban background [6, 7]. This important study is now several decades old and since its publication, the US Hispanic community has changed dramatically and continues to do so (it is the second fastest growing segment of the population feeding on a dynamic immigration pattern), a fact that must be taken into account when analyzing health-related information and reaching conclusions in this group. Although the Multiethnic Study of Atherosclerosis (MESA) study accounted for White, African American/Black, Hispanic, and Asian (of Chinese descent) categories, the Hispanic sample included was

modest with certain Hispanic origin subgroups (such as Cubans) clearly underrepresented [8, 9].

The Hispanic Communities Health Study-Study of Latinos (HCHS/SOL), from now on referred to as SOL, constitutes the largest, multi-center, prospective study that has focused on the CV risk profile of Hispanics. It was launched in the context of the already mentioned very much needed characterization of this group's current health status. Sponsored by the National Institute of Health (NIH)/National Heart, Lung and Blood Institute (NHLBI), SOL is a population-based study designed to evaluate risk and protective factors and to prospectively measure morbidity and mortality [10].

As a longitudinal cohort study, SOL enrolled 16,415 Hispanics from 2008 to 2011; during the baseline visit, participants were aged 18–74 years, of Cuban, Dominican, Mexican, Puerto Rican, Central American, and South American origin recruited in the Bronx (New York), Chicago (Illinois), Miami (Florida), and San Diego (California) areas that hold the largest urban Hispanic communities in the nation [10, 11]. The multistage population-based sampling design of SOL allows for all descriptive statistics and modeling to be weighted for inferences to apply to all Hispanics/Latinos living in the SOL sampled regions (a population of ~600,000 individuals). At baseline, individuals underwent clinical examination and documentation of already present CV disease and traditional CV risk factors rigorously defined: hypertension, diabetes, dyslipidemia, tobacco use, obesity, and sleep-disordered breathing, as well as anthropometry; electrocardiography; socio-demographic data; health behaviors and psychosocial factors; ankle-brachial index; audiometry; oral examination; lung function; sleep studies; physical activity monitoring; oral glucose load, biospecimen collection, medical history, medication use, dietary and physical activity patterns; and sociocultural (acculturation) factors. Annual follow-up data collection was also anticipated.

This chapter will summarize SOL results and discuss lessons learned contextualizing them in respect to the American Heart Association (AHA) Science Advisory document on the status of CV disease and Stroke in Hispanics published by Rodriguez et al. several years ago [12]. The authors hope that the comments included here provide insight in this era of precision medicine of the need for inclusive, socially conscious, and culturally sensitive interventions that relate to the rapidly growing Hispanic population living in the US.

Cultural and Psychosocial Spectrum

Sociodemographic Factors

In addition to access to appropriate medical care services and technologies, the health of a population is also influenced, perhaps as importantly, by socioeconomic and cultural factors; the process of globalization has brought with it an even more relevant role for those considerations particularly in light of mid and late twentieth century immigration to the United States, a scenario that often confronts dietary habits, religious and cultural beliefs as well as the adoption of aspects of a new life otherwise common occurrence among the rest of the American population.

In spite of the previously mentioned differences among Hispanics, important social, cultural, and demographic factors are generally shared by its various ethnic groups and nations: *familism*, defined as placing one's family above oneself and deemphasizing independence over interdependence and as such, family members becoming reliable sources of financial and emotional support; *personalism* and respect, concepts that imply tightly knitted family and spousal interconnections particularly from the elders that will become important when Hispanics interact with health care providers. Unique aspects of gender roles where both men (heads of the family) and mothers (single or not) represent figures of responsibility, hierarchy, and engagement when health-related matters surface; and importantly, faith and spiritual values that become key factors in a community with an overwhelming embracement of religion and with it, potentially harmful practices (such as fatalistic destiny-mandated health outcomes) and simultaneously

potentially useful opportunities of engagement (such as the use of the church for targeted interventions).

Language

Language and health literacy are key determinants of an individual societal participation, adaptation, and health care resource utilization in any community. This is particularly more relevant among those individuals, like Hispanics, who after migrating tend to retain their native language and at the same time perhaps due to economic and educational disadvantages, have lower likelihood of fully adopting the new language. Note, that historically, language has been recognized as a great modifier to education and access to health care, and, that education has been clearly shown to be the most reliable socioeconomic predictor for CV disease [13].

Hispanics predominately speak Spanish, and over 70% do so as their primary language at home. Fifty-seven percent of Spanish-speaking Hispanics report that they also speak English "very well," whereas others recognize having limited proficiency in the English language [11]. When considering Hispanics of relatively recent immigrant status, language can be a barrier to enjoy workforce opportunities and if that limitation remains, it may also hinder their ability to obtain and use health insurance and subsequently further impacts negatively their access to the system.

It is well known that non-English-speaking Hispanics are far less likely to be knowledgeable of heart attack and stroke symptoms than English-speaking Hispanics, non-Hispanic Blacks (NHBs), and non-Hispanic Whites (NHWs) [14]. In addition, even after controlling for socioeconomic status and demographic characteristics, non-English-speaking Hispanics report perceived differences in the quality of information and care that clinicians provide them and also note that the health education information they receive is less detailed and empathetic and even consider that non-Spanish speaking physicians spend less time with them and respect less their treatment decisions [15].

This language and cultural dissonance can affect patient–provider relations and make Hispanics feel as if they are not receiving a correct diagnosis or treatment through conventional medical practice making them at risk by their seeking and using unproven alternative medicines. In one report, 29% cited failure by medical professionals to diagnose their problem as the reason for pursuing alternative medicine instead, while others cited being unhappy with previous medical advice (21%) [16].

Acculturation

Acculturation is defined as the process of adaptation to a new culture assessed by the integration into the new country's cultural values, behaviors, beliefs, and attitudes. In the context of this review, proxy markers for acculturation can be years of residence in the United States, generational status, and language preference, although gaining access to English, surprisingly, may not only imply positive effects. It could also promote the sense of not belonging or not identifying with the new culture and therefore rejecting some or most of its aspects including health care access.

Acculturation may also lead to improvement in socioeconomic status and enhanced access to health care, but it is not without disadvantages since the integration to the adopted culture does not necessarily provide benefits health-wise. As an example, it has been shown that second- and third-generation Hispanics have incorporated behavioral and nutritional habits into their lives that are more "typical" of the new culture and that can be deleterious such as sugary drinks and fast-food consumption [17].

The SOL study showed that those who prefer to speak English and have more acculturation had statistically significant more CV disease risk factors (≥ 3) (18.7% vs. 13.5%), coronary heart disease (2% vs.1.3%), and stroke (1.4% vs. 0.8%). In general, more acculturated participants exhibited markedly higher rates of current smoking and suffer from more obesity than the less acculturated subjects indicating that migrant health tends to worsen with increased duration of living in the United States [12]. Greater acculturated Hispanics also have worse cardiac structure and function [18].

Further secondary analysis of SOL data demonstrated that the strongest predictor of moderate and extreme obesity was the length of residency in the United States. Individuals reporting eating Hispanic and American foods in equal amounts (as a sign of greater acculturation) were more likely to have extreme obesity, compared to those eating mostly Hispanic foods [19]. As Rodriguez et al. have pointed out it needs to be kept in mind that there are other important aspects to acculturation beyond language: resilience, vulnerability and stress, lack of social support, isolation, and financial burden, among others, are relevant concepts that may make conclusions on acculturation research quite challenging [12].

Education

As far as education is concerned, Hispanics have the lowest rates of holding a high school diploma (72%; 2017) compared with NHWs (93%; 2017), NHBs (87%; 2017), and Asians (91%; 2017) [20]. Discussing how education impacts health is a subject beyond the scope of this document; however, as an example of its relevance is worth mentioning that participants with lower household income or education enrolled in SOL had higher rates of smoking, diabetes, obesity, and hypercholesterolemia [12].

As previously mentioned, education can be a reliable socioeconomic predictor for the development of CV disease: lack of formal education limits the Hispanic population's understanding of how modifiable disease risk factors (e.g., smoking, high-fat diets) can contribute to their health. Not only is their decision-making power limited by this information/education bias, but also their wealth inequity restricts access to nutrient-rich-balanced diets and the leisure time necessary to engage in other healthy habits such as exercise or meditation.

Unhealthy carbohydrate-containing diets are cheaper and more easily accessible to minorities living in low socioeconomic environments; in addition, disadvantaged Hispanics are more likely to live in densely populated urban communities with less availability of fresh foods, health care providers, and facilities, as opposed to Hispanics living in more diverse and affluent neighborhoods.

In summary, to understand the burden of CV disease among Hispanics living in the US, one must acknowledge that it cannot "boil down" to the scientific adage of *"Nature versus nurture."* For future research and public policy making, the factors described above are essential components in the process of understanding this group's CV health status and with it, the nation's CV health as whole.

Cardiovascular Risk Factors Among Hispanics

When compared with other ethnic groups in the US, Hispanic individuals are disproportionately affected by CV risk factors, but often have a lower burden of CV disease. Nonetheless, from the epidemiological point of view, these differences are more complex in their origin and perpetuation than in other races/ethnicities as there are multiple social and cultural modifiers at play, including access to health care providers/facilities, health literacy, and language barrier.

The AHA 2020 health strategy aims at reducing CV deaths by 20% and improving CV health by 20% among all Americans by 2020; this includes Hispanics of course, a group showing the lower prevalence of ideal health than NHWs even after adjusting for age and gender [12, 13, 21, 22].

Findings in SOL demonstrated that most Hispanic men and women (80% and 71%, respectively) had adverse levels of at least one major CV disease risk factor. The prevalence of three or more of those differed across subgroups with Puerto Ricans showing the highest burden and 25% of the entire population having at least three risk factors [10].

As described by Daviglus et al., large prospective cohort follow-up studies of young and middle-aged non-Hispanics have demonstrated that favorable levels of all major CV disease risk

factors (i.e., low risk [LR]) are associated with important age-specific CV disease and total mortality rates, higher life expectancy, better quality of life, and lower health care-related costs. According to those reports, the prevalence of LR among US NHWs was 8.2% with few data available on LR rates among Hispanics except for those of Mexican background until SOL data were analyzed [23]. Among all participants, the age-adjusted prevalence of LR status was low, particularly for men (5%) vs. women (11%) with some noticeable variation among ethnic groups (highest in Central Americans and lowest in Dominicans and Mexicans).

The intervariability of risk factors among Hispanic subgroups according to sex uncovered by SOL has shed new light into the understanding of contemporary cardiovascular health among this ethnic group never appreciated before [10]. In addition, the disturbing rates of LR status have brought this important epidemiological endpoint to the table underlining the urgency of developing and establishing comprehensive public health strategies both ethnic-based and gender-driven for Hispanics living in the United States.

Hypercholesterolemia

According to SOL, hypercholesterolemia was defined as low-density lipoprotein-cholesterol levels ≥ 130 mg/dL and/or total cholesterol ≥ 240 mg/dL or use of cholesterol-lowering medication. Almost half (49%) of Hispanics with high cholesterol were aware of their condition; less than a third (29%) were under treatment; and among those receiving drug therapy, less than two-thirds (64%) had lipids levels that were adequately controlled [24]. SOL investigators reported an overall prevalence of hypercholesterolemia of 52% among men, ranging from 48% (Dominicans and Puerto Ricans) to 55% (Central Americans). In women, the prevalence of hypercholesterolemia was 37% and it ranged from 31% (South Americans) to 41% (Puerto Ricans) [10]. In the MESA study, on the other hand, Mexicans as a group had the highest prevalence of dyslipidemia (45%) although this finding may be related to methodological factors in the sampling of Hispanics [9].

In the Northern Manhattan Study, Rodriguez found a higher prevalence of low HDL-C or high triglycerides among elderly Hispanics compared with NHBs and NHWs. Dyslipidemia defined as high total or LDL-C, low HDL-C, and/or high triglycerides is highly prevalent in US Hispanics (~65%) with significant variations seen by Hispanic heritage groups [25]. Among participants of the Insulin Resistance Atherosclerosis Study, Hispanics had lower HDL-C and higher triglyceride levels than African Americans and NHWs. This potentially translates to a more atherogenic phenotype of small, dense LDL [26] more likely to cross into the vascular endothelium to promote atherosclerosis. This high-risk pattern of dyslipidemia among Hispanics may be better accounted for by nontraditional lipid markers such as apoB and Lp(a) as LDL alone does not seem to paint the complete picture of CV risk among Hispanics.

Hypertension

As with hypercholesterolemia, the prevalence of hypertension in Hispanics in the SOL varied significantly across their ethnic backgrounds with a total age-adjusted prevalence slightly lower than that seen in NHWs 25.5% vs. 27.4% [27]. Nonetheless, in this study there was overlap between both populations in confidence intervals, meaning that comparison between groups could not be objectively drawn. Among National Health Interview Survey (NHIS) respondents, in multivariate-adjusted analyses, odds of self-reported hypertension were 67% higher among Dominicans and 20–27% lower among Mexican Americans and Central/South Americans than NHWs [28]. Among Northern Manhattan Study participants (predominantly Dominican), objectively measured prevalent hypertension was similarly significantly higher in Hispanics (59%) than in NHWs (42%) [29]. Among foreign-born Hispanics who responded to the NHIS, those of Puerto Rican and Dominican origin had significantly higher hypertension prevalence than those of Mexican origin [30]. Collectively, these currently available data suggest that Hispanics of Caribbean origin are at a particularly high risk of hypertension and it's morbidity and mortality. This prompts the question as to the relation of African ancestry and hypertension, a poorly studied phenomena in Hispanics.

SOL found that 25.4% of Hispanic men had hypertension with the highest prevalence seen among Dominicans (32.6%) compared to any other Hispanic background group, findings consistent with those of MESA participants [9, 10]. In SOL, Dominican men also had the highest mean systolic and diastolic blood pressure readings (129.4 mmHg and 77.2 mmHg) compared to any other Hispanic background group despite the highest rates of drug treatment for it (18.4%); this finding prompts the question as to the potential heterogeneity of specific drugs on different ethnicities, poorly studied phenomena in Hispanics.

In SOL, overall hypertension prevalence among women was 23.5%, ranging from 16% (South Americans) to 29% (Puerto Ricans); rates of drug treatment for hypertension were highest for women of Dominican and Puerto Rican backgrounds (18.8% each) while South American men and women subgroups (17.2%) had the lowest sex-specific rates of hypertension [10, 27].

In SOL, of those participants with hypertension, 74.1% were aware and 63.4% were receiving treatment; most concerning, only 37.5% of those treated had readings under control. These findings underline the importance of insight and awareness on hypertension in reference to drug adherence and ultimately, blood pressure control [27].

Future research will be required to explore how cultural factors, including perceived mistrust and provider–patient relationships, may influence hypertension control in addition to insurance, low socioeconomic and immigrant status, and access to the health care system.

Obesity, BMI, Physical Activity, and Nutrition

National data confirm what has been long suspected: the dangerous upward trend of obesity (defined as body mass index [BMI] ≥ 30 kg/m^2)

among all races and ethnic groups in the US, Hispanics not being the exception. This worrisome finding is coupled with an additional concern: the fact that the proportion of obese individuals grows in parallel with socioeconomic disadvantage [31, 32]. Hispanics disproportionately live in low socioeconomic conditions and have been particularly vulnerable to this trend and generally have had higher rates of obesity than NHWs (37.9% vs. 31.9%) although less than NHBs (44.1%). Puerto Rican women and more so Mexican American women have the highest obesity rates among all Hispanic groups [33].

NHANES data from 1999 showed that the overall prevalence of obesity in the US was 32.2% among adult men and 35.5% among adult women [33]. Twenty years later, obesity prevalence among some of the Hispanic groups in SOL was similar to the one reported among Hispanic participants enrolled in that earlier cohort of NHANES. This finding calls into question whether public health policies over time have truly made a dent in this epidemic [10]. In SOL, men were less likely to be obese than women (36% vs. 43%) and less likely to meet criteria for obesity class II (BMI $\geq$ 35 kg/m^2) or III (BMI $\geq$ 40 kg/m^2). Obesity rates according to the Hispanic subgroup were the lowest in participants of South American background (27% men, 31% women) and highest among the Puerto Rican population (41% men, 51% women). As opposed to NHANES results, Mexican Americans were not the Hispanic group with the highest obesity prevalence [10, 34].

SOL uncovered that obesity among Hispanics was associated with a considerable excess of CVD risk factors including diabetes, hypertension, low-density lipoprotein cholesterol levels, hypertriglyceridemia, and increased inflammation as demonstrated by levels of high C-reactive protein. In addition, it must be remembered that at the highest BMI levels CVD risk factors often emerge during the earliest decades of adulthood affecting men more often than women [10, 34, 35].

Remarkably, SOL showed that despite higher obesity rates, participants of Puerto Rican and Dominican background had the most minutes/day of moderate-to-vigorous physical activity (MVPA) (32.1 and 29.1, respectively), whereas those of Cuban origin had the fewest. (15.3) Puerto Rican subjects had the most leisure-time specific MVPA and transportation-related physical activity compared to other Hispanics of different backgrounds [36]. These are important facts since there was little mention of physical activity among Hispanics in previously published surveys.

Furthermore, and despite having a more active lifestyle, individuals of Puerto Rican ancestry were not able to offset their obesity risk due to nutrition. Correspondingly to obesity rates, participants of Puerto Rican origin showed higher intakes of foods and nutrients associated with CVD risks such as total and saturated fat, sodium, refined carbohydrates, and red meats, as well as lower intake of foods associated with reduced CV disease risks including fibers, fish, and fruits.

The Puerto Rican subgroup also proved to have a higher consumption of sugar-sweetened beverages than any other, whereas South Americans reported a lower intake of nutrients associated with higher CVD risk, except for refined grains. South Americans, perhaps related to geographical and cultural factors, had the highest fish intake and were second in fruit and poultry consumption [37].

Hispanics face a greater number of chronic stressors and report greater levels of perceived stress, facts that are known to correlate with a higher total energy intake and lower diet quality. Compared to those with no stressors, Hispanics with $\geq$3 stressors carried higher odds of being obese, particularly among participants of Puerto Rican ancestry who reported much higher chronic and perceived stress compared to other groups [38].

Diabetes Mellitus and Metabolic Syndrome

Diabetes was defined in SOL as a fasting plasma glucose $\geq$126 mg/dL, or impaired glucose tolerance as indicated by a glucose level $\geq$ 200 mg/dL after a 2-h oral glucose tolerance test, or elevated glycosylated hemoglobin (A1c $\geq$ 6.5%; 48 mmol/

mol), or documented (scanned) use of hypoglycemic agents [10, 39]. The prevalence of diabetes varies within the different Hispanic backgrounds; in SOL, overall, one in six enrollees had diabetes, morbidity strongly associated with increased prevalence of both coronary heart disease and stroke [10].

Prevalence of diabetes in SOL ranged from 10% among South American men and women, 13.5% in Cubans to 17% in Central Americans, 18% in Dominicans and Puerto Ricans, and highest in Mexicans, 19%. Overall prevalence among Mexicans was consistent with previous MESA and NHANES findings. These differences in diabetes prevalence as a function of ethnic background remained significant even after controlling for age, sex, BMI, field center, and years living in the US, findings that warrant further investigation as to the potential roles of diet vs. genetics among Mexican Americans [39].

Among SOL participants with diabetes, 58.7% indicated awareness of their condition, 48% displayed adequate control (A1C <7%; 53 mmol/mol), and 52.4% reported having health insurance coverage [39]. Moreover, the association between diabetes awareness and low total and added sugar intake was observed in individuals of Mexican and Puerto Rican backgrounds but not in other subgroups; among those with known diabetes, participants with an HbA1c ≥ 7% consumed more total fats, more saturated fats, and more cholesterol-rich foods [40]. In summary, the discord between awareness and remediation, as seen in Hispanics with hypertension, is also displayed among those affected by diabetes.

Diabetes, as a true cardiovascular equivalent condition represents an important departing point when analyzing cardiovascular health among Hispanics since most, if not all of the comorbidities linked to diabetes are coresponsible for the majority of adult deaths. Diabetes in Hispanics is also closely linked to socioeconomic status such that in SOL diabetes prevalence was inversely related to household income and level of education [35].

The prevalence of metabolic syndrome (MeS), and that of the cardiometabolic abnormalities that are components of this entity, is quite high among Hispanics and varies by sex and across backgrounds. In SOL, MeS was present in 36% of women and 34% of men. As with obesity, the overall prevalence of MeS was highest among Puerto Ricans (37% overall, but higher on women than men); not statistically significantly different from other Hispanic groups among men, but significantly lower among South Americans (27%) compared with other Hispanic groups overall as well as in women [41].

The most common components of the MeS among participants in SOL were abdominal obesity (73%), hyperglycemia (73%), and hypertriglyceridemia (73%) for men, and abdominal obesity (96%) followed by low high-density lipoprotein cholesterol (75%) for women [41]. It is therefore obvious that in the next decades Hispanics will undoubtedly represent the highest at-risk community in the country, and perhaps one with a prevalence of CV disease at least as high as that of NHWs or NHBs literally negating the existence of the so-called "Hispanic paradox."

Smoking

Cigarette smoking has been previously poorly described or under-reported in the Hispanic population. In 2012, the CDC published a 19% rate of cigarette smoking in the US population with Hispanics (12.9%) showing lower rates than NHBs (19.4%) and NHWs (20.6%) [42]. A recent landmark report by the CDC published in 2017 revealed that 14% of adults are currently engaged in cigarette smoking with Hispanics showing significantly lower rates than NHBs and NHWs: 9.9% vs. 14.9% vs. 15.2% respectively [43]. This decrease has been consistent with worldwide efforts to reduce tobacco abuse—a good example of the success that joint efforts on public health policies and medical interventions can achieve.

Interestingly, there are clear racial/ethnic disparities in reports of smoking cessation advice. Among those that do smoke, Hispanics as less likely of being advised to quit by health care practitioners or offered nicotine replacement therapy or antidepressant adjunct therapy for cessation than NHWs and NHBs or other non-Hispanic groups [44, 45].

SOL found higher levels of self-reported cigarette smoking among Hispanics than the CDC's 2012 & 2017 surveys—25% for men and 15% for women [10]. Smoking behavior also varied widely across Hispanics with other risk factors: prevalence was highest among Puerto Ricans and Cubans, with particularly pronounced smoking intensity noted among Cuban men as measured by pack-years and cigarettes/day. Dominicans, on the other hand, had the lowest smoking prevalence, halving that of any other high prevalence group. A substantial number of individuals in SOL who were current smokers reported that they smoked cigarettes only on some days rather than daily, with Hispanics of Mexican backgrounds being the most prevalent intermittent smokers. The likelihood of being a current smoker was independently associated with male gender, age below 60 years, lower income, and lower level of education. Smoking was more common among individuals who were born in the US and had a higher level of acculturation, particularly among women [46].

As with obesity, adaptation to US cultural influences appears to promote smoking. Furthermore, the likelihood of quitting was higher among older people with higher socioeconomic status (income and education) [46]. Over 90% of female and male former smokers reported quitting on their own without cessation aids or therapy. Smoking cessation without aids remains a subject of study particularly in Hispanics, where sociocultural factors such as familism, spiritualism, and less acculturation may play a potentially important yet undetermined role.

Household smoking exposure was an independent risk factor for adult current cigarette smoking among Hispanics making it harder for former smokers to remain abstinent. At the risk of being redundant, it is worth mentioning that smoking practices, like other habits, are largely influenced by social behaviors. As such, since the prevalence of childhood second-hand exposure to household smoking was 40% among Hispanics, with Cubans, and Puerto Ricans having the highest rates, one wonders about the efficacy of current cigarette smoking cessation practices among these groups compared with non-Hispanic groups and those with less childhood exposure [47, 48].

Established Cardiovascular Disease

Coronary Heart Disease (CHD)

SOL showed that the overall prevalence of self-reported CHD was 4% for Hispanic men and 2% for women. Prevalence was reported to be higher in Puerto Rican men and women (5%) than any other subgroup except men of Cuban background who also showed similar percentages with overlapping confidence intervals [10].

Stroke

Among Hispanics of different backgrounds, self-reported stroke prevalence in SOL was 2% for men and 1% for women, the highest among Dominican men (3.9%) and Puerto Rican women (2.2%). Age and sex-adjusted prevalence of both CHD and stroke were significantly higher among men, older participants (aged 65–74 years), second- or third-generation immigrants, and those who preferred English [10].

Peripheral Vascular Disease (PVD)

It has been known that rates of lower extremity revascularization procedures are lower in Hispanics than in NHWs, and that admission rates for limb-amputation are higher for Hispanics [49]. However, until recently there were no data on PVD variability among the diverse Hispanic subgroups. A subanalysis of SOL by Allison et al. showed an overall 6% prevalence of PVD among Hispanics as defined by an Ankle-Brachial index (ABI) < 0.90 [50]. However, most notably, participants of Cuban (27.1%) and Mexican (30.3%) ancestries had the highest rates of PVD, and those with PVD were older, had more evidence of macro and microvascular injury, higher levels of systolic blood pressure, fasting glucose, and pack-years of cigarette smoking while having lower eGFR's. Interestingly, these findings were independent of educational attainment, immigrant generation, and traditional CV risk factors other than diabetes, raising the possibility that not only environmental factors are at play but also genetically mediated predisposition to PVD given the over threefold differential increase in these subgroups' PVD prevalence [50].

Lessons Learned from SOL

This landmark long-awaited study has undoubtedly placed the largest ethnic minority of the United States at the center of the Public Health and CV Epidemiology arena; SOL's clinical and socioeconomic relevance, rigorous design, and scientific scope have allowed gathering robust and highly pertinent data never known before. Here summarized are what we believe are the key findings provided by SOL to the medical community. The process of how we will use this information looking towards the future is only beginning.

- The finding that contemporary Hispanics/ Latinos carry a significant burden of CV disease risk factors provides a new benchmark for the dissemination of their health status to the public, lawmakers, and providers.
- As a diverse group, Hispanics/Latinos demonstrate very different CV risk profiles among their various ethnic and geographical backgrounds.
- In descending order, the most prevalent CV risk factors among Hispanics/Latinos include hypercholesterolemia, obesity, hypertension, diabetes, and tobacco use.
- A definitive answer as to the role played by acculturation in health and disease among Hispanics/Latinos remains elusive.
- The question of a Hispanic paradox brings an opportunity to better study commonly ignored CV health-related issues such as literacy, social support, and family structures.
- Long-term follow-up of the HCHS/SOL cohorts will provide information as to the

effectiveness of education and preventive interventions in rates of CV disease.

We now have a clearer picture of the CV health of self-identified Hispanics from multiple ethnic backgrounds, varied age groups, US birth rates, and duration of residence: their sociodemographic profiles, adverse nutritional and exercise habits, traditional lifestyle and cardiometabolic risk factors, medication use, anthropomorphic phenotypes, periodontal health status, and self-reported CV disease prevalence have all been uncovered. Several contributions to the understanding of CV health among Hispanics provided by SOL deserve special attention.

First, the substantial variation in the adverse profile of several measurable risk factors among different Hispanic subgroups uncovered by this study, a clear reflection of their diverse genetic background, lifestyles, and acculturation in the new society. While individuals of Central American origin showed the "healthiest" profile, Mexican and Dominicans exhibited the least, with disparities seen across genders and age groups mostly among Puerto Rican women and younger subjects, the latter appearing to have the highest rates of unhealthy low CV risk profiles.

Second, the findings just described challenge the now antiquated notion that extrapolation of old data obtained from registries that included exclusively or predominantly Mexican participants to that of other ethnic Hispanics is acceptable; third, except among younger women, SOL acculturation indices did not show a consistent relationship with CV risk factors profiles leaving unanswered questions as to the role, if any, played by the length of US residence or language preference in their behavior.

Finally, and perhaps most importantly, SOL paints a clearer picture as to the reality and challenge of Hispanics being able to reach the AHA cardiovascular health goals (aka, Life's Simple 7, LS7); this score, which includes diet, physical activity, smoking, BMI, BP, cholesterol and fasting glucose, was established with the hope of improving the health of all Americans while reducing CV deaths by 20% [51]. For better or worse, SOL found that LS7 profiles among

Hispanics were not particularly different than the general population with two important exceptions: the prevalence of a higher BMI and excess obesity particularly among women, and the presence of unhealthy dietary patterns across most subgroups [52]. One can only wonder if LS7 may not represent the best index of Hispanic cardiovascular risk.

In summary, the whole of the information detailed here has shed light on the complex heterogeneous definition of Hispanics; has raised important ethical questions about how should the country address the CV health of its largest class of immigrants in the context of the historically mixed and foreign composition of the US; has shown a similar pervasive unfavorable CV risk factor profile among Hispanics compared to the general population; and most importantly, SOL's results have begun to question how will governmental institutions incorporate these data into Public Health planning, educational initiatives, policymaking, and resource allocation.

The Hispanic Paradox

As we have discussed, Hispanics, compared to NHWs, are known to have a similar or greater prevalence of most CV risk factors, including obesity and diabetes, perhaps except for tobacco use among women. In general, Hispanics achieve lower levels of education; have less access to health care, and lower socioeconomic status, therefore remaining as one of the groups with the highest poverty rates in the US. Despite this unfavorable picture, Hispanics show lower rates of CV disease mortality and overall mortality than age-matched non-HWs and enjoy a longer life expectancy [5, 53–57]. For decades, this complex and intriguing epidemiological finding has been known as the "Hispanic paradox," a term first coined in the 1990s [58–64]. The notion of the Hispanic paradox has been challenged by some reports, including the San Antonio Heart Study and the Corpus Christi Heart Project both of which showed that CV mortality was similar and even greater among the largely Mexican cohort analyzed in these prospective studies [65, 66]. The Northern Manhattan study supported the existence of the Paradox only partially, and other studies found disparate results when separating Hispanics by national subgroups with only Mexicans and Central/South Americans demonstrating lower mortality rates [55, 63, 67].

In the only meta-analysis performed to systematically study the body of evidence published on the issue of the Hispanic paradox to date, Cortes-Bergoderi et al. reviewed 17 papers that included over 22 million Hispanics compared with more than 88 million non-HWs enrolled between 1950 and 2009 [68]. The data showed a statistically significant association between Hispanic ethnicity and lower CV mortality (OR 0.67; 95% CI, 0.57–0.78; $p = < 0.001$) and lower all-cause mortality (0.72; 95% CI, 0.63–0.82; $p < 0.001$). The authors concluded that these results indeed confirm the existence of a Hispanic paradox regarding CV mortality, but this notion is not conclusive. There are the known limitations of a meta-analysis, the heterogeneity of studies combined, how is the supposed "Paradox" impacted by low or high SES, by low or high acculturation. Does the supposed "Paradox" apply to every Hispanic background group equally? Does the "Paradox" apply to every form of CV disease (CHD, arrhythmias, heart failure, congenital heart disease) equally?

It is fair to say that regardless of the strength or weaknesses of this paradox or whether it truly exists or not, several important issues must be kept in mind: That (1) prospective studies will be needed to better understand the true nature of this conundrum; that (2) there should be no distraction or unfounded confidence when it comes to attribution of Hispanics' presumed protection by this paradox; education and preventive measures against CV disease should be heightened and enhanced because after all, CV disease is the leading cause of death among all Hispanics and their various subgroups. One must not rely on the notion that Hispanics have lower CV death as this may result in a less aggressive stand when it comes to screening and early detection of CV disease; and lastly, that (3) if indeed such paradox exists, it is imperative to understand the mechanisms that explain it whether genetic, psychosocial, sociocultural or nutritional. US Hispanics, their descendants, and other race-ethnic groups may all benefit from these answers.

A Call for Action

New data are emerging demonstrating that achieving a better CV health profile can lead to an equally important reduction in the rates of adverse events among all and any ethnic groups, including Hispanics. Dong et al. showed that in a contemporary urban community the presence of ideal CV health is an exceedingly rare occurrence, particularly among Hispanics, as demonstrated by the dismal rates of the cardiovascular health of metrics among participants enrolled in the Northern Manhattan Study [55]. Nonetheless, achieving a healthier CV profile conveys significant protection from morbidity and mortality, a fact that should stimulate the urgent implementation of comprehensive public health interventions.

In addition, it must be emphasized that culturally sensitive health promotion policies directed at Hispanic communities, particularly to the younger generations aiming at lifestyle modification such as enhanced physical activity, reduction of unhealthy food consumption, smoking cessation, and weight reduction, are as important as improving "hard" metrics of blood pressure, glycemia or lipid levels.

It should be recognized that important barriers to the betterment of CV health among Hispanics within the system itself remain prevalent: not all physicians feel comfortable caring for underrepresented minority patients and many cardiologists consider that health disparities do not even exist [69]. Although newer generations of physicians may have a different understanding of these matters, there is no doubt that we must continue to underline the need to increase awareness of the unique CV health characteristics shared by Hispanic groups.

The distinguished humanist, essayist, and scholar Pedro Henriquez Ureña, Dominican-born of mixed racial parenthood and an immigrant himself to the US, once said that the similarities in the History of the Americas and the common political and intellectual goals of their nations make this continent a magnificent Homeland as a group of peoples destined to come together closer and closer time after time. In that context, as scientists, we must set aside political views and embrace the fact that the US is not only the land of "opportunities for all," but also the epitome of a nation that has grown to become the giant it is today by not only accepting but embracing the diversity of all of its inhabitants, newly arrived or long established.

With that in mind, we should continue to work alongside our scientific colleagues and our policymakers toward the betterment of the CV health of Hispanics and all Americans for years to come. Starting with improving access to health care, culturally sensitive education geared toward the younger generations of Hispanics, engaging communities and local organizations very much like what the successful African American initiatives have achieved, and as importantly, sensitizing and educating non-Hispanic health care providers about the uniqueness of cardiac health is this group.

Last, it must be recognized that further research is needed. The SOL is a prospective study and over many years to come it will continue to shed light on the concept of a Hispanic paradox; the lack of Hispanic representation on the AHA Pooled Cohort equation for CV risk assessment; on the influence of family support, migration and acculturation on the CV status of future generations of Hispanics; and on finding the best clinical, community-based sociocultural and psychosocial interventions for the Hispanic community.

References

1. U.S. CENSUS BUREAU. Projections of the Size and Composition of the U.S. Population: 2014 to 2060. 2015. U.S. CENSUS BUREAU, 8–11. Accessed April 27, 2019 at: https://www.census.gov/content/dam/Census/library/publications/2015/demo/p25-1143.pdf

2. Cowie CC, Rust KF, Byrd-Holt DD, et al. Prevalence of diabetes and impaired fasting glucose in adults in the U.S. population: National Health and Nutrition Examination Survey 1999-2002. Diabetes Care. 2006;29(6):1263–8. https://doi.org/10.2337/dc06-0062.

3. Delgado JL, Johnson CL, Roy I, Treviño FM. Hispanic health and nutrition examination survey: methodological considerations. Am J Public Health. 1990;80(Suppl):6–10. https://doi.org/10.2105/ajph.80.suppl.6.

4. Caballero AE. Type 2 diabetes in the Hispanic or Latino population: challenges and opportunities. Curr Opin Endocrinol Diabetes Obes. 2007;14(2):151–7. https://doi.org/10.1097/MED.0b013e32809f9531.

5. Behavioral Risk Factor Surveillance System: BRFSS 2002 survey data and documentation. Centers for Disease Control and Prevention Web site. http://www.cdc.gov/brfss/annual_data/annual_2002.htm. Accessed September 25, 2020.

6. Marks G, Garcia M, Solis JM. Health risk behaviors of Hispanics in the United States: findings from HHANES, 1982-84. Am J Public Health. 1990;80(Suppl):20–6. https://doi.org/10.2105/ajph.80.suppl.20.

7. Flegal KM, Carroll MD, Kit BK, Ogden CL. Prevalence of obesity and trends in the distribution of body mass index among US adults, 1999-2010. JAMA. 2012;307(5):491–7. https://doi.org/10.1001/jama.2012.39.

8. Kramer H, Han C, Post W, et al. Racial/ethnic differences in hypertension and hypertension treatment and control in the multi-ethnic study of atherosclerosis (MESA). Am J Hypertens. 2004;17(10):963–70. https://doi.org/10.1016/j.amjhyper.2004.06.001.

9. Allison MA, Budoff MJ, Wong ND, Blumenthal RS, Schreiner PJ, Criqui MH. Prevalence of and risk factors for subclinical cardiovascular disease in selected US Hispanic ethnic groups: the multi-ethnic study of atherosclerosis. Am J Epidemiol. 2008;167(8):962–9. https://doi.org/10.1093/aje/kwm402.

10. Daviglus ML, Talavera GA, Avilés-Santa ML, et al. Prevalence of major cardiovascular risk factors and cardiovascular diseases among Hispanic/Latino individuals of diverse backgrounds in the United States. JAMA. 2012;308(17):1775–84. https://doi.org/10.1001/jama.2012.14517.

11. United States Census Bureau. Facts for Features: Hispanic Heritage Month 2017. American Community Survey (ACS) – 2016. 2017. Accessed April 27, 2019 at: https://www.census.gov/newsroom/facts-for-features/2017/hispanic-heritage.html

12. Rodriguez CJ, Allison M, Daviglus ML, et al. Status of cardiovascular disease and stroke in Hispanics/Latinos in the United States: a science advisory from the American Heart Association. Circulation. 2014;130(7):593–625. https://doi.org/10.1161/CIR.0000000000000071.

13. Winkleby MA, Jatulis DE, Frank E, Fortmann SP. Socioeconomic status and health: how education, income, and occupation contribute to risk factors for cardiovascular disease. Am J Public Health. 1992;82(6):816–20. https://doi.org/10.2105/ajph.82.6.816.

14. DuBard CA, Garrett J, Gizlice Z. Effect of language on heart attack and stroke awareness among U.S. Hispanics. Am J Prev Med. 2006;30(3):189–96. https://doi.org/10.1016/j.amepre.2005.10.024.

15. Wallace LS, DeVoe JE, Heintzman JD, Fryer GE. Language preference and perceptions of healthcare providers' communication and autonomy making behaviors among Hispanics. J Immigr Minor Health. 2009;11(6):453–9. https://doi.org/10.1007/s10903-008-9192-9.

16. Trangmar P, Diaz VA. Investigating complementary and alternative medicine use in a Spanish-speaking Hispanic community in South Carolina. Ann Fam Med. 2008;6(Suppl 1):S12–5. https://doi.org/10.1370/afm.736.

17. Bolstad AL, Bungum T. Diet, acculturation, and BMI in Hispanics living in southern Nevada. Am J Health Behav. 2013;37(2):218–26. https://doi.org/10.5993/AJHB.37.2.9.

18. Burroughs Peña M, Swett K, Schneiderman N, et al. Cardiac structure and function with and without metabolic syndrome: the echocardiographic study of Latinos (Echo-SOL). BMJ Open Diabetes Res Care. 2018;6(1):e000484. https://doi.org/10.1136/bmjdrc-2017-000484.

19. Isasi CR, Ayala GX, Sotres-Alvarez D, et al. Is acculturation related to obesity in Hispanic/Latino adults? Results from the Hispanic community health study/study of Latinos. J Obes. 2015;2015:186276. https://doi.org/10.1155/2015/186276.

20. United States Census Bureau. Educational Attainment in the United States: 2017. Current Population Survey, 2017 Annual Social and Economic Supplement, 2017. Accessed May 1, 2019 at: https://www.census.gov/data/tables/2017/demo/education-attainment/cps-detailed-tables.html

21. Folsom AR, Yatsuya H, Nettleton JA, et al. Community prevalence of ideal cardiovascular health, by the American Heart Association definition, and relationship with cardiovascular disease incidence. J Am Coll Cardiol. 2011;57(16):1690–6. https://doi.org/10.1016/j.jacc.2010.11.041.

22. Yang Q, Cogswell ME, Flanders WD, et al. Trends in cardiovascular health metrics and associations with all-cause and CVD mortality among US adults. JAMA. 2012;307(12):1273–83. https://doi.org/10.1001/jama.2012.339.

23. Daviglus ML, Pirzada A, Durazo-Arvizu R, et al. Prevalence of low cardiovascular risk profile among diverse Hispanic/Latino adults in the United States by age, sex, and level of acculturation: the Hispanic community health study/study of Latinos. J Am Heart Assoc. 2016;5(8):e003929. Published 2016 Aug 20. https://doi.org/10.1161/JAHA.116.003929.

24. Rodriguez CJ, Cai J, Swett K, et al. High cholesterol awareness, treatment, and control among

Hispanic/Latinos: results from the Hispanic community health study/study of Latinos. J Am Heart Assoc. 2015;4(7):e001867. https://doi.org/10.1161/JAHA.115.001867.

25. Willey JZ, Rodriguez CJ, Carlino RF, et al. Race-ethnic differences in the association between lipid profile components and risk of myocardial infarction: the northern Manhattan study. Am Heart J. 2011;161(5):886–92. https://doi.org/10.1016/j.ahj.2011.01.018.

26. Haffner SM, D'Agostino R Jr, Goff D, et al. LDL size in African Americans, Hispanics, and non-Hispanic whites: the insulin resistance atherosclerosis study. Arterioscler Thromb Vasc Biol. 1999;19(9):2234–40. https://doi.org/10.1161/01.atv.19.9.223.

27. Sorlie PD, Allison MA, Avilés-Santa ML, et al. Prevalence of hypertension, awareness, treatment, and control in the Hispanic community health study/study of Latinos. Am J Hypertens. 2014;27(6):793–800. https://doi.org/10.1093/ajh/hpu003.

28. Borrell LN, Crawford ND. Disparities in self-reported hypertension in Hispanic subgroups, non-Hispanic black and non-Hispanic white adults: the national health interview survey. Ann Epidemiol. 2008;18(10):803–12. https://doi.org/10.1016/j.annepidem.2008.07.008.

29. Rodriguez CJ, Sciacca RR, Diez-Roux AV, et al. Relation between socioeconomic status, race-ethnicity, and left ventricular mass: the Northern Manhattan study. Hypertension. 2004;43(4):775–9. https://doi.org/10.1161/01.HYP.0000118055.90533.88.

30. Pabon-Nau LP, Cohen A, Meigs JB, Grant RW. Hypertension and diabetes prevalence among U.S. Hispanics by country of origin: the National Health Interview Survey 2000-2005. J Gen Intern Med. 2010;25(8):847–52. https://doi.org/10.1007/s11606-010-1335-8.

31. Siddiqi A, Brown R, Nguyen QC, Loopstra R, Kawachi I. Cross-national comparison of socioeconomic inequalities in obesity in the United States and Canada. Int J Equity Health. 2015;14:116. Published 2015 Oct 31. https://doi.org/10.1186/s12939-015-0251-2.

32. Jiwani SS, Carrillo-Larco RM, Hernández-Vásquez A, et al. The shift of obesity burden by socioeconomic status between 1998 and 2017 in Latin America and the Caribbean: a cross-sectional series study [published correction appears in Lancet Glob Health. 2020 Mar;8(3): e340]. Lancet Glob Health. 2019;7(12):e1644–54. https://doi.org/10.1016/S2214-109X(19)30421-8.

33. Flegal KM, Carroll MD, Ogden CL, Curtin LR. Prevalence and trends in obesity among US adults, 1999-2008. JAMA. 2010;303(3):235–41. https://doi.org/10.1001/jama.2009.2014.

34. Kaplan RC, Avilés-Santa ML, Parrinello CM, et al. Body mass index, sex, and cardiovascular disease risk factors among Hispanic/Latino adults: Hispanic community health study/study of Latinos. J Am Heart Assoc. 2014;3(4):e000923. Published 2014 Jul 9. https://doi.org/10.1161/JAHA.114.000923.

35. Schneiderman N, Chirinos DA, Avilés-Santa ML, Heiss G. Challenges in preventing heart disease in hispanics: early lessons learned from the Hispanic Community Health Study/Study of Latinos (HCHS/SOL). Prog Cardiovasc Dis. 2014;57(3):253–61. https://doi.org/10.1016/j.pcad.2014.08.004.

36. Arredondo EM, Sotres-Alvarez D, Stoutenberg M, et al. Physical activity levels in U.S. Latino/Hispanic adults: results from the Hispanic community health study/study of Latinos. Am J Prev Med. 2016;50(4):500–8. https://doi.org/10.1016/j.amepre.2015.08.029.

37. Siega-Riz AM, Sotres-Alvarez D, Ayala GX, et al. Food-group and nutrient-density intakes by Hispanic and Latino backgrounds in the Hispanic Community Health Study/Study of Latinos. Am J Clin Nutr. 2014;99(6):1487–98. https://doi.org/10.3945/ajcn.113.082685.

38. Isasi CR, Parrinello CM, Jung MM, et al. Psychosocial stress is associated with obesity and diet quality in Hispanic/Latino adults. Ann Epidemiol. 2015;25(2):84–9. https://doi.org/10.1016/j.annepidem.2014.11.002.

39. Schneiderman N, Llabre M, Cowie CC, et al. Prevalence of diabetes among Hispanics/Latinos from diverse backgrounds: the Hispanic Community Health Study/Study of Latinos (HCHS/SOL). Diabetes Care. 2014;37(8):2233–9. https://doi.org/10.2337/dc13-2939.

40. Wang X, Jung M, Mossavar-Rahmani Y, et al. Macronutrient intake, diagnosis status, and glycemic control among US Hispanics/Latinos with diabetes. J Clin Endocrinol Metab. 2016;101(4):1856–64. https://doi.org/10.1210/jc.2015-3237.

41. Heiss G, Snyder ML, Teng Y, et al. Prevalence of metabolic syndrome among Hispanics/Latinos of diverse background: the Hispanic community health study/study of Latinos. Diabetes Care. 2014;37(8):2391–9. https://doi.org/10.2337/dc13-2505.

42. Centers for Disease Control and Prevention (CDC). Current cigarette smoking among adults – United States, 2011. MMWR Morb Mortal Wkly Rep. 2012;61(44):889–94.

43. Wang TW, Asman K, Gentzke AS, et al. Tobacco product use among adults – United States, 2017. MMWR Morb Mortal Wkly Rep. 2018;67(44):1225–32. Published 2018 Nov 9. https://doi.org/10.15585/mllmwr.mm6744a2. External or Accessed May 3, 2019 at: https://www.cdc.gov/mmwr/volumes/67/wr/mm6744a2.htm?s_cid=mm6744a2_w

44. Lopez-Quintero C, Crum RM, Neumark YD. Racial/ethnic disparities in report of physician-provided smoking cessation advice: analysis of the 2000 National Health Interview Survey. Am J Public Health. 2006;96(12):2235–9. https://doi.org/10.2105/AJPH.2005.071035.

45. Levinson AH, Pérez-Stable EJ, Espinoza P, Flores ET, Byers TE. Latinos report less use of pharmaceutical aids when trying to quit smoking. Am J Prev Med. 2004;26(2):105–11. https://doi.org/10.1016/j.amepre.2003.10.012.

46. Kaplan RC, Bangdiwala SI, Barnhart JM, et al. Smoking among U.S. Hispanic/Latino adults: the Hispanic community health study/study of Latinos. Am J Prev Med. 2014;46(5):496–506. https://doi.org/10.1016/j.amepre.2014.01.014.

47. Merzel CR, Isasi CR, Strizich G, et al. Smoking cessation among U.S. Hispanic/Latino adults: findings from the Hispanic Community Health Study/Study of Latinos (HCHS/SOL). Prev Med. 2015;81:412–9. https://doi.org/10.1016/j.ypmed.2015.10.006.

48. Navas-Nacher EL, Kelley MA, Birnbaum-Weitzman O, et al. Association between exposure to household cigarette smoking behavior and cigarette smoking in Hispanic adults: findings from the Hispanic Community Health Study/Study of Latinos. Prev Med. 2015;77:35–40. https://doi.org/10.1016/j.ypmed.2015.04.011.

49. Morrissey NJ, Giacovelli J, Egorova N, et al. Disparities in the treatment and outcomes of vascular disease in Hispanic patients. J Vasc Surg. 2007;46(5):971–8. https://doi.org/10.1016/j.jvs.2007.07.021.

50. Allison MA, Gonzalez F 2nd, Raij L, et al. Cuban Americans have the highest rates of peripheral arterial disease in diverse Hispanic/Latino communities. J Vasc Surg. 2015;62(3):665–72. https://doi.org/10.1016/j.jvs.2015.03.065.

51. Lloyd-Jones DM, Hong Y, Labarthe D, et al. Defining and setting national goals for cardiovascular health promotion and disease reduction: the American Heart Association's strategic impact goal through 2020 and beyond. Circulation. 2010;121(4):586–613. https://doi.org/10.1161/CIRCULATIONAHA.109.192703.

52. González HM, Tarraf W, Rodríguez CJ, et al. Cardiovascular health among diverse Hispanics/Latinos: Hispanic community health study/study of Latinos (HCHS/SOL) results. Am Heart J. 2016;176:134–44. https://doi.org/10.1016/j.ahj.2016.02.008.

53. Centers for Disease Control and Prevention, National Center for Health Statistics. Compressed mortality data. Series 20 No. 2P. CDC WONDER Online Database [database online]. Released January 2013. http://wonder.cdc.gv/cmf-icd10.html. Accessed February 12, 2014.

54. Askim-Lovseth M, Aldana A. Looking beyond "affordable" health care: cultural understanding and sensitivity-necessities in addressing the health care disparities of the U.S. Hispanic population. Health Mark Q. 2010;27:354–87.

55. Dong C, Rundek T, Wright CB, et al. Ideal cardiovascular health predicts lower risks of myocardial infarction, stroke, and vascular death across whites, blacks, and Hispanics: the Northern Manhattan Study. Circulation. 2012;125:2963–4.

56. Murphy SL, Xu J, Kochanek KD. Deaths: preliminary data for 2010. National Vital Statistics Reports. Vol 60, No 4. Hyattsville: National Center for Health Statistics; 2012.

57. Hoyert DL, Kung HC, Smith BL. Deaths: preliminary data for 2003. National Vital Statistics Reports. Vol 53, No 15. Hyattsville: National Center for Health Statistics; 2005.

58. Sorlie PD, Backlund E, Johnson NJ, Rogot E. Mortality by Hispanic status in the United States. JAMA. 1993;270:2464–8.

59. Friis R, Nanjundappa G, Prendergast TJ, et al. Coronary heart disease mortality and risks among Hispanics and non-Hispanics in Orange County. Calif Public Health Rep. 1981;96:418–22.

60. Iribarren C, Darbinian JA, Fireman BH, et al. Birthplace and mortality among insured Latinos: the paradox revisited. Ethn Dis. 2009;19:185–91.

61. Swenson CJ. Cardiovascular disease mortality in Hispanics and non-Hispanic whites. Am J Epidemiol. 2002;156:919–28.

62. Wei M, Mitchell BD, Haffner SM, et al. Effects of cigarette smoking, diabetes, high cholesterol, and hypertension on all-cause mortality and cardiovascular disease mortality in Mexican Americans. The San Antonio Heart Study. Am J Epidemiol. 1996;144:1058–65.

63. Willey JZ, Rodriguez CJ, Moon YP, et al. Coronary death and myocardial infarction among Hispanics in the Northern Manhattan Study: exploring the Hispanic paradox. Am J Epidemiol. 2012;22:303–9.

64. Palaniappan L, Wang Y, Fortmann SP. Coronary heart disease mortality for six ethnic groups in California, 1990-2000. Ann Epidemiol. 2004;14:499–506.

65. Hunt KJ, Resendez RG, Williams K, et al. All-cause and cardiovascular mortality among Mexican American and non-Hispanic White older participants in the San Antonio Heart Study: evidence against the "Hispanic paradox". Am J Epidemiol. 2003;158:1048–57.

66. Pandey DK, Labarthe DR, Goff DC, et al. Community-wide coronary heart disease mortality in Mexican Americans equals or exceeds that in non-Hispanic whites: the Corpus Christy Heart Project. Am J Med. 2001;110:81–7.

67. Hummer RA. Adult mortality differentials among Hispanic subgroups and non-Hispanic whites. Soc Sci Q. 2000;81:459–76.

68. Cortes-Bergoderi M, Goel K, Murad MH, et al. Cardiovascular mortality in Hispanics compared to non-Hispanic whites: a systematic review and meta-analysis of the Hispanic paradox. Eur J Intern Med. 2013;24(8):791–9. https://doi.org/10.1016/j.ejim.2013.09.003.

69. Lurie N, Fremont A, Jain AK, et al. Racial and ethnic disparities in care: the perspectives of cardiologists. Circulation. 2005;111:1264–9.

Lessons Learned from the Jackson Heart Study

Ervin R. Fox, Solomon K. Musani,
Frances C. Henderson, Adolfo Correa,
and Herman A. Taylor, Jr.

Abbreviations

AA	African Americans
BMI	Body mass index
BNP	B-type natriuretic peptide
BP	Blood pressure
CHF	Congestive heart failure
CRP	C-reactive protein
CVD	Cardiovascular disease
DM	Diabetes mellitus
GWAS	Genome-wide association study
HDL	High-density lipid
JHS	Jackson heart study
METS	Metabolic syndrome
SES	Socioeconomic status

E. R. Fox (✉)
Division of Cardiovascular Diseases, Department of
Medicine, University of Mississippi Medical Center,
Jackson, MS, USA
e-mail: efox@umc.edu

S. K. Musani
University of Mississippi Medical Center, Statistical
Geneticist, Jackson Heart Study, Jackson, MS, USA
e-mail: smusani@umc.edu

F. C. Henderson
Jackson Heart Study, Jackson, MS, USA

A. Correa
Jackson Heart Study, Jackson, MS, USA

Department of Medicine, University of Mississippi
Medical Center, Jackson, MS, USA
e-mail: acorrea@umc.edu

H. A. Taylor, Jr.
Cardiovascular Research Institute, Morehouse School
of Medicine, Atlanta, GA, USA
e-mail: htaylor@msm.edu

Introduction

The Jackson Heart Study (JHS) began to evolve in 1994. It was related to a family of similar studies that started in 1948 with the Framingham Heart Study. It was a logical progression of the all-African American (AA) Jackson cohort of the Atherosclerosis Risk in Communities Study which began in 1987. A group of physician and epidemiologist researchers from the National Institutes of Health, National Heart, Lung, and Blood Institute then led by Dr. Claude Lenfant, the then Office of Research on Minority Health led by Dr. John Ruffin, and administrators of three educational institutions in the Jackson, Mississippi area all worked together to shape the idea. The result was funding from the National Heart, Lung, and Blood Institute for a Planning and Feasibility Phase for the JHS 1996–1999. In 1997, a JHS Scientific Planning Group convened to explore the topic of "Research Priorities for the Study of Cardiovascular Disease (CVD) in AAs." The Planning Group derived seven potential research questions that addressed hypertension, congestive heart failure (CHF), renovascular disease, traditional CVD risk factors, genetic

© Springer Nature Switzerland AG 2021
K. C. Ferdinand et al. (eds.), *Cardiovascular Disease in Racial and Ethnic Minority Populations*,
Contemporary Cardiology, https://doi.org/10.1007/978-3-030-81034-4_10

epidemiology, newer imaging techniques, and sociodemographic factors (see Table 10.1).

Using these research priorities and other substantive data, the National Heart, Lung, and Blood Institute leaders posed four objectives for the initial funding period of the JHS 1999–2004.

- Establish a single-site epidemiological study of CVD in AA men and women by including and expanding the Jackson Atherosclerosis Risk in Communities Study.
- Identify risk factors or factors for the development and progression of CVD disease in AAs, with an emphasis on manifestations related to hypertension, such as left ventricular hypertrophy, coronary heart disease, CHF, stroke, and renovascular disease.

Table 10.1 Selected original JHS research questions, 1998

1. *Hypertension:* Can and should the JHS be designed to look at the risk factors for the development of high blood pressure, e.g., sodium, potassium, obesity, and diabetes?
2. *Left Ventricular Hypertrophy and Heart Failure:* What is the importance of left ventricular hypertrophy and congestive heart failure to coronary heart disease risk in African Americans? How should it be studied to best understand its role?
3. *Renovascular Diseases:* What is the importance of renovascular disease and its precursors to cardiovascular disease risk in African Americans? Can they and/or their precursors be studied effectively in a prospective study?
4. *Traditional CVD Risk Factors:* Do we know the relationship of the traditional risk factors, i.e., age, high blood pressure, serum cholesterol, low-density lipids, high-density lipids, smoking, obesity, and diabetes to the risk of heart disease in African American men and women? Should they be studied in the Jackson Heart Study? If so, how?
5. *Newer Methodologies, Genetics Epidemiology:* How can the study of genetic epidemiology be incorporated into the Jackson Heart Study?
6. *Newer Methodologies, Imaging Techniques:* What are the key non-invasive imaging techniques that should be incorporated into the Jackson Heart Study?
7. *Sociodemographic Factors:* What is the impact of social forces, e.g., discrimination, socioeconomic status, urban/rural differences, residential mobility, on cardiovascular disease risk in African Americans? Can and should they be studied in the Jackson Heart Study?

- Build research capabilities in minority institutions at the undergraduate and graduate level by developing partnerships between minority and majority institutions and enhancing the participation of minority investigators in large-scale epidemiological studies.
- Develop programs to attract minority students and prepare them for careers in public health and epidemiology [1].

The study design was flexible enough to accommodate the addition of bioimaging and biomarkers as opportunities to collect these data from a large AA cohort as the opportunities became available.

Rationale Supporting the Decision to Establish the Jackson Heart Study

The JHS Planning and Feasibility Team documented at least three decades of troubling CVD trends: CVD remained the number one cause of death in the United States, death rates for CVD in the United States were considerably higher among AAs, CVD death rates among AAs in Mississippi were among the highest in the nation, and the decline in CVD death rates had been slowest among AA men and women in Mississippi relative to other groups in the state and nation [2]. Ten trends were noted that documented the rising levels of CVD mortality in Mississippi (see Table 10.2).

The authors affirmed that there were many unanswered questions and concerns that provided the basis for recommendations for research, as well as more effective use of currently available strategies for reducing CVD risk. They were concerned that, when all the known or understandable links were accounted for, significant gaps in the understanding of racial and regional differences in CVD mortality remained.

As further justification for the JHS, the groundbreaking 1985 Report of the Secretary's Task Force on Black and Minority Health included the following recommendation: "Population-based, prospective, observational

Table 10.2 Ten trends documenting the rising levels of cardiovascular disease in Mississippi (before the launch of the Jackson Heart Study)

1. The 1995 age-adjusted cardiovascular mortality rate in Mississippi was the highest in the country; it was approximately 37% higher than the rate for the United States as a whole.
2. In the United States and Mississippi, African American men had the highest age-adjusted cardiovascular disease mortality rates.
3. The age-adjusted mortality rates in Mississippi for African American women were 70% percent higher than those for White women.
   1. The age-adjusted cardiovascular mortality rate for African American men was 46% higher than those for White men.
   2. The three leading causes of cardiovascular disease mortality were heart disease, stroke, and hypertension.
   3. In 1995, Mississippians had the highest heart disease mortality rate in the country, the fourth highest stroke rate, and the third highest hypertension rate.
   4. The African American /White differentials in Mississippi for heart disease were even higher for women, whereas similar differentials were found for stroke and hypertension. Heart disease mortality rates were 62% higher in African American women than those in White women. Differences between races were most pronounced in young adults.
   5. Between 1979 and 1995, cardiovascular disease mortality rates in Mississippi were slowly diverging from those in the United States, and these rates for African Americans in Mississippi were increasing significantly as rates in the nation as a whole were decreasing.
   6. From 1979 to 1995, the divergence in mortality rates resulted in an estimated 19,400 excess deaths from cardiovascular disease in Mississippi.
   7. African American men in Mississippi in the 45–54 age groups had a 3.5-fold greater chance of dying from cardiovascular disease than their White United States counterparts. For African American women, the relative risk was 4.2 times greater than that for White women."

studies of coronary heart disease (similar to the Framingham study) are needed for minority populations. A key component of this research would be the validation in minorities of the major established and/or suspected biological and psychological risk factors for CVD that have been identified for the White American population" [3]. In addition to studies to compare the AA population to other populations, within-population studies were recognized as needed to explore heart, lung, blood, and sleep risk factors for CVD within the AA population. Furthermore, while substantial evidence was emerging linking racism, discrimination, and hypertension, there had been few population-based epidemiological studies of perceived discrimination and hypertension [4]. Other aspects of psychosocial and sociocultural factors' influence on the incidence of CVD were significantly underexplored.

Against the national backdrop, Mississippi stood out as particularly hard-hit and a natural site to investigate to gain insight into the national CVD epidemic among AAs. Prior to the JHS, no study had comprehensively evaluated the combined contributions of traditional risk factors, novel risk factors (e.g., biomarkers, endothelial function, psychosocial and sociocultural influences) and noncardiac target-organ-disease to the risk of CVD, cardiac remodeling, and CHF in an African American (AA) community-based group. Lessons learned related to CVD in the JHS follow.

Lessons Learned Related to Cardiovascular Disease in the Jackson Heart Study

A major priority of the JHS is to study traditional risk factors for CVD more expansively and uncover novel CVD risk factors in the AA community. The JHS is optimally poised to better understand how the overall set of CVD risks translates to the higher rates of CVD events quoted in AA. Learning from the longitudinal study of JHS equips the scientific community with a guide to better address the growing racial disparity in CVD outcomes, which appears to be out of proportion to the degree of traditional CVD risk burden alone.

Traditional and Novel Risk Factors in the Jackson Heart Study

Traditional risk factors of CVD are those modifiable risks that increase the likelihood of heart attack and stroke such as hypertension, obesity,

DM, dyslipidemia, smoking, physical inactivity, and diet. Biomarkers (mediators in biological pathways including the neuroendocrine, renin-angiotensin, and natriuretic peptide pathways) and vascular endothelial dysfunction represent relatively novel factors under study for their potential roles in identifying or causing excess CVD risk. In this section, we review selected investigations in these areas of study in the JHS all-AA cohort.

Hypertension

In the JHS, the prevalence of hypertension is high; 62.9% of participants in Exam I, conducted 2000–2004, were hypertensive and its prevalence has increased substantially since then. Factors impacting the control of diagnosed hypertension have been a JHS focus. Approximately 87% of the hypertensive participants are aware of having hypertension, 83% of participants are on medication, and 66% are controlled [5]. JHS data show that hypertensive men on medication are less likely to be at their blood pressure (BP) goal compared to women; adherence to antihypertensive regimens appears to be the most prominent contributor to this difference [6]. Among those in Exam I and II conducted 2005–2009, approximately 27% of participants were nonadherent with their antihypertensive medications and these individuals were more likely to have higher systolic and diastolic BP and higher rates of uncontrolled BP [7]. In the JHS treatment-resistant hypertension is more common in those with nocturnal hypertension (defined as a mean nighttime systolic BP ≥ 120 mm Hg or diastolic BP ≥ 70 mm Hg) and/or non-dipping BP (defined as a mean nighttime to daytime systolic BP ratio >0.90) [8]. Diuretic therapy is associated with BP dipping at night; a potential mechanism for this is through the effect of diuretics on the renal sodium-chloride transporter. The potential for diuretic therapy in managing treatment-resistant hypertension is particularly important in AA as their hypertension is more often due to salt sensitivity and therefore may be more likely to be responsive to this approach [9, 10].

In the JHS, vigorous exercise and high-level sports during leisure time are associated with a lower likelihood of developing high BP [11]. However, physical activity on the job or while performing housework does not appear to lower the risk of development of hypertension suggesting a need to differentiate the contribution of these different forms of physical activity to hypertension prevention in AA. Weight loss was not a mediator between physical activity and the lower incidence of hypertension in recent studies. Potential mechanisms through which physical exercise may help in lowering the incidence of hypertension include the impact of exercise on improving endothelial function and on attenuating the renin-angiotensin system [12–15]. Further there is a graded relationship between incident hypertension and the number of Life's Simple 7 components achieved. Lowering hypertension risk in AA is optimal when the number of achieved components of the simple 7 is maximized.

Further, a comparison of JNC 7 vs JNC 8 guidelines on the treatment of hypertension among those with hypertension >60 years old found that individuals in this age group with a BP of 140–149/<90 mm Hg were at a higher risk for adverse CVD outcomes (HR: 2.61) compared to those without hypertension in this age group, [16, 17] supporting the current consensus that the therapeutic target for patients >60 years old should a blood pressure of <140/90.

Obesity

In the JHS cohort, the overall prevalence of obese and overweight participants is extremely high. At the baseline exam, approximately 60% of women and 40% of men were obese and approximately 28% of women and 40% of men were overweight [18]. Beyond body mass index (BMI), findings from the JHS emphasize the importance of the *distribution* of adiposity [19]. Participants with greater visceral adiposity are at higher risk of developing metabolic derangement and subsequently atherosclerosis [19]. Visceral adiposity volumes in the JHS are related to cardiometabolic risk factors such as cholesterol, triglycerides, BP, and fasting blood glucose. Further, in women visceral adiposity is related to lower levels of adiponectin a modulator of cardiometabolic risk factors [19]. Overall, obesity in the JHS cohort is associated with adverse CVD outcomes including cardiac hypertrophy, systolic and diastolic dysfunction, the risk of incident HF and HF hospitalization [20].

The relevance of social and behavioral determinants of obesity in the AA community is underscored in JHS. Those with higher income are less likely to be obese whereas those with lower income and those with higher stress levels are more likely to be obese [21]. Behaviors such as sleep duration, sleep quality, and physical activity in the JHS cohort are significantly associated with BMI [18, 22]. The lack of sleep and lower total physical activity are associated with higher rates of obesity whereas longer sleep duration, good sleep quality, and higher total physical activity are associated with lower BMI and smaller waist circumference [18, 22].

Diabetes and Metabolic Syndrome

In the JHS, there is a high prevalence of both metabolic syndrome (MetS) and DM. Approximately 17% of the cohort has a diagnosis of DM, 25% of the cohort has MetS (without DM) [23]. Compared to those without DM or MetS, those with MetS and DM are older, more likely female, more likely to have subclinical disease, and at greater risk of adverse clinical outcomes compared to those without metabolic derangement. In terms of subclinical disease, JHS participants with MetS and/or DM, have higher coronary artery calcification scores, are more likely to have cardiac hypertrophy on echocardiogram and microalbuminuria (a marker of kidney disease) compared to those without MetS or DM [23]. Additionally, those with DM are more likely to have peripheral artery disease. The relation of DM to chronic kidney disease (CKD) is already well known; however, through the JHS we now know that in AA, greater MetS severity is also associated with higher likelihood of developing CKD among women but not men [24]. Further, among JHS participants, having MetS confers a twofold greater risk of CVD events and > fourfold greater risk of adverse CVD events in those with DM compared to those without metabolic derangement. This risk of CVD events in those with DM and MetS is greater still in those with subclinical disease. In the presence of subclinical disease, there is a fourfold greater risk of CVD in those with MetS and a sevenfold greater risk in those with DM compared to those without metabolic derangement [23].

The JHS also provides several lessons on how social context influences the prevalence and incidence of DM in AA. For example, in the JHS, socioeconomic status is strongly associated with the prevalence of DM, and among women in the cohort socioeconomic status is also significantly related to awareness and treatment [25]. Further among JHS women, upward mobility from a socioeconomic perspective over the life course is associated with a lower incidence of DM [26]. The JHS also provides important information on the impact of social networks and support on the presence of DM in AA. In the JHS, high social networks and high social support are associated with lower prevalence of DM in women and men [27].

Hypercholesterolemia

JHS has taught us how important it is to keep total cholesterol concentration as a priority in optimizing the cardiovascular risk factor profile of AA. Overall, less than half of the JHS cohort had ideal total cholesterol at the baseline exam and that percentage decreased significantly over an approximate 8-year follow-up period from the baseline exam across all ages [28].

Further, it is well accepted that low levels of high-density lipoprotein (i.e., "low HDL") cholesterol are a major contributor to CVD in all Americans. An important lesson learned in the JHS is that there exists a high prevalence of low HDL in the cohort despite studies prior to the first examination suggesting overall high concentrations of HDL in the AA community [29]. In the baseline examination, low HDL cholesterol concentrations (defined as HDL <40 mg/dL in men and <50 mg/dl in women) were present in approximately 37% of those with MetS identifying low HDL as one of the primary risk factors contributing to the high prevalence of MetS in the JHS. Moreover, low HDL is more common in women compared to men and is equally distributed across all age groups [29]. Given these findings from JHS, early screening and management of low HDL in AA are underscored as a significant and perhaps under-utilized strategy to remove the racial disparity in heart disease and stroke, particularly among women.

Cigarette Smoking

Among JHS participants approximately 68% have never smoked, 19% are past smokers and 13% are current smokers [30]. Current smokers are more likely to be men and to also drink alcohol compared to those who never smoked. Past smokers are more likely to be men, have DM, and have hypertension compared to those who never smoked [30].

Investigations in the JHS allow the opportunity to better understand how cigarette smoking relates to cardiovascular morbidity in AA. As seen in previous studies identifying risk factors for heart disease in the population, investigators have found that in JHS cigarette smoking is significantly related to incident all-CVD (heart attack, stroke, and CHF) [31, 32]. An important lesson learned from JHS is that current cigarette smokers demonstrate a significantly higher incidence of kidney function decline compared to those who never smoked. There may be a role of systemic inflammation linking cigarette smoking and kidney function decline in this group as those in the JHS who are current smokers have a significantly higher C-reactive protein (CRP) level [33]. Further, in the JHS among AA in the cohort cigarette smoking is related to the development of DM and the progression of peripheral artery disease [30, 34]. Those smoking more than 20 cigarettes (1 pack) daily (defined as high-intensity smoking) have an approximately 80% higher likelihood of developing DM than never smokers and a higher likelihood of developing subclinical peripheral artery disease [30].

Physical Inactivity and Diet

Through JHS, we have learned to what extent physical inactivity and diet contribute to the less than optimal cardiovascular risk profile that prevails in the AA community. The overall low proportion of participants in the JHS that achieved an ideal cardiovascular health score at the baseline exam was largely due to the high proportion of participants failing to achieve ideal status for these two modifiable risk factors [28]. Less than 20% of participants at the baseline exam adhered to ideal physical activity recommendations and less than 1% met recommendations for an ideal diet [28]. Over an 8-year follow-up, there was a small improvement in the proportion of participants achieving ideal physical activity in the cohort. An extraordinarily high percentage of participants did not meet recommendations for salt intake (<1.5 g/day) and/or whole-grain intake [28]. These findings related to physical activity and diet noted in the JHS underscore the need for community-based interventions that concentrate on modifying exercise and dietary behaviors to improve risk profiles within a vulnerable population. Further there is evidence that life course and neighborhood socioeconomic position impact dietary behaviors in this group [35]. These findings suggest that critical attention needs to be directed at increasing information about, availability of, and access to quality affordable food options in order to improve dietary behaviors in the AA community.

Cardiovascular Health Score in the Jackson Heart Study

In the JHS, clustering of risk factors is associated with a significant impact on heart disease in AA. This is most evident in evaluating MetS in earlier studies and in a more recent study using the new American Heart Association Life's

Simple Seven to define ideal cardiovascular health [23, 24, 36]. Using the cardiovascular health score, JHS investigators have been able to identify in what ways and to what extent the totality of modifiable lifestyle behaviors contributes to cardiovascular morbidity in the community. Lessons learned from investigations in the JHS using Life's Simple Seven show that cardiovascular health practices in mid-life in AA influence the incidence of cardiovascular risk factors such as hypertension and DM and the incidence of CVD outcomes specifically cardiac remodeling and HF development [36]. Specifically, among the risk factors in Life's Simple 7, hypertension, glucose metabolism, physical inactivity, and cigarette smoking are related to HF development. BMI and glucose level are associated with less adverse cardiac remodeling and systolic function as seen on cardiac magnetic resonance imaging [36].

Biomarkers Relation to Cardiovascular Disease Risk Factors and Subclinical Disease

Using available biomarkers, the JHS allows for a novel approach to identifying biological pathways that potentially contribute to disease in AA. Investigators have shown from analysis using B-type natriuretic peptide (BNP) that the natriuretic peptide pathway plays an important role in the longitudinal increase in systolic and diastolic blood pressure and to the progression to a higher BP category across examinations [37]. Additionally, lower BNP levels showed a significant relation to higher BMI [38]. Importantly, in later studies, BNP showed a U-shaped relation with MetS. It is thought that the rising limb of the U-shape represents the direct impact of the natriuretic peptide pathway on blood pressure, while the falling limb reflects the indirect relation of the natriuretic peptide pathway to obesity [39].

Similarly, CRP as a marker of systemic inflammation has been studied in the JHS. Without adjusting for obesity, smoking and statin therapy, CRP concentrations are significantly higher in the JHS compared to those reported in non-Hispanic White populations. However, after adjusting for these risk factors, CRP concentrations are similar between the two ethnic groups [40]. In the JHS, CRP was significantly related to subclinical disease, including kidney disease and peripheral artery disease [41, 42].

Further, studying a panel of biomarkers (including BNP and CRP), JHS investigators have identified potential pathophysiological mechanisms for the pathogenesis of MetS in AAs. In a panel of seven biomarkers representing systemic inflammation (C-reactive protein—CRP), adiposity (leptin), natriuretic pathway (BNP), adrenal pathway (cortisol and aldosterone), and endothelial function (endothelin and homocysteine) investigators showed that MetS is associated with the adrenal, natriuretic peptide and inflammatory pathways in the JHS [39].

Using a similar panel of nine biomarkers (same panel as in the analysis with MetS however including adiponectin and renin activity and mass), investigators identified that in the JHS cohort aldosterone and leptin are associated with incident CKD [43]. Leptin, adiponectin, and CRP are associated with rapid kidney function decline. Together these findings implicate adiposity, adrenal, and systemic inflammation pathways in the development of kidney disease in AA. Though overall, the biomarker panel contributed at most modestly to the prediction of incident kidney disease above traditional risk factors alone, this research adds to lessons learned from the JHS by providing significant insight into the pathophysiology of chronic kidney disease progression in this high-risk population [43].

In the JHS, troponin has also proven to be a very informative biomarker particularly as a marker of subclinical myocardial injury that identifies a malignant form of left ventricular hypertrophy [44]. Those in the JHS with the combination of left ventricular hypertrophy and subclinical myocardial injury based on elevated troponin levels identify a phenotype with a five-fold increased risk of development of clinical HF compared to those with left ventricular hypertrophy or elevated troponin alone. This phenotype appears particularly malignant among men in the cohort [44].

Aortic Stiffness and Endothelial Dysfunction

Recent work in the JHS confirms that aortic stiffness as determined by pulse wave velocity (PWV) and endothelial function are novel markers that are relevant to cardiovascular risk in AA [45–47]. Prior to JHS, studies on aortic stiffness and endothelial function had been conducted in predominantly White cohorts; how they relate to disease in AA had not been comprehensively studied. In the JHS, aortic stiffness is significantly associated with multiple cardiovascular risk factors that include age, mean arterial pressure, total/HDL cholesterol ratio, and glucose control [48]. Further, preliminary studies in the cohort show that aortic stiffness is significantly associated with chronic kidney disease (defined by microalbuminuria and urine albumin-to-creatinine ratio) and to prevalent CVD.(unpublished work). Findings in the JHS support the theory that aortic stiffening and resulting impedance matching between the aorta and conduit vessels lead to microvascular dysfunction and damage and subsequent target organ damage.

Another lesson learned from the JHS is that there are sex-specific differences in the relation of aortic stiffness to cardiovascular risk factors. In JHS women, the relation between age and aortic stiffness is stronger than in men and there is a stronger association between total/HDL cholesterol ratio and aortic stiffness. Moreover, there is a steeper relation of mean arterial pressure with stiffness in women [48]. Finally, the protective effect of female sex on microvascular integrity and reserve is no longer seen after middle age [47]. These sex differences may partially explain the greater risk for CVD, CHF, and dementia in older women.

Subclinical Disease Prevalence and Associated Risk of Cardiovascular Events

In the JHS, the prevalence of subclinical disease defined by the presence of one or more components (peripheral artery disease, left ventricular hypertrophy, low LV ejection fraction, microalbuminuria, or high coronary artery calcium score) is approximately a third of the cohort [23]. Despite a lower prevalence of these measures in AAs of Jackson relative to the Framingham Heart Study (FHS) participants, the strength of the association with incident CVD was more robust (HR 3.16 vs. 1.90 in Framingham) [49]. Further, the presence of subclinical disease in JHS participants confers a substantial increased risk of CVD events (including myocardial infarction, stroke, and CHF) compared to those absent of subclinical disease [23]. Specifically, the presence of a high coronary artery calcium score (Agatston score >100) or echocardiographic cardiac hypertrophy increased the risk of incident CVD two- to four-fold.) [23]. This investigation particularly highlights the need to not only aggressively manage risk factors for heart disease but to also consider the early assessment of subclinical disease in AA as an integrated approach to lower the risk of CVD events in the population.

Predictors of Left Ventricular Mass Progression and Cardiovascular Outcomes

The high prevalence of echocardiographic left ventricular hypertrophy and its associated risk of CVD events and mortality are well studied. In the JHS, we have learned more about the factors that contribute to the progressive increase in left ventricular mass over time in this high-risk population. Baseline left ventricular mass, baseline BMI, baseline systolic BP, and change in systolic BP are all significant independent contributors to the progression of left ventricular mass over an 8-year follow-up period among participants [50]. Further, progression in left ventricular mass between visits is significantly associated with incident CVD in the JHS cohort [50]. Findings from the study underscore the need for greater control of BP and weight in AA to prevent the progression of LV mass and subsequent risk of CVD events including CHF.

Predictive Models for Cardiovascular Events Based on the JHS Cohort

Based on findings from JHS relating risk factors and subclinical disease to CV outcomes over the first 15 years, JHS investigators conducted a study generating multiple all CVD (CHD and CHF) risk prediction models using a combination of standard risk factors, biomarkers, and subclinical disease components in the JHS cohort [32]. The rationale for undertaking this project stemmed from the fact that previous risk models were developed in predominantly White populations and validated in AA populations. Investigators sought the most accurate estimate for CVD in the Black population that has a disproportionately higher risk for CVD events including HF compared to other ethnic groups [51]. A total of six all CVD risk models were generated: one with traditional risk factors alone, one with traditional risk factors and biomarkers, two with traditional risk factors and subclinical disease markers and two incorporating all three risk domains (traditional risk factors, biomarkers and subclinical disease). Both biomarkers and subclinical disease markers improved model prediction beyond the traditional risk factor model. Among the biomarkers used in the analysis for risk prediction, BNP proved statistically significant. This most likely is due to the inclusion of CHF in the definition of all CVD; however, others may relate to its roles in the natriuretic peptide pathway and in lipid and glucose metabolism [52].

The traditional risk factor model and a model incorporating traditional risk factors, BNP, and ankle-brachial index were the two selected based on their ease of use in a primary care setting. Both models selected were validated in external AA cohorts. In a comparison with the ACC/AHA Pooled Cohort Risk Assessment Equation for CVD, there was no substantial improvement in risk prediction classification however the effort remains an important contribution to the literature [32, 52]. The study confirms that existing equations are not easily improved upon in their assessment of CVD risk

in AA. Further, it illustrates the importance of adding CHF in risk assessment in the definition of all CVD given in JHS CHF accounted for 1/3 all CVD events [32, 52].

Social Determinants of Cardiovascular Disease in the Jackson Heart Study

Social conditions are increasingly recognized as the most potent determinants of population health and disease. The COVID-19 pandemic of 2020 heightened awareness of the health effects of social structure and conditions within which people live, work, and play, and how those conditions can impact health disparities. The JHS has a particular focus on social determinants and African American's CV health and disease.

A notable example is found in the JHS data demonstrating the relationship between social variables and high BP. Among AAs, hypertension is associated with a larger proportion of CVD than other traditional risk factors, including DM, hypercholesterolemia, obesity, and smoking [53]; a study pooling data from JHS and the REGARDS study showed a population attributable risk of >30% of hypertension for major CVD outcomes among AAs [54]. Hypertension is linked to poor outcomes for AA in HF, stroke, chronic kidney and myocardial infarction, left ventricular hypertrophy, and mortality. But in addition to the primordial factors usually associated with hypertension, the JHS has shown consistently that social conditions contribute significantly. Analysis of JHS data at baseline revealed a strong association between the stress of lifetime discrimination and the prevalence of hypertension [55]. Recent publications have strengthened this association. Using prospectively ascertained data, these recent analyses show that the incidence of new-onset hypertension among the people normotensive at baseline is strongly related to the stress of discrimination [55]. The toxicity of these negative interpersonal interactions may be compounded by other more impersonal systemic/structural social factors. For instance, JHS data have shown that social position, education, and household median income influence the diurnal pattern of 24-hour BP [56]. Significant blunting of nocturnal dipping—a worrisome indicator of excess CVD risk—was associated with lower levels of educational attainment and income among AAs. Neighborhood socioeconomic status, estimated by validated metrics, is negatively associated with heavy alcohol use, a primordial risk for the development of hypertension [57]. Such stressors—neighborhood conditions, proximity to physical and or environmental toxins, educational attainment, are distinct from day-to-day discriminatory or racist interactions experienced by AAs, but they are no less real in their individual and population-level health consequences. These health-damaging realities are significantly determined by discriminatory and racist practices and policies (e.g., residential segregation policies which have concentrated AA citizens in toxic physical environments near major roadways or industrial pollutants), which have had a transgenerational impact.

Beyond hypertension, other important CVD consequences of social context have been documented by the JHS. Higher prevalence of peripheral vascular disease and elevated carotid intima-media thickness were found among AAs living within 150 of heavily traveled roads compared with participants living greater than 300 m away, after adjustment for likely confounders [58]. Among women, neighborhood safety significantly influences visceral adiposity, a major cardiometabolic risk [59]. Neighborhood disadvantage (an index inclusive of eight indicators of disadvantage from US Census data) was related to the incidence of major cardiovascular events, even after adjustment of individual levels of socioeconomic status (SES)—suggesting a powerful influence of context at all levels of individual economic prosperity [56].

The JHS has been particularly productive in verifying and extending observations of other groups as well as documenting new areas of concern relating to social determinants of CVD. The work of the JHS has implications for further research as well intervention at individual, neighborhood, and policy levels.

Genomics and Proteomics Studies

Introduction

Genetic research in the Jackson Heart Study (JHS) began with the NHLBI's Candidate Gene Association Resource (NHLBI CARe) consortium a decade ago [60, 61]. Until then genetic research in individuals of African Ancestry had been scarce. The NHLBI's main motivation, which coincided with the completion of the human genome project a few years prior, was to discover new variants that are associated with disease traits using candidate gene and genome-wide association (GWAS) mapping approaches in AAs. Thus, JHS has been part of several consortia designed to enhance the capacity for gene discovery. Examples include Continental Origins and Genetic Epidemiology Network (COGENT) [62], Cohorts for Heart and Aging Research in Genomic Epidemiology (CHARGE) [63, 64], Genetics of Obesity and Liver related Diseases (GOLD) [65], and Genetic Consortium on Asthma among African-ancestry Populations in the Americas (CAAPA) [66] Yet, the motivation has remained the same. In this review, we highlight some of the lessons learned by JHS's participation in genetic research for the last two decades. We will categorize our results into the proportion of genetic ancestry, admixture mapping, GWAS, exome analysis, and candidate gene analysis.

Genome of JHS Participants

AAs in the JHS and indeed most of the United States and the Caribbean are admixed, i.e., their chromosomes are a mosaic of blocks of DNA that descended from West African and European ancestral populations. These two previously divergent populations, subjected to differing demographic history (e.g., drift and selective pressures) leading to differences in allelic frequencies and patterns of linkage disequilibrium [67, 68], came together because of the trans-Atlantic slave trade. As such, the prevalence of many simple and complex diseases varies with genetic ancestry, more so probably due to genetic and/or environmental factors rather than genetic differences, which are typically known to represent only a small fraction of genetic variation [69, 70]. This finding has been confirmed in several genetic studies in JHS such as Deo and colleagues who found that on average the proportion of African genetic ancestry among JHS participants is 84% (interquartile range: 77.9–88.7) [71]. Traits that have been reported to be associated with the proportion of ancestry in JHS include DM [72], hemoglobin A1c [73], adiponectin [74, 75] and subclinical atherosclerosis [76, 77]. Importantly, the African proportion of genetic ancestry has been found to be correlated (inversely) with socioeconomic status in the JHS. A similar finding has been reported in studies of Latinx groups, [69] underscoring the potency of SES as a potential confounder in such analyses.

Most recently, JHS became part of efforts under the CAAPA consortium to leverage the high-coverage whole-genome data to: summarize genetic variation resulting from the African Diaspora across the Americas and into the Caribbean; refine estimates on the burden of deleterious variants carried across populations; and to appreciate how these estimates vary with African ancestry [76]. This is particularly important in medical genetics where failure to account for fine-scale population structure resulting from lower linkage disequilibrium and decreased genome-wide array coverage in these populations can lead to spurious results [78, 79].

Admixture Mapping and Discovery of Genetic Variants Associated with CVD Traits in AA

Admixture mapping is the preferred method for discovering genetic variants that contribute to interethnic variation in certain traits. It uses genetic markers whose alleles show frequency differential between ancestral populations. Admixture mapping using a panel of ancestry informative markers [68, 71, 80] has enabled investigation of the genetic basis for several

CVD-related traits, including hematological traits [68, 81], serum lipids [83] blood pressure [84, 85], DM [72], iron, and traits [82].

Neutropenia

Individuals of African ancestry often exhibit "benign ethnic" neutropenia—characterized by low white blood cell (WBC) and neutrophil counts. This is due to a regulatory variant in the Duffy antigen receptor for chemokines (DARC) gene [86]. Studies at JHS have provided unambiguous evidence for the genetic basis of this variation. First, Nalls and colleagues used admixture mapping to identify a locus on chromosome 1q that was strongly associated with WBC [80]. Individuals with two copies of the West African allele had lower mean WBC of 4.9 (SD 1.3) compared to individuals with two European alleles [mean WBC of 7.1 (SD 1.3)]. Up to 20% of population variation in WBC is attributed to this variant. In a follow-up study [68], it was demonstrated that the causal variant for the association was at least 91% different in frequency between West Africans and European Americans and that the Duffy Null polymorphism (SNP rs2814778 at chromosome 1q23.2) was the ideal candidate. This SNP is in a genomic region known to be so differentiated in frequency and is already known to protect against Plasmodium vivax malaria.

JHS along with other cohorts recruiting people of African ancestry in the COGENT consortium later identified several variants associated with WBC and WBC subtypes by GWAS. Some of the regions such as CXCL2, CDK6, and PSMD3-CSF3 have been validated in individuals of European, Asian, and Hispanic ancestry, suggesting the association is present in other ancestries as well.

Lipoprotein Lipase Lp(a)

Lipoprotein lipase (a) [(Lp(a)] is another CVD-related trait that has been investigated using admixture in the JHS. Lp(a) is highly variable, with 80% of the variance in Lp(a) levels in AAs attributable to variation within LPA gene but the corresponding proportion in European Americans is over 90%. By employing admixture and dense fine-mapping, we discovered genetic variants that are responsible for this difference in Lp(a) [83]. Indeed, effect sizes for 12 of the risk variants discovered in European populations were lower than in African local ancestry background observed in JHS. This finding highlighted the need for caution in the use of genetic variants for risk assessment across different populations. Follow-up research work using GWAS and exome array has narrowed the region further and confirmed that ancestry-specific causal risk variant(s) reside in or near LPA [87]. In an earlier study, Deo et al. [68, 71] reported that genetic background matters for lipoprotein lipase LPL locus. A "gain-of-function" S447X mutation at LPL, which is known to be a determinant for the strong LPL-TG genetic association had a significantly diminished strength of biological effect when it is found on a background of African rather than European ancestry.

Blood Pressure

Efforts involving combined admixture mapping and GWAS to discover variants associated with BP have also provided opportunities to glean some lessons from genetic research in JHS. In the first-ever GWAS study for blood pressure in people of African ancestry done under NHLBI CARe initiative, Fox et al. [84] found several suggestive signals of variants associated with BP. In a follow-up study, the same group conducted admixture mapping followed by association analysis [85]. They found one novel variant (rs7726475) located near natriuretic peptide receptor c (NPR3) genes known to play an important role in blood pressure regulation [88–91]. This risk variant was replicated in five independent cohorts of AAs including a cohort from Nigeria [85] and in populations of European and East Asian ancestry [92–94]. This finding highlights the fact that for admixed populations such as AAs, a combination of admixture mapping and GWAS may be more powerful than either of the approaches alone.

GWAS findings that have suggested traits that might have universal effects across populations of multiple ancestries include BP [62], BNP [95], platelet and mean platelet volume [96], cardiac structure [97]. There is also evidence for unique and shared genetic architecture for example CRP [98, 99].

Gene–Lifestyle Interactions

JHS participation in the CHARGE Consortium's Gene-Lifestyle working Group has paved way for studies that incorporate gene-by-lifestyle interactions as a novel approach to identifying new variants modulated by lifestyle factors to influence cardiovascular traits. Lifestyle factors such as smoking, alcohol drinking, sleep, physical activity, and psychosocial factors have proven to be critical in the discovery of genetic variants for complex traits [64]. Several novel loci for BP identified by accounting for lifestyle factors such as smoking behavior [100] and alcohol drinking and the majority in African ancestry [101]. Similar findings reported for lipids when accounting for smoking [102], alcohol drinking [103], physical activity [104], and sleep [105]. These findings demonstrate the importance of including diverse populations, particularly in studies of interactions with lifestyle factors, where genomic and lifestyle differences by ancestry may contribute to novel findings. Additionally, it also demonstrates the need for careful consideration of ancestry because it may be a proxy for both genomic and environmental context.

Selected Candidate Gene Analysis

Analysis of selected candidate genes (e.g., sickle cell trait (SCT) and APOL1) widely known to have high frequency in individuals of African ancestry due to positive selection has also been tested for their association with CVD traits. For instance, the APOL1 alleles G1 and G2 are known to enhance lysis of Trypanosoma brucei rhodesiense, conveying resistance to the African sleeping sickness [106]. However, in a study on increased burden of CVD in carriers of *APOL1* genetic variants, Ito and colleagues observed that *APOL1* variants contribute to atherosclerotic CVD risk and also revealed a genetic component to cardiovascular health disparities in individuals of African ancestry [107]. This finding was confirmed recently in a meta-analysis of 21,305 AAs from eight large cohorts [108]. The considerable population of AA with two *APOL1* risk alleles may benefit from intensive interventions to reduce CVD.

Replication of Genetic Variants with High Impact Findings

Investigations of somatic mutations in the blood of persons not known to have hematologic disorders in JHS for their relations with cardiovascular events and survival have been conducted [109]. Findings have shown that the presence of somatic mutations can depend on age [109], being rare in younger (i.e., less 40 years old) but more frequently found in older participants. In addition, investigations revealed that most variants of high impact were in *DNMT3A*, *TET2*, and *ASXL1* genes and increased risk of incident coronary heart disease (hazard ratio, 2.0; 95% CI, 1.2–3.4) and ischemic stroke (hazard ratio, 2.6; 95% CI, 1.4–4.8). From these results, we learned that while age-related clonal hematopoiesis may be a common condition associated with increases in the risk of hematologic cancer and in all-cause mortality, the increased risk at advanced age might be due to higher risk of CVD. We also learned that the risk of somatic mutations was universal across persons of multiple ancestries.

For the past two decades, JHS has played a crucial role as a source of genetic data in minority populations for investigators to explore in search of answers to specific questions. Key among them being whether there are genetic influences on racial health disparities. While much remains to be investigated, so far, we have learned at least one thing from genomic research in JHS. Genetic background is important in gene discovery, thus the previous and current focus of the field on populations derived principally from

Northwestern Europe has severe limitations. Inclusion of individuals of African ancestry in genomic research is paramount if we are to broaden the possibilities of novel insights into human biology, a broadening that will benefit the entire human family, as well as offer an improved understanding of health disparities.

Future Directions

The future directions of the Jackson Heart Study are guided by 20 years of gathering, analyzing data, and disseminating findings related to epidemiological observations. The vision of the Jackson Heart Study—to transform a history of African American's excess heart disease into a legacy of heart health—has remained constant though approaches have adapted to advances in technology, imaging, computational and genomics science, and other methodologies. Jackson Heart Study investigators and collaborators have explored traditional and novel risk factors, subclinical disease, cardiac structure and function, vascular function, visceral and abdominal adiposity, and social determinants of health. They have initiated and contributed to consortia studying numerous -omics aspects of heart disease and health since 2000.

From 2018 to 2024, the JHS will prioritize topics such as: (1) comprehensive understanding of the role that risk factors play in systolic and diastolic CHF; (2) the prevalence and cardiometabolic correlate of cognitive impairment and brain structure; (3) the interplay between environmental, behavioral, and social drivers of obesity, DM, and hypertension on CVD and chronic kidney disease; (4) masked hypertension and its correlation with sleep disorders; (5) the true incidence and psychosocial risk factors of atrial fibrillation in AAs; and (6) the social determinants of health in AA. The JHS will be well poised to investigate how social construct impacts the relation between CVD risk factors, genes, and the environment to increase the allostatic load. Conversely, factors contributing to resilience in participants who do well despite high allostatic load will also be a focus.

Further, we will continue to harmonize phenotypic and genotypic data across multiple cohorts to answer broad questions that impact multiple ethnicities across different geographic regions. Analysis of harmonized data will also allow for across population comparisons. We will use findings generated in the JHS to drive translational research and implementation science that can have measurable impact on population health.

The JHS future will embrace the use of multiple technology-assisted approaches for collecting and analyzing data and disseminating findings such as mobile phones and wearable devices to collect data on heart rate variability, body temperature, sleep pattern, blood pressure, and physical activity, and other data. An exciting prospect for the cohort would be to consider telehealth-based interventions that can build on lessons learned to improve risk factor profiles and behaviors. Through monitoring participants' risk factors and providing feedback and educational information on findings in-between visits, we can improve healthy behavior and adherence to medication regimens to achieve better risk factor control.

The JHS is charting its future direction based on a longitude of exploring risk factors and cardiovascular health disparities and a latitude of uncovering new approaches to reduce or eliminate them. It will continue to concentrate on establishing a platform that brings an array of disciplines together to solve the complex challenges that race-associated CVD disparities produce. If successful, it will increasingly lay the groundwork for lasting change—a change that must be pursued with energy and urgency.

References

1. Sempos CT, Bild DE, Manolio TA. Overview of the Jackson Heart Study: a study of cardiovascular diseases in African American men and women. Am J Med Sci. 1999;317(3):142–6.
2. Jones DW, Sempos CT, Thom TJ, et al. Rising levels of cardiovascular mortality in Mississippi, 1979-1995. Am J Med Sci. 2000;319(3):131–7.
3. Report of the secretary's task force on black and minority health volume IV, cardiovascular and cerebrovascular disease, part I and part II, Department of Health and Human Services 1986.
4. Payne TJ, Wyatt SB, Mosley TH, et al. Sociocultural methods in the Jackson Heart Study: conceptual and descriptive overview. Ethn Dis. 2005;15(4 Suppl 6):S6–48.
5. Wyatt SB, Akylbekova EL, Wofford MR, et al. Prevalence, awareness, treatment, and control of hypertension in the Jackson Heart Study. Hypertension. 2008;51(3):650–6.
6. Ferdinand KC. Improving approaches to hypertension treatment in African Americans: lessons learned from the Jackson Heart Study. J Clin Hypertens (Greenwich). 2013;15(6):362–4.
7. Butler MJ, Tanner RM, Muntner P, et al. Adherence to antihypertensive medications and associations with blood pressure among African Americans with hypertension in the Jackson Heart Study. J Am Soc Hypertens. 2017;11(9):581–8. PMCID: PMC5603252
8. Irvin MR, Booth JN III, Sims M, et al. The association of nocturnal hypertension and nondipping blood pressure with treatment-resistant hypertension: the Jackson Heart Study. J Clin Hypertens (Greenwich). 2018;20(3):438–46. PMCID: PMC5907922
9. Aviv A. Cellular calcium and sodium regulation, salt-sensitivity and essential hypertension in African Americans. Ethn Health. 1996;1(3):275–81.
10. Morris RC Jr, Sebastian A, Forman A, Tanaka M, Schmidlin O. Normotensive salt sensitivity: effects of race and dietary potassium. Hypertension. 1999;33(1):18–23.
11. Diaz KM, Booth JN III, Seals SR, et al. Physical activity and incident hypertension in African Americans: the Jackson Heart Study. Hypertension. 2017;69(3):421–7. PMCID: PMC5302780
12. Aizawa K, Shoemaker JK, Overend TJ, Petrella RJ. Metabolic syndrome, endothelial function and lifestyle modification. Diab Vasc Dis Res. 2009;6(3):181–9.
13. Ashor AW, Lara J, Siervo M, et al. Exercise modalities and endothelial function: a systematic review and dose-response meta-analysis of randomized controlled trials. Sports Med. 2015;45(2):279–96.
14. Dod HS, Bhardwaj R, Sajja V, et al. Effect of intensive lifestyle changes on endothelial function and on inflammatory markers of atherosclerosis. Am J Cardiol. 2010;105(3):362–7.
15. Rush JW, Aultman CD. Vascular biology of angiotensin and the impact of physical activity. Appl Physiol Nutr Metab. 2008;33(1):162–72.
16. Chobanian AV, Bakris GL, Black HR, et al. The seventh report of the joint national committee on prevention, detection, evaluation, and treatment of high blood pressure: the JNC 7 report. JAMA. 2003;289(19):2560–72.
17. Nayor M, Duncan MS, Musani SK, et al. Incidence of cardiovascular disease in individuals affected by recent changes to US blood pressure treatment guidelines. J Hypertens. 2018;36(2):436–43. PMCID: PMC6062206

18. Dubbert PM, Robinson JC, Sung JH, et al. Physical activity and obesity in African Americans: the Jackson Heart Study. Ethn Dis. 2010;20(4):383–9. PMCID: PMC5074338

19. Liu J, Fox CS, Hickson DA, et al. Impact of abdominal visceral and subcutaneous adipose tissue on cardiometabolic risk factors: the Jackson Heart Study. J Clin Endocrinol Metab. 2010;95(12):5419–26. PMCID: PMC2999970

20. Pandey A, Kondamudi N, Patel KV, et al. Association between regional adipose tissue distribution and risk of heart failure among blacks. Circ Heart Fail. 2018;11(11):e005629.

21. Gebreab SY, Diez-Roux AV, Hickson DA, et al. The contribution of stress to the social patterning of clinical and subclinical CVD risk factors in African Americans: the Jackson Heart Study. Soc Sci Med. 2012;75(9):1697–707. PMCID: PMC3580180

22. Jefferson T, Addison C, Sharma M, Payton M, Jenkins BC. Association between sleep and obesity in African Americans in the Jackson Heart Study. J Am Osteopath Assoc. 2019;119(10):656–66.

23. Xanthakis V, Sung JH, Samdarshi TE, et al. Relations between subclinical disease markers and type 2 diabetes, metabolic syndrome, and incident cardiovascular disease: the Jackson Heart Study. Diabetes Care. 2015;38(6):1082–8. PMCID: PMC4439537

24. DeBoer MD, Filipp SL, Musani SK, Sims M, Okusa MD, Gurka M. Metabolic syndrome severity and risk of CKD and worsened GFR: the Jackson Heart Study. Kidney Blood Press Res. 2018;43(2):555–67. PMCID: PMC6037309

25. Sims M, Diez Roux AV, Boykin S, et al. The socioeconomic gradient of diabetes prevalence, awareness, treatment, and control among African Americans in the Jackson Heart Study. Ann Epidemiol. 2011;21(12):892–8. PMCID: PMC3192269

26. Beckles GL, McKeever BK, Saydah S, Imperatore G, Loustalot F, Correa A. Life course socioeconomic position, allostatic load, and incidence of type 2 diabetes among African American adults: the Jackson Heart Study, 2000-04 to 2012. Ethn Dis. 2019;29(1):39–46. PMCID: PMC6343544

27. Glover LM, Bertoni AG, Golden SH, et al. Sex differences in the association of psychosocial resources with prevalent type 2 diabetes among African Americans: the Jackson Heart Study. J Diabetes Complicat. 2019;33(2):113–7. PMCID: PMC6554648

28. Djousse L, Petrone AB, Blackshear C, et al. Prevalence and changes over time of ideal cardiovascular health metrics among African-Americans: the Jackson Heart Study. Prev Med. 2015;74:111–6. PMCID: PMC4397893

29. Taylor H, Liu J, Wilson G, et al. Distinct component profiles and high risk among African Americans with metabolic syndrome: the Jackson Heart Study. Diabetes Care. 2008;31(6):1248–53. PMCID: PMC3209804

30. White WB, Cain LR, Benjamin EJ, et al. High-intensity cigarette smoking is associated with incident diabetes mellitus in black adults: the Jackson Heart Study. J Am Heart Assoc. 2018;7(2):e007413. PMCID: PMC5850161

31. Kamimura D, Cain LR, Mentz RJ, et al. Cigarette smoking and incident heart failure: insights from the Jackson Heart Study. Circulation. 2018;137(24):2572–82. PMCID: PMC6085757

32. Fox ER, Samdarshi TE, Musani SK, et al. Development and validation of risk prediction models for cardiovascular events in Black adults: the Jackson Heart Study Cohort. JAMA Cardiol. 2016;1(1):15–25. PMCID: PMC5115626

33. Hall ME, Wang W, Okhomina V, et al. Cigarette smoking and chronic kidney disease in African Americans in the Jackson Heart Study. J Am Heart Assoc. 2016;5(6):e003280. PMCID: PMC4937270

34. Clark D III, Cain LR, Blaha MJ, et al. Cigarette smoking and subclinical peripheral arterial disease in blacks of the Jackson Heart Study. J Am Heart Assoc. 2019;8(3):e010674. PMCID: PMC6405586

35. Gao Y, Hickson DA, Talegawkar S, et al. Influence of individual life course and neighbourhood socioeconomic position on dietary intake in African Americans: the Jackson Heart Study. BMJ Open. 2019;9(3):e025237. PMCID: PMC6429841

36. Spahillari A, Talegawkar S, Correa A, et al. Ideal cardiovascular health, cardiovascular remodeling, and heart failure in blacks: the Jackson Heart Study. Circ Heart Fail. 2017;10(2):e003682. PMCID: PMC5319800

37. Fox ER, Musani SK, Singh P, et al. Association of plasma B-type natriuretic peptide concentrations with longitudinal blood pressure tracking in African Americans: findings from the Jackson Heart Study. Hypertension. 2013;61(1):48–54. PMCID: PMC3521855

38. Fox ER, Musani SK, Bidulescu A, et al. Relation of obesity to circulating B-type natriuretic peptide concentrations in blacks: the Jackson Heart Study. Circulation. 2011;124(9):1021–7. PMCID: PMC3318977

39. Musani SK, Vasan RS, Bidulescu A, et al. Aldosterone, C-reactive protein, and plasma B-type natriuretic peptide are associated with the development of metabolic syndrome and longitudinal changes in metabolic syndrome components: findings from the Jackson Heart Study. Diabetes Care. 2013;36(10):3084–92. PMCID: PMC3781556

40. Fox ER, Benjamin EJ, Sarpong DF, et al. Epidemiology, heritability, and genetic linkage of C-reactive protein in African Americans (from the Jackson Heart Study). Am J Cardiol. 2008;102(7):835–41. PMCID: PMC3733442

41. Fox ER, Benjamin EJ, Sarpong DF, et al. The relation of C--reactive protein to chronic kidney disease in African Americans: the Jackson Heart Study. BMC Nephrol. 2010;11:1. PMCID: PMC2826325

42. Sung JH, Lee JE, Samdarshi TE, et al. C-reactive protein and subclinical cardiovascular disease among African-Americans: (the Jackson Heart Study). J Cardiovasc Med (Hagerstown). 2014;15(5):371–6. PMCID: PMC4353570

43. Mwasongwe SE, Young B, Bidulescu A, Sims M, Correa A, Musani SK. Relation of multi-marker panel to incident chronic kidney disease and rapid kidney function decline in African Americans: the Jackson Heart Study. BMC Nephrol. 2018;19(1):239. PMCID: PMC6147037

44. Pandey A, Keshvani N, Ayers C, et al. Association of cardiac injury and malignant left ventricular hypertrophy with risk of heart failure in African Americans: the Jackson Heart Study. JAMA Cardiol. 2019;4(1):51–8. PMCID: PMC6439681

45. McClendon EE, Musani SK, Samdarshi TE, et al. The relation of digital vascular function to cardiovascular risk factors in African-Americans using digital tonometry: the Jackson Heart Study. J Am Soc Hypertens. 2017;11(6):325–33.

46. Tripathi A, Benjamin EJ, Musani SK, et al. The association of endothelial function and tone by digital arterial tonometry with MRI left ventricular mass in African Americans: the Jackson Heart Study. J Am Soc Hypertens. 2017;11(5):258–64.

47. Cooper LL, Musani SK, Washington F, et al. Relations of microvascular function, cardiovascular disease risk factors, and aortic stiffness in blacks: the Jackson Heart Study. J Am Heart Assoc. 2018;7(20):e009515. PMCID: PMC6474961

48. Tsao CW, Washington F, Musani SK, et al. Clinical correlates of aortic stiffness and wave amplitude in black men and women in the community. J Am Heart Assoc. 2018;7(21):e008431. PMCID: PMC6404204

49. Ingelsson E, Sullivan LM, Murabito JM, et al. Prevalence and prognostic impact of subclinical cardiovascular disease in individuals with the metabolic syndrome and diabetes. Diabetes. 2007;56(6):1718–26.

50. Fox ER, Musani SK, Samdarshi TE, et al. Clinical correlates and prognostic significance of change in standardized left ventricular mass in a community-based cohort of African Americans. J Am Heart Assoc. 2015;4(2):e001224. PMCID: PMC4345860

51. Virani SS, Alonso A, Benjamin EJ, et al. Heart disease and stroke statistics-2020 update: a report from the American Heart Association. Circulation. 2020;141(9):e139–596.

52. Goff DC Jr, Lloyd-Jones DM. The pooled cohort risk equations-black risk matters. JAMA Cardiol. 2016;1(1):12–4.

53. Howard G, Cushman M, Kissela BM, et al. Traditional risk factors as the underlying cause of racial disparities in stroke: lessons from the half-full (empty?) glass. Stroke. 2011;42(12):3369–75. PMCID: PMC3226886

54. Clark D III, Colantonio LD, Min YI, et al. Population-attributable risk for cardiovascular disease associated with hypertension in black adults.

JAMA Cardiol. 2019;4(12):1194–202. PMCID: PMC6813577

55. Sims M, Diez-Roux AV, Dudley A, et al. Perceived discrimination and hypertension among African Americans in the Jackson Heart Study. Am J Public Health. 2012;102(Suppl 2):S258–65. PMCID: PMC3477918

56. Barber S, Hickson DA, Wang X, Sims M, Nelson C, Diez-Roux AV. Neighborhood disadvantage, poor social conditions, and cardiovascular disease incidence among African American adults in the Jackson Heart Study. Am J Public Health. 2016;106(12):2219–26. PMCID: PMC5105010

57. Wang X, Auchincloss AH, Barber S, et al. Neighborhood social environment as risk factors to health behavior among African Americans: the Jackson Heart Study. Health Place. 2017;45:199–207. PMCID: PMC5546244

58. Wang Y, Wellenius GA, Hickson DA, Gjelsvik A, Eaton CB, Wyatt SB. Residential proximity to traffic-related pollution and atherosclerosis in 4 vascular beds among African-American adults: results from the Jackson Heart Study. Am J Epidemiol. 2016;184(10):732–43. PMCID: PMC5141947

59. Pham DQ, Ommerborn MJ, Hickson DA, Taylor HA, Clark CR. Neighborhood safety and adipose tissue distribution in African Americans: the Jackson Heart Study. PLoS One. 2014;9(8):e105251. PMCID: PMC4148311

60. Keating BJ, Tischfield S, Murray SS, et al. Concept, design and implementation of a cardiovascular gene-centric 50 k SNP array for large-scale genomic association studies. PLoS One. 2008;3(10):e3583. PMCID: PMC2571995

61. Musunuru K, Lettre G, Young T, et al. Candidate gene association resource (CARe): design, methods, and proof of concept. Circ Cardiovasc Genet. 2010;3(3):267–75. PMCID: PMC3048024

62. Franceschini N, Fox E, Zhang Z, et al. Genome-wide association analysis of blood-pressure traits in African-ancestry individuals reveals common associated genes in African and non-African populations. Am J Hum Genet. 2013;93(3):545–54. PMCID: PMC3769920

63. Psaty BM, O'Donnell CJ, Gudnason V, et al. Cohorts for Heart and Aging Research in Genomic Epidemiology (CHARGE) Consortium: design of prospective meta-analyses of genome-wide association studies from 5 cohorts. Circ Cardiovasc Genet. 2009;2(1):73–80. PMCID: PMC2875693

64. Rao DC, Sung YJ, Winkler TW, et al. Multiancestry study of gene-lifestyle interactions for cardiovascular traits in 610 475 individuals from 124 cohorts: design and rationale. Circ Cardiovasc Genet. 2017;10(3):e001649. PMCID: PMC5476223

65. Palmer ND, Musani SK, Yerges-Armstrong LM, et al. Characterization of European ancestry nonalcoholic fatty liver disease-associated variants in indi-

viduals of African and Hispanic descent. Hepatology. 2013;58(3):966–75. PMCID: PMC3782998

66. (CAAPA), genetic consortium on asthma among African-ancestry populations in the Americas 2012. Retrieved from https://www.caapa-project.org/

67. Lohmueller KE, Indap AR, Schmidt S, et al. Proportionally more deleterious genetic variation in European than in African populations. Nature. 2008;451(7181):994–7. PMCID: PMC2923434

68. Reich D, Nalls MA, Kao WH, et al. Reduced neutrophil count in people of African descent is due to a regulatory variant in the Duffy antigen receptor for chemokines gene. PLoS Genet. 2009;5(1):e1000360. PMCID: PMC2628742

69. Florez JC, Price AL, Campbell D, et al. Strong association of socioeconomic status with genetic ancestry in Latinos: implications for admixture studies of type 2 diabetes. Diabetologia. 2009;52(8):1528–36. PMCID: PMC3113605

70. Smith MW, O'Brien SJ. Mapping by admixture linkage disequilibrium: advances, limitations and guidelines. Nat Rev Genet. 2005;6(8):623–32.

71. Deo RC, Reich D, Tandon A, et al. Genetic differences between the determinants of lipid profile phenotypes in African and European Americans: the Jackson Heart Study. PLoS Genet. 2009;5(1):e1000342. PMCID: PMC2613537

72. Chen Z, Tang H, Qayyum R, et al. Genome-wide association analysis of red blood cell traits in African Americans: the COGENT Network. Hum Mol Genet. 2013;22(12):2529–38. PMCID: PMC3658166

73. Echouffo-Tcheugui JB, Mwasongwe SE, Sims M, et al. Sickle cell trait, European ancestry, and longitudinal tracking of HbA1c among African Americans: the Jackson Heart Study. Diabetes Care. 2019;42(10):e166–7. PMCID: PMC6754235

74. Bidulescu A, Choudhry S, Musani SK, et al. Associations of adiponectin with individual European ancestry in African Americans: the Jackson Heart Study. Front Genet. 2014;5:22. PMCID: PMC3918651

75. Riestra P, Gebreab SY, Xu R, et al. Gender-specific associations between ADIPOQ gene polymorphisms and adiponectin levels and obesity in the Jackson Heart Study cohort. BMC Med Genet. 2015;16:65. PMCID: PMC4593213

76. Mathias RA, Taub MA, Gignoux CR, et al. A continuum of admixture in the Western hemisphere revealed by the African Diaspora genome. Nat Commun. 2016;7:12522. PMCID: PMC5062574

77. Gebreab SY, Riestra P, Khan RJ, et al. Genetic ancestry is associated with measures of subclinical atherosclerosis in African Americans: the Jackson Heart Study. Arterioscler Thromb Vasc Biol. 2015;35(5):1271–8. PMCID: PMC4523273

78. McKeigue PM. Prospects for admixture mapping of complex traits. Am J Hum Genet. 2005;76(1):1–7. PMCID: PMC1196412

79. Tishkoff SA, Kidd KK. Implications of biogeography of human populations for 'race' and medicine. Nat Genet. 2004;36(11 Suppl):S21–7.

80. Nalls MA, Wilson JG, Patterson NJ, et al. Admixture mapping of white cell count: genetic locus responsible for lower white blood cell count in the health ABC and Jackson Heart studies. Am J Hum Genet. 2008;82(1):81–7. PMCID: PMC2253985

81. Reiner AP, Lettre G, Nalls MA, et al. Genome-wide association study of white blood cell count in 16,388 African Americans: the continental origins and genetic epidemiology network (COGENT). PLoS Genet. 2011;7(6):e1002108. PMCID: PMC3128101

82. Li J, Lange LA, Duan Q, et al. Genome-wide admixture and association study of serum iron, ferritin, transferrin saturation and total iron binding capacity in African Americans. Hum Mol Genet. 2015;24(2):572–81. PMCID: PMC4334839

83. Deo RC, Wilson JG, Xing C, et al. Single-nucleotide polymorphisms in LPA explain most of the ancestry-specific variation in Lp(a) levels in African Americans. PLoS One. 2011;6(1):e14581. PMCID: PMC3025914

84. Fox ER, Young JH, Li Y, et al. Association of genetic variation with systolic and diastolic blood pressure among African Americans: the Candidate Gene Association Resource study. Hum Mol Genet. 2011;20(11):2273–84. PMCID: PMC3090190

85. Zhu X, Young JH, Fox E, et al. Combined admixture mapping and association analysis identifies a novel blood pressure genetic locus on 5p13: contributions from the CARe consortium. Hum Mol Genet. 2011;20(11):2285–95. PMCID: PMC3090198

86. Haddy TB, Rana SR, Castro O. Benign ethnic neutropenia: what is a normal absolute neutrophil count? J Lab Clin Med. 1999;133(1):15–22.

87. Li J, Lange LA, Sabourin J, et al. Genome- and exome-wide association study of serum lipoprotein (a) in the Jackson Heart Study. J Hum Genet. 2015;60(12):755–61.

88. Matsukawa N, Grzesik WJ, Takahashi N, et al. The natriuretic peptide clearance receptor locally modulates the physiological effects of the natriuretic peptide system. Proc Natl Acad Sci U S A. 1999;96(13):7403–8. PMCID: PMC22098

89. Nakayama T. The genetic contribution of the natriuretic peptide system to cardiovascular diseases. Endocr J. 2005;52(1):11–21.

90. Pitzalis MV, Sarzani R, Dessi-Fulgheri P, et al. Allelic variants of natriuretic peptide receptor genes are associated with family history of hypertension and cardiovascular phenotype. J Hypertens. 2003;21(8):1491–6.

91. Sarzani R, Dessi-Fulgheri P, Salvi F, et al. A novel promoter variant of the natriuretic peptide clearance receptor gene is associated with lower atrial natriuretic peptide and higher blood pressure in obese hypertensives. J Hypertens. 1999;17(9):1301–5.

92. Ehret GB, Munroe PB, Rice KM, et al. Genetic variants in novel pathways influence blood pressure and cardiovascular disease risk. Nature. 2011;478(7367):103–9. PMCID: PMC3340926

93. Johnson T, Gaunt TR, Newhouse SJ, et al. Blood pressure loci identified with a gene-centric array. Am J Hum Genet. 2011;89(6):688–700. PMCID: PMC3234370

94. Kato N, Takeuchi F, Tabara Y, et al. Meta-analysis of genome-wide association studies identifies common variants associated with blood pressure variation in east Asians. Nat Genet. 2011;43(6):531–8. PMCID: PMC3158568

95. Musani SK, Fox ER, Kraja A, et al. Genome-wide association analysis of plasma B-type natriuretic peptide in blacks: the Jackson Heart Study. Circ Cardiovasc Genet. 2015;8(1):122–30. PMCID: PMC4426827

96. Qayyum R, Snively BM, Ziv E, et al. A meta-analysis and genome-wide association study of platelet count and mean platelet volume in African Americans. PLoS Genet. 2012;8(3):e1002491. PMCID: PMC3299192

97. Fox ER, Musani SK, Barbalic M, et al. Genome-wide association study of cardiac structure and systolic function in African Americans: the Candidate Gene Association Resource (CARe) study. Circ Cardiovasc Genet. 2013;6(1):37–46. PMCID: PMC3591479

98. Ellis J, Lange EM, Li J, et al. Large multiethnic Candidate Gene Study for C-reactive protein levels: identification of a novel association at CD36 in African Americans. Hum Genet. 2014;133(8):985–95. PMCID: PMC4104766

99. Schick UM, Auer PL, Bis JC, et al. Association of exome sequences with plasma C-reactive protein levels in >9000 participants. Hum Mol Genet. 2015;24(2):559–71. PMCID: PMC4334838

100. Sung YJ, Winkler TW, de Las FL, et al. A large-scale multi-ancestry genome-wide study accounting for smoking behavior identifies multiple significant loci for blood pressure. Am J Hum Genet. 2018;102(3):375–400. PMCID: PMC5985266

101. Feitosa MF, Kraja AT, Chasman DI, et al. Novel genetic associations for blood pressure identified via gene-alcohol interaction in up to 570K individuals across multiple ancestries. PLoS One. 2018;13(6):e0198166. PMCID: PMC6005576

102. Bentley AR, Sung YJ, Brown MR, et al. Multi-ancestry genome-wide gene-smoking interaction study of 387,272 individuals identifies new loci associated with serum lipids. Nat Genet. 2019;51(4):636–48. PMCID: PMC6467258

103. de Vries PS, Brown MR, Bentley AR, et al. Multiancestry genome-wide association study of lipid levels incorporating gene-alcohol interactions. Am J Epidemiol. 2019;188(6):1033–54. PMCID: PMC6545280

104. Kilpelainen TO, Bentley AR, Noordam R, et al. Multi-ancestry study of blood lipid levels identifies four loci interacting with physical activity. Nat Commun. 2019;10(1):376. PMCID: PMC6342931

105. Noordam R, Bos MM, Wang H, et al. Multi-ancestry sleep-by-SNP interaction analysis in 126,926 individuals reveals lipid loci stratified by sleep duration. Nat Commun. 2019;10(1):5121. PMCID: PMC6851116

106. Genovese G, Friedman DJ, Ross MD, et al. Association of trypanolytic ApoL1 variants with kidney disease in African Americans. Science. 2010;329(5993):841–5. PMCID: PMC2980843

107. Ito K, Bick AG, Flannick J, et al. Increased burden of cardiovascular disease in carriers of APOL1 genetic variants. Circ Res. 2014;114(5):845–50. PMCID: PMC3982584

108. Grams ME, Surapaneni A, Ballew SH, et al. APOL1 kidney risk variants and cardiovascular disease: an individual participant data meta-analysis. J Am Soc Nephrol. 2019;30(10):2027–36. PMCID: PMC6779370

109. Jaiswal S, Fontanillas P, Flannick J, et al. Age-related clonal hematopoiesis associated with adverse outcomes. N Engl J Med. 2014;371(26):2488–98. PMCID: PMC4306669

Cardiovascular Disease Risk Factors in the Hispanic/Latino Population

11

Leonor Corsino and Jonathan D. Velez-Rivera

Introduction

In this chapter, we summarize new and emerging data pertaining to the difference in cardiovascular risk factors in the increasingly diverse and heterogeneous Hispanic/Latino population in the United States. Over the last decade, available data provided an array of information that allowed us to better understand the impact of Hispanic/Latino heritage as it relates to cardiovascular risk factors. Previously, evidence focused mainly on the Mexican heritage subgroup. However, with the increasing representation of Hispanic/Latino heritage subgroups from the Caribbean region and Central and South America, further understanding the differences in risk factors by subgroups has gained significant importance. The burden of cardiovascular disease and cardiovascular disease risk factors in the Hispanic/Latino population remains a major health disparity in the United States, but its impact is significantly greater among certain Hispanic/Latino subgroups. Although there have been significant advances in the treatment and management of cardiovascular disease risk factors in the United States, the Hispanic/Latino population experiences a significant burden that is further perpetuated by the historically limited understanding of the different factors influencing each heritage subgroup.

To better inform decisions that will have a major impact on the prevention and treatment of cardiovascular disease in the US Hispanic/Latino population, it is important to better understand how Hispanics/Latinos are not a homogenous group. In Chap. 8, we learned how the National Institute of Health (NIH) sponsored Hispanic Community Health Study/Study of Latinos (HCHS/SOL) provided significant information that provided a better understanding of how Hispanics/Latinos from different heritage groups are affected in unique and different ways by cardiovascular disease and cardiovascular risk factors. Our goal is to provide information beyond that learned from HCHS/SOL and to summarize and review emerging data informing and enhancing our understanding of the differences in cardiovascular disease risk factors, such as metabolic syndrome, hypertension, dyslipidemia, diabetes, and obesity in the diverse US Hispanic/Latino population.

Metabolic Syndrome

Metabolic syndrome encompasses cardiovascular disease risk factors such as central obesity, hyperglycemia, dyslipidemia, hypertension, and

L. Corsino (✉) · J. D. Velez-Rivera
Duke University School of Medicine, Division of Endocrinology, Metabolism, and Nutrition, Durham, NC, USA
e-mail: corsi002@mc.duke.edu;
Jonathan.velez.rivera@duke.edu

© Springer Nature Switzerland AG 2021
K. C. Ferdinand et al. (eds.), *Cardiovascular Disease in Racial and Ethnic Minority Populations*, Contemporary Cardiology, https://doi.org/10.1007/978-3-030-81034-4_11

elevated proinflammatory/prothrombotic markers [1–3]. Figure 11.1 depicts a proposed model of interactions between cardiovascular disease risk factors leading to metabolic syndrome [4]. The pathophysiology of metabolic syndrome has been studied extensively. Multiple mechanisms have been proposed which range from abnormalities in fatty acid metabolism leading to insulin resistance to oxidative stress and low-grade inflammation [5, 6].

Multiple definitions of metabolic syndrome exist using different criteria and cutoff values [7–10]. In 2009, the National Cholesterol Education Program (NCEP) Adult Treatment Panel III (ATP-III) attempted to unify existent definitions of metabolic syndrome [11, 12]. Since the publication of their consensus statement, the International Diabetes Foundation (IDF)/ATP-III 2009 definition is the most widely used. Numerous publications have emerged that attempt to reanalyze previous population studies using this newer definition. Using the IDF/ATP-III criteria, a reanalysis of participants in the

Framingham Heart Study (the year 1990, mostly white population), who were followed for 8 years, showed that the prevalence of metabolic syndrome increased by 56% and 47% among men and women, respectively, compared with original reports from the study. Of those identified with metabolic syndrome, a high prevalence of established cardiovascular disease and diabetes was noted on follow-up (~30% and ~50%, respectively) [13].

In the IDF/ATP-III 2009 definition of waist circumference, the cutoffs used were those identified by the IDF in 2004 for certain ethnic groups. These waist circumference cutoffs include population- and country-specific definitions, which highlights the role that ethnicity plays in defining metabolic syndrome [9]. For example, the IDF threshold for abdominal obesity in ethnic Central/South Americans irrespective of where they are living should be ≥90 cm in men and ≥80 cm in women; but, if the ATP-III criteria are used for foreign-born Mexicans living in the United States then the thresholds

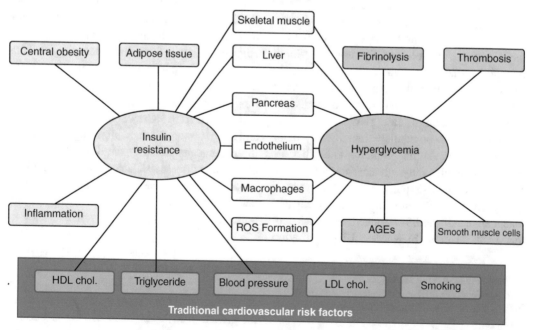

Fig. 11.1 Cardiovascular risk factors and atherogenic processes clustered around insulin resistance and hyperglycemia. HDL = high-density lipoprotein, LDL = low-density lipoprotein, AGEs = advanced glycosylated end products, ROS = reactive oxygen species. (Reproduce with permission from Stančáková and Laakso [4])

could change to ≥102 cm in men and ≥88 cm for women if the ethnic background is not considered by the investigators. This concept is something very important to consider when analyzing data from different time periods using different criteria and definitions to define obesity by means of waist circumference. Other risk factors not considered as criteria for metabolic syndrome but highly suspected to play a role in its development include family history, smoking, increasing age, low socioeconomic status, Mexican American ethnicity, postmenopausal status, physical inactivity, sugary drink and soft drink consumption, excessive alcohol consumption, Western dietary patterns, low cardiorespiratory fitness, excessive television watching, use of antiretroviral drugs in human immunodeficiency virus infection, and atypical antipsychotic drug use (e.g., clozapine) [11].

Most authorities agree that metabolic syndrome usually precedes the development of type 2 diabetes mellitus. But not all patients with diabetes have metabolic syndrome and vice versa [13]. The risk of acute myocardial infarction and stroke can be three times higher in patients who fulfill criteria for metabolic syndrome, irrespective of diabetes status [14, 15]. In patients with diabetes, the more risk factors present the higher the risk of micro- and macrovascular complications [16]. Furthermore, the prevalence of coronary artery disease was higher in patients with both conditions than in those with diabetes alone [17, 18].

An important question arises regarding metabolic syndrome—is there a genetic component? And if so, can it be transmitted from generation to generation? We are starting to understand that metabolic syndrome risk factors have a certain degree of genetic heritability that might be as high as 70% [19–21]. Studies have shown that having one obese parent throughout childhood increases the odds of adult obesity [22]. High-density lipoprotein (HDL) had the highest heritability, followed by dysglycemia and obesity; systolic blood pressure had the lowest heritability but was still present. Similar results were found in the San Antonio Family Heart Study [23] and the Northern Manhattan Family Study [21], both

studies mostly with Hispanic/Latino participants. However, results have shown too many gene associations but very few consistently reproducible findings. The exact genes involved in metabolic syndrome might also be influenced by ethnicity, age, sex, lifestyle, and epigenetic factors that are impossible to control in vivo [24, 25]. As in many hereditary conditions, we might never identify one exact gene responsible for the development of the metabolic syndrome. However, if we are able to determine genetic patterns and interactions common to specific ethnic populations, potential therapeutic agents might be developed or risk assessments could identify people at higher risk of developing the cardiometabolic disease. The Genetics Underlying Diabetes in Hispanics/Latinos (GUARDIAN) Consortium is a large group of researchers focused on determining genetic patterns of diabetes in people with Mexican heritage [26]. Thus far, they have found more than 70 susceptibility loci that might be related to the pathophysiology of diabetes in this Hispanic/Latino subgroup.

A systematic review by Stančáková & Laakso [4] collected the available evidence regarding the genetics of metabolic syndrome. Only four genome-wide association studies (GWAS) were found. In brief, most of the gene variants found to have some association with the development of metabolic syndrome were mostly linked to genes involved in lipid homeostasis (APOA1/C3/A4/A5, LPL, CETP, APOB, APOC1, LIPC, GCKR, ABCB11, TRIB1). They do reiterate that this finding must be analyzed with caution since elevated triglycerides and low HDL cholesterol represent 40% of the criteria needed for metabolic syndrome.

Metabolic Syndrome in US Hispanics/Latinos

The HCHS/SOL, the largest epidemiologic study ever conducted in the United States with the heterogeneous Hispanic/Latino population, provided valuable information regarding the difference in the prevalence of metabolic syndrome by Hispanic/Latino heritage subgroup living in the United States. The study included individuals from Cuba, Dominican Republic, Mexico, Puerto Rico, Central America, and South America and enrolled participants aged 18–74 years from 2008 to 2011. Using the 2009 ATP-III definition, Heiss et al. found that metabolic syndrome was present in 36% and 34% of Hispanic/Latino women and men, respectively, and the prevalence of metabolic syndrome proportionally increased with age [3]. Their group concluded that their analysis of HCHS/SOL data revealed a much higher prevalence of metabolic syndrome in Hispanics/Latinos living in the United States that found in the previously published Assessment of cardiovascular risk in seven Latin American cities (CARMELA) study (27–32% vs. 14–27%) [27]

The CARMELA study assessed the prevalence of cardiovascular disease risks in Hispanics/Latinos living in seven Latin American cities: Barquisimeto, Venezuela; Bogota, Colombia; Buenos Aires, Argentina; Lima, Peru; Mexico City, Mexico; Quito, Ecuador; and Santiago, Chile. Between the years 2003 and 2005, the study enrolled approximately 1600 participants aged 25 to 64 years. An important difference is that the age cutoff in the Heiss et al. analysis was up to 74 years. Higher prevalence of metabolic syndrome and risk factor burden was seen in the 60- to 74-year age groups. Therefore, this could have potentially confounded the higher prevalence of metabolic syndrome found in HCHS/SOL.

In 2009, the prevalence of metabolic syndrome in Caribbean Hispanic/Latino women living in Northern Manhattan was assessed by Yale and colleagues. Participants enrolled in the Northern Manhattan study were predominantly of Dominican and Puerto Rican heritage subgroups [28]. Study participants from Dominican, Cuban, and Puerto Rican heritage subgroups were compared with non-Hispanic/Latino White/Black participants. In brief, a higher prevalence of metabolic syndrome was found in Caribbean Hispanic/Latino women (63.3%) versus non-Hispanic Whites (29.6%). This higher prevalence was associated with a lower education level. Women reporting some high school education or

less had almost double the prevalence of metabolic syndrome than those reporting completion of high school and college graduates.

Unfortunately, trends might suggest that the prevalence of the metabolic syndrome is worsening [1]. A recent study aimed at exploring the prevalence of metabolic syndrome among two Hispanic/Latino heritage subgroups (Central and South Americans) living in Washington DC showed that from 1993 to 2009 the prevalence increased from 19.7% to 28%. Obesity and dyslipidemia were the most abnormal cardiometabolic risk factors in the studied population [29].

Data for three time periods from the National Health and Nutrition Examination Survey (NHANES) (1988–1994, 1999–2006, and 2007–2012) reveal that metabolic syndrome prevalence increased from 25% to 34% in two decades, almost a 35% change [30]. Unlike in the HCHS/SOL data, Mexican Americans are overrepresented in the NHANES data and those in this Hispanic/Latino heritage subgroup are known to have higher rates of cardiometabolic risks and diabetes than their other Hispanic/Latino counterparts (excluding Puerto Ricans) [31]. Similar results were observed by others using different definitions of metabolic syndrome [32–34]. It continues to be of major concern that the prevalence of metabolic syndrome remains a major health issue for the diverse Hispanic/Latino population, independent of the heritage subgroup.

Hypertension

The main goal of screening, diagnosing, and treating hypertension is to decrease the risk of future cardiovascular events. Different guidelines offering a multitude of recommendations exist worldwide [35–38]. We will discuss how hypertension is currently affecting the Hispanic/Latino population in the United States. Further, we will discuss and summarize how Hispanics/Latinos are represented in the most recent major hypertension trials.

Data gathered from NHANES (1999–2002) and NHANES III (1988–1994) revealed that the prevalence of hypertension in African Americans was the highest within the US population (41.4%), despite increased awareness and treatment [39]. From 2011 to 2012, the prevalence of hypertension in non-Hispanic Blacks, non-Hispanic Whites, Hispanics/Latinos, and non-Hispanic Asians was estimated to be 42.1%, 28%, 26%, and 24.7%, respectively [18]. However, data collected 5 years later (2015 to 2016) showed that these numbers shifted unfavorably for Hispanics/Latinos, with the prevalence of hypertension increasing from 26% to 27.8% [40]. Further, in the HCHS/SOL, the age-adjusted prevalence of hypertension in men ranged from 19.9% in South Americas to 32.6% in Dominicans. Among women, South Americans had the lowest prevalence of hypertension (15.9%) and Puerto Ricans has the highest (29.1%) [41]. The prevalence of hypertension in the United States seems to be similar to the prevalence reported in parts of Latin America [42].

The INTERHEART study, a case-control study that included participants from 52 countries, aimed to identify modifiable risk factors associated with acute myocardial infarction [43]. A comparison of the INTERHEART Latin American population with the rest of the world showed that hypertension contributed a 32.9% population-attributable risk for ischemic heart disease to Hispanics/Latinos versus a 22% population-attributable risk in the rest of the world. The Latin American countries included in the study were Argentina, Brazil, Colombia, Chile, Guatemala, and Mexico. Collectively they accounted for almost 9% of the total worldwide sample. A subanalysis by country of population-attributable risk for acute myocardial infarction due to hypertension revealed that Brazil had the highest population-attributable risk followed by Argentina, Chile, and Colombia (43.2%, 33.4%, 32%, and 25.5%, respectively) [44].

The NHANES and more recently the HCHS/SOL have shown a gradual improvement in hypertension awareness, treatment, and control among the US population; however, they have also shown a persistent burden among Hispanics/Latinos when compared with non-Hispanic Whites and non-Hispanic Blacks. This burden is likely related to multiple factors such as less

access to health care, lower-income level, less insurance coverage, language barriers, and possibly genetic factors.

Treatment of hypertension in Hispanics/Latinos has been less studied than in non-Hispanic Blacks and non-Hispanic Whites [1]. The Antihypertensive and Lipid-Lowering Treatment to Prevent Heart Attack Trial (ALLHAT) was a multicenter, double-blind, parallel group, randomized controlled trial aimed at investigating the effect of blood pressure medications in lowering the incidence of cardiovascular events [45]. Enrollment occurred from 1994 to 1998 at 623 centers in North America, including Puerto Rico. The Hispanic/Latino population accounted for 16% of the total population sample (~32,000 participants of which 1090 were Black Hispanic/Latino and 5239 were White Hispanic/Latino). The ALLHAT trial provided access to personalized continuous lifestyle education, therapy titration, and medication at no cost to participants. After 4 years of follow-up, Hispanics/Latinos had the best therapeutic response to intensively monitored therapy despite more than 90% of this subgroup reporting use of hypertension treatment at enrollment and simultaneously being the subgroup with the most uncontrolled blood pressure at baseline. Blood pressure control was achieved in ~70% of Hispanics/Latinos, 67% of non-Hispanic Whites, and 59% of non-Hispanic Blacks. The results of ALLHAT demonstrate that hypertension control in Hispanics/Latinos can be effectively achieved if access to care, education, and medications are appropriately delivered. In this study, chlorthalidone led to similar positive outcomes in Hispanics/Latinos as in non-Hispanic Blacks and non-Hispanic Whites in terms of decreasing cardiovascular events.

The International Verapamil-Trandolapril (INVEST) study included a large Hispanic/Latino population. Researchers reported that Hispanics/Latinos treated with atenolol or verapamil sustained release (SR), alone or in a combination of trandolapril or hydrochlorothiazide achieved better hypertension control with fewer medications when compared to non-Hispanics. They also had lower cardiovascular events. And, when comparing the atenolol versus verapamil SR strategies, the verapamil SR strategies appeared to confer a lower risk of developing new-onset diabetes mellitus in Hispanics/Latinos. Therefore, the researchers postulated that treatment of arterial hypertension in Hispanics/Latinos should probably include the combination of an ACEI with calcium-channel blocker [46]. As in ALLHAT, similar rates of hypertension prevalence and uncontrolled hypertension despite treatment were found upon enrollment.

The Systolic Blood Pressure Intervention Trial (SPRINT) was a randomized controlled trial that showed that lower systolic blood pressure (<120 mm Hg) reduced cardiovascular events in patients without diabetes. A subgroup analysis by Still et al. confirmed these findings by race/ethnicity. In the SPRINT study, approximately 984 of 9185 participants self-identified as Hispanics/Latinos (11%) [47]. In SPRINT, the authors concluded that achieving a blood pressure goal of <120/80 mm Hg was equally beneficial among all ethnic groups. Furthermore, they did not found evidence of Hispanic/Latino paradox—improved cardiovascular mortality despite a high cardiovascular disease risk burden. However, 59% of Hispanics/Latinos enrolled in SPRINT were from Puerto Ricans heritage. Interestingly, baseline blood pressure control (prior to being enrolled in SPRINT) was similar among Hispanics/Latinos and non-Hispanics. However, mainland Hispanics/Latinos had better baseline blood pressure control than Hispanics/Latinos in Puerto Rico, likely because the subgroup from Puerto Rico had higher rates of beta-blocker use compared with the other Hispanic/Latino subgroups [48]. This finding might expose differences in terms of prescription and treatment practices among mainland/island physicians.

Similar to SPRINT, the Action to Control Cardiovascular Risk in Diabetes blood pressure trial (ACCORD-BP) aimed to determine whether a blood pressure goal of 120/80 mm Hg could be beneficial to patients with diabetes. In ACCORD-BP, targeting blood pressure of 120/80 mm Hg did not reduce fatal and nonfatal cardiovascular events. However, it did result in an increased rate of adverse events. Although they included 330 (7% of participants) Hispanics/Latinos, to date no subgroup analysis has been performed evaluating outcomes in this subgroup.

A subgroup analysis of the Northern Manhattan Study contradicted the 2014 Eighth Joint National Committee's recommendations of targeting systolic blood pressure in persons aged >60 years to less than 150 mm Hg. In this study, an analysis looking Hispanics/Latinos without any history of stroke, diabetes mellitus, or chronic kidney disease suggested that doing so increases the risk of stroke among Hispanics/Latinos and non-Hispanic Blacks [51].

Nicolas Guzman [52] published a comprehensive review article aimed at investigating the safety, efficacy, and outcomes of antihypertensive medications in Hispanics/Latinos. He generated a list of the landmark trials and described in detail their outcomes in Hispanics/Latinos. The list included: ACQUIRE, ALLHAT, ASCENT, ATTAIN, EVALUATE, INCLUSIVE, INVEST, TRINITIY, Val-MARC, and 10 other randomized-controlled trials. The enrollment of Hispanics/Latinos in these studies ranged on average from 30 to 200 participants. The highest Hispanic/Latino enrollment rates (>1000 participants) were seen in ALLHAT and INVEST. Given the paucity of data investigating appropriate therapy for hypertension management in Hispanics/Latinos, Guzman theorized that considering the high prevalence of diabetes, metabolic syndrome, obesity, and chronic kidney disease in Hispanics/Latinos, the mainstay treatment should always include a renin-angiotensin-aldosterone system inhibitor, which includes angiotensin-converting enzyme inhibitors and angiotensin II receptor blockers. If the patient has none of these risk factors or has a contraindication for such, then a thiazide diuretic could be considered.

Finally, Hispanics/Latinos have been shown to have a good response to overall pharmacological therapies during clinical trials. However, despite the increasing representation of Hispanics/Latinos in hypertension trials, the description of Hispanic/Latino heritage subgroups is usually not included as part of the study results making it challenging to further determine the impact of heritage subgroup on major outcomes. Therefore, subgroup descriptions of the composition of Hispanics/Latinos within Hispanic/Latino ethnicity should always be considered [53].

Dyslipidemia

There is a high prevalence of dyslipidemia in Hispanics/Latinos in the United States [1]. NHANES 2013 data showed that Hispanics/Latinos had higher levels of low-density lipoprotein (LDL) cholesterol and lower levels of high-density lipoprotein (HDL) cholesterol as compared to non-Hispanic Whites [54]. Using the HCHS/SOL database, Rodriguez et al. found that among Hispanics/Latinos subgroups in the United States the overall prevalence of any dyslipidemia, high LDL, high triglycerides, and low HDL was 65% [55]. Cubans had the highest prevalence of elevated LDL levels, Central Americans had the highest prevalence of elevated triglyceride levels, and Dominicans tended to have the lowest prevalence of any dyslipidemia. Interestingly, low HDL was similarly prevalent among all Hispanic/Latino subgroups.

The mainstay treatment for dyslipidemia is the same as with other ethnic groups: lifestyle modification followed by medical therapy. With regard to medical therapy in Hispanics/Latinos, very few studies have been published investigating the efficacy of any particular therapy. The STudy Assessing RosuvaStatin in HIspanic Population (STARSHIP) enrolled 696 Hispanic/Latino participants meeting ATP-III criteria for dyslipidemia. Participants were assigned to receive atorvastatin or rosuvastatin and the results indicated that both medications were equally effective in achieving lipid parameter goals with a similar incidence of side effects, regardless of treatment assignment [57]. Finally, it is of utmost importance to recognize that the atherosclerotic CVD (ASCVD) risk estimator has not been validated in Hispanic/Latino populations [58]. It might overestimate the risk in Mexican Americans but underestimate it in Puerto Ricans and other Hispanic/Latino heritage subgroups [54]. The current recommendations suggest that utilizing race/ethnicity and country of origin in combination with socioeconomic status and acculturation should be discussed and can potentially explain the ASCVD burden better than using the more generic term Hispanic/Latino while assessing risk in this heterogeneous population [59].

Type 2 Diabetes Mellitus

Diabetes mellitus was the fifth leading cause of death in 2016 for Hispanics/Latinos [60]. Centers for Disease Control and Prevention (CDC) data reveal that Mexicans have the highest prevalence (13.8%), followed by Puerto Ricans (12%), Cubans (9%), and Central/South Americans (8%) [61]. Innumerable studies have shown that Hispanics/Latinos have a higher prevalence of cardiovascular disease risk factors than non-Hispanic/Latinos which includes diabetes which leads to a higher prevalence of cardiovascular disease morbidity [1, 52, 62, 63]. Additionally, recent studies have shown that diabetes, hypertension, and lipid control in this subgroup are suboptimal [64, 65]. Only 8.4% of Hispanics/Latinos in the HCHS/SOL achieved all three recommended targets. Diabetes-related mortality seems to be highest among non-Hispanic Blacks and American Indian/Alaskan natives compared with other racial and ethnic groups. Within the Hispanic/Latino population, Mexican Americans have the highest diabetes-related mortality rate [66].

Daviglus et al. [31] reported a study looking at metabolic syndrome risk factors, they also considered smoking and diabetes prevalence among the Hispanics/Latinos enrolled in HCHS/SOL. They found the following prevalence (%) of diabetes in men and women by Hispanic/Latino subgroup: Mexican (19.3/18.5), Dominican (18.2/18), Puerto Rican (16.2/19.2), Central American (16.3/17.9), Cuban (13.2/13.9), South American (10.1/9.8), and all combined (16.7/17.2). Using the National Health Interview Survey from 2000 to 2005, Pabon-Nau found great variability in the prevalence of diabetes and hypertension among the subgroups of Hispanics/Latinos living in the United States, including among foreign and US-born Hispanic/Latinos. Interestingly, the prevalence of diabetes and hypertension was higher in foreign-born Puerto Ricans when compared to other US-born and foreign-born Hispanics/Latinos, even after adjusting for confounders [67]. Larissa Aviles-Santa et al. [42] published an extensive list of population-based epidemiological studies that have provided data about the incidence, prevalence (Table 11.1), and outcomes of those with

Table 11.1 Prevalence of type 2 diabetes and prediabetes among Hispanic/Latino populations in the United States (selected studies)

Study (reference)	Study period	Sample size	Age range (years)	Glycemic criteria	Key findings
Puerto Rico Heart Health Program [57, 58]	1965–1980	2567 rural and 6190 urban Puerto Rican men	45–64	FPG ≥ 126 mg/dL, self-reports of physician-diagnosed diabetes, or use of inulin or hypoglycemic agents	3.6% in rural men and 9% in urban men
Laredo Project [59]	1979	389 Mexican Americans	40–74	Fasting hyperglycemia defined as FPG > 140 mg/dL	Age-adjusted prevalence was 10.9% in men and 10.1% in women
Starr County Study, Texas [68]	1981	2498 Mexican Americans	≥15	Zero-hour (fasting) plasma glucose level ≥140 mg/dL or a 2-h level ≥200 mg/dL.	6.9% males and 6.7% females
Albuquerque New Mexico [69]	1964–1986	1175 Hispanics	≥18	Self-reported diagnosis	Prevalence increased with age: Men: 1.9% in 25–34 to 13.8% in ≥75. Women: 0.6% in 25–34 to 16.1% in ≥75
San Luis Valley Diabetes Study, Colorado [64, 70]	1984	607 Hispanics without prior history of DM 343 Hispanics with previously diagnosed DM	20–74	History of previously diagnosed CM with confirmation using FPG ≥ 140 mg/dL or 2-h OGTT ≥200 mg/dL	Age-adjusted prevalence of previously diagnosed DM: 3.3% in men and 4.9% in women Newly diagnosed DM: 2.2% in men and 4.3% in women
San Antonio Heart Study, Texas [60, 61, 71]	First phase: 1979–1982 Second phase: 1984–1988	3302 Mexican Americans	25–64	2-h OGTT	Age-adjusted prevalence for men was 14.0% in the barrio vs. 6.5% in the suburbs and for men was 18.0% in the barrio vs. 4.3% in the suburbs Prevalence was two to three times higher in Mexican Americans than in NHWs
Puerto Rico Household Health Interview Survey [72]	1975–1986	Minimum sample size of 2696 in 1983 Maximum sample size of 12,212 in 1976	All ages	Self-reported diagnosis	3.1% in 1975 to 5.1% in 1986 4.5% of males and 58% of females reported a history of DM

Table 11.1 (continued)

Study (reference)	Study period	Sample size	Age range (years)	Glycemic criteria	Key findings
HHANES [11]	1982–1984	6588 Hispanics	20–74 years	OGTT administered to subsample of 1326	Cubans 45–74: 15.8% Mexican Americans 45–74: 23.9% Puerto Ricans 45–74: 26.1% Cubans 20–44: 2.4% Mexican Americans 20–44:3.8% Puerto Ricans 20–44:4.1%
Mexico City Diabetes Study [73]	1979–1982	2282 individuals of Mexican descent in San Antonio and Mexicans in Mexico City	35–64	FPG ≥ 126 mg/dL	San Antonio: 178% in men and 23% in women Mexico City: 12.3% in men and 18.5% in women
NHANES [74]	1999–2000	915 Mexican Americans, NHBs, and NHWs	12–19	IFG: 100–125 mg/dL	Prevalence of IFG was 13.0, 4.2, and 7% in Mexican Americans, NHBs, and NHWs, respectively
NHANES [49]	1999–2002	1802 adolescents without DM (672 Mexican American)	12–19	HOMA-IR	Mexican American children had higher HOMA-IR levels than white children
NHANES [75]	1988–1994 1999–2002	1988–1994: 31,638 Mexican American, NHW and NHB adults 1999–2002: 17,217 Mexican American, NHW and NHB adults	≥20	Previously diagnosed DM undiagnosed DM: FPG ≥ 126 mg/dL IFG: 100–125 mg/dL	Among Mexican Americans: Previously diagnosed DM: 9.6 and 10.6% Undiagnosed DM: 4.7 and 3.5% FG: 32.9 and 33.0%
MESA [76]	2000–2002	1437 Hispanics	45–84	FPG ≥ 126 mg/dL or use of hypoglycemic medication	Age-adjusted prevalence of diabetes Mexican Americans: 22.3% Dominicans: 16.1% Puerto Ricans: 19.7% Other Hispanics: 15.2%
NHANES [77]	2005–2006	2806 Mexican American, NHW and NBH adults	≥20	FPG, OGTT	Mexican Americans Diagnosed DM: 12.6% Undiagnosed DM: 7.5% Total DM: 20.1% Percent undiagnosed DM 35.9% Prediabetes: 32.0% Prediabetes/CM: 52.0%
NHANES [78]	2005–2006	277 Mexican Americans 257 NHBs 198 NHWS	12–19	FPG and 2-h OGTT ADA 1998	Prevalence of IFG, FT, and prediabetes among Mexican Americans were 14.3, 3.5, and 16.9%, respectively

(continued)

Table 11.1 (continued)

Study (reference)	Study period	Sample size	Age range (years)	Glycemic criteria	Key findings
Study of Women's Health Across the Nation (SWAN) [79]	1996–1997	3302 women in seven sites; analysis based on 420 women recruited in the New Jersey site	42–52	FPG ≥ 126 mg/dL or self-reported use of insulin	33% in Caucasians, 5.9% in Dominicans, 8.3% in Central Americans, 9.8% in Cubans, 13.5% in Puerto Ricans, 15.6% in South Americans
Phase I of the US–Mexico Border Diabetes Prevention and Control Project [80]	2001–2002	4027: 2120 Hispanics from Mexico, 1437 Hispanics from the United States, and 470 non-Hispanics from the United States	≥18	Self-reported diagnosis FPG ≥ 126 mg/dL	Age-adjusted prevalence of self-reported and unrecognized DM was 16.6% of the Mexican side and 14.7% on the US side; age-adjusted prevalence of IFG was similar on both sides of the border (14.1% on the Mexican side and 13.6% on the US side)
BRFSS [81]	1995–2010	1995: 1193 in Montana to 5107 in Maryland 2010: 1964 in Alaska to 35,109 in Florida	≥18	Self-reported diagnosis	In 1995, age-adjusted prevalence was >6% in only three states, Washington, DC, and Puerto Rice In 2010, age-adjusted prevalence was highest (>10%) in Alabama, Mississippi, Puerto Rice, South Carolina, Tennessee, Texas, and West Virginia
NHANES [82]	1999–2008	22,621 Mexican American, NHW and NHB adults, of whom 551 had undiagnosed DM	≥20	Undiagnosed DM was defined as HbA1c ≥ 6.5% without a serf-report of physician-diagnosed DM	Overall prevalence of undiagnosed DM of 1.5% in NHWs, 3.1% in NHBs, and 2.7% in Mexican Americans Overall prevalence of diagnosed DM of 6.7% in NHWs, 11.3% in NHBs, and 7.6% in Mexican Americans
California Health Interview Survey [83]	2001, 2003, 2005, and 2007	33,633 Hispanics and 126,488 NHWs	≥18	Self-report of physician-diagnosed DM	Mexicans: 9% Central Americans: 1% South Americans: 0.5% 2 or more countries of origin: 7% Other Hispanics: 13% NHWs 7%
NHANES [84]	1999–2002 2003–2006 2007–2010	19,182 Mexican American. NHW and NHB adults	≥12	HbA1c: 5.7–6.4% FPG: 100–125 mg/dL	Prevalence of prediabetes among Mexican Americans 34.4, 30.3, and 37.8%

Table 11.1 (continued)

Study (reference)	Study period	Sample size	Age range (years)	Glycemic criteria	Key findings
HCHS/SOL [12, 85]	2008–2011	16,415 Hispanics	18–74	FPG, 2-h OGTT, HbA1c	Overall prevalence of DM was 16.9% South Americans: 10.2% Cubans: 13.4% Central Americans: 17.7% Dominicans 18.1% Puerto Ricans: 18.1% Mexicans/'Mexican Americans: 18.3%
SEARCH study [86, 87]	2001–2009	3,345,783 youths in 2001 and 3,458,974 in 2009	<20	Physician-diagnosed DM	Prevalence of type 2 DM among Hispanic youth aged 10–19 years was 0.45 per 1000 in 2001 and 0.79 per 1000 in 2009, representing a relative increase of 76% over the 8- year period
NHANES [88]	1988–1994 1999–2004 2005–2010	1988–1994: 4201 1999–2004: 2860 2005–2010: 2766 Mexican Americans	≥20	Based on HbA1c	Diagnosed DM: 7.6 (0.57), 8.8 (1.06), 11.9 (1.01) Undiagnosed DM: 1.8 (0.17), 2.3 (0.40), 2.9 (0.32) Prediabetes: 5.6 (0.64), 10.6 (0.68), 12.7 (0.76)
NHANES [8]	1968–2012	2011–2012: 2623 (561 all Hispanics)	≥20	Self-reported diagnosis undiagnosed DM based on FPG, 2-h OGTT, HbA1c	All Hispanics Total DM: 22.6% Diagnosed DM: 12,5% Undiagnosed DM: 10.1% Prediabetes: 36.8% Mexican Americans Total DM: 23.8% Diagnosed DM: 14.4% Undiagnosed DM: 9.4% Prediabetes: 38.0%
NHS [89]	1997–2012	427,975 (367,292 non-Hispanics and 60,683 Hispanics)	≥18	Self-reported diagnosis	Less than high school education: 17.6% for Puerto Ricans, 134% for Cubans, and 9.7% for Mexicans High school diploma/GED: 9.8% for Puerto Ricans, 8.2% for Cubans, and 6.3% for Mexicans More than high school education: 6.8% for Puerto Ricans, 6.0% for Cubans, and 6.7% for Mexicans
HCHS/SOL [13]	2008–2011	15,507 Hispanics	18–74	FPG, 2-h OGTT, HbA1c	6.7% met at least one diagnostic criterion of probable DM – 39.4% of total DM (self-reported plus probable DM)

(continued)

Table 11.1 (continued)

Study (reference)	Study period	Sample size	Age range (years)	Glycemic criteria	Key findings
HCHS/SOC [90]	2012–2014	1466 Hispanics	8–16	FPG and HbA1c ADA 2015	Prevalence of prediabetes/DM was 16.5%, being higher in boys (20.9%) than in girls (11.8%)
Starr County, Texas [50]	2002–2014	5230 Mexican American adults	≥20	FPG, OGTT, HbA1c	Previously identified DM: 11.8% in men and 14.4% in women Newly identified DM: 11.9% in men and 12.3% in women Total DM: 23.7% in men and 26.7% in women prediabetes: 32.8% in men and 31.9% in women
NHANES [89]	2005–2014	2606 NHWs, NHBs, and Hispanics	12–19	FPG, 2-h OGTT, HbA1c	Prevalence of total DM, prediabetes, and percent undiagnosed DM: All Hispanics: 0.76, 22.9, and 39.5% Mexican Americans: 0.85, 22.4, and 43.9%
HCHS/SCL [91]	2008-2011	15,507 Hispanics	18–74	FPG, 2-h OGTT, HbA1c	Prediabetes: 36.3% Total IFG: 18.1% Total IGT: 15.4% Total impaired HbA1c: 21.2% IFG + impaired HbA1c: 8.6% IFG + IGT + impaired HbA1c: 3.8%

From Avilés-Santa et al. [42]

diabetes and other cardiovascular disease risk factors in the heterogeneous group of Hispanics/Latinos living in the United States.

The ACCORD trial showed that intensive control of diabetes to a target hemoglobin A1c (HbA1c) of <6% was associated with increased overall mortality compared with standard of care targeting an HbA1c of 7.0–7.9%; however, progression of microvascular events and occurrence of nonfatal acute myocardial infarction decreased among those with an HbA1c <6% [92]. Hispanics/Latinos in this trial composed about 7% of the participants: 243 Mexicans, 199 Puerto Ricans, and 150 Dominicans. Subgroup analysis revealed that Mexicans were most likely than other Hispanic/Latino subgroups to achieve the target HbA1c in the intensive arm. Puerto Ricans and Dominicans were the least likely of the Hispanic/Latino subgroups to do so [93]. This reinforces the idea that Hispanics/Latinos represent a very heterogeneous group.

Like ACCORD, the Veterans Affairs Diabetes Trial (VADT) did not find any benefits of intensive glycemic control in terms of mortality, macrovascular, or microvascular endpoints in type 2 diabetes mellitus [94]. However, a subgroup analysis of Hispanics/Latinos in the VADT found that this population did benefit from intensive glycemic therapy [95]. Although the Hispanic/Latino participants in the VADT were less heterogeneous than those in ACCORD, the findings from the VADT subgroup analysis lend support to the idea that further studies are needed to assess whether Hispanics/Latinos from different heritage groups will benefit the same from such control.

Obesity

Obesity is likely one of the most rapidly increasing modifiable cardiovascular disease risk factors worldwide, irrespective of race and ethnicity. It is closely linked to the development of metabolic syndrome, usually (but not always) preceding the onset of such. Since Hispanics/Latinos have some of the highest incidence and prevalence of metabolic syndrome in the United States, it is also expected that Hispanics/Latinos have a greater incidence and prevalence of obesity [1, 34]. NHANES data from 2015 to 2017 published by the CDC's Division of Nutrition, Physical Activity, and Obesity revealed that obesity prevalence among racial/ethnic US populations was higher in non-Hispanic Blacks (38.4%), followed by Hispanics/Latinos (32.6%), and non-Hispanic Whites (28.6%). Differences in these outcomes are likely driven by socioeconomic disparities [68–70]. Despite ongoing initiatives intended to curb this growing epidemic [1, 42], the prevalence keeps increasing among Hispanics/Latinos in the United States as evidenced by Fig. 11.2. A similar trend was noticed by Bermudez & Tucker [71], showing that the prevalence of overweight/obesity among Mexican Americans interviewed during NHANES (1982 to 1984) and NHANES III (1988 to 1994) rose from around 60% to 68% in both men and women aged 20 to 74 years. More worrisome is the fact that childhood obesity trends are also showing racial disparities with higher rates in Hispanics/Latinos as shown in Fig. 11.3 [68].

Obesity is classically measured as a function of body mass index (BMI) as an alternative way to estimate body fat levels. The World Health Organization (WHO) provided a framework in which obesity could be classified as: (1) overweight (BMI 25–29.9 kg/m²) and (2) obesity (BMI >30 kg/m²). However, it is increasingly recognized that BMI must also be correlated with other measurements such as waist circumference and waist-to-hip ratio [1, 9, 11, 12, 32]. The reason for this is that BMI cannot distinguish between weight from muscle tissues or adipose tissues. For instance, muscular body builders can be mistakenly classified as obese when they are not. Alternatively, BMI can also underestimate fat and cardiovascular disease risks in people with a normal weight for their height but with a higher body fat (visceral) composition [74]. The latter concept was illustrated in the Massachusetts Hispanic Elders Study (MAHES) conducted among Hispanics/Latinos and non-Hispanic Whites aged 60 to 92 years in Massachusetts. Anthropometric measurements and medical history were obtained in a total of 457 Puerto Ricans, 139 Dominicans, and 239 non-Hispanic Whites (other Hispanics/Latinos were excluded in order to avoid aggregation bias due to their low sample size) [48–50, 71]. The objective was to identify a correlation between BMI, waist circumference, and type 2 diabetes mellitus. In brief, the prevalence of type 2 diabetes was overall higher in all participants with higher BMI and waist circumference. However, unlike non-Hispanic Whites, Hispanics/Latinos had a higher prevalence of type 2 diabetes even among participants with a normal BMI. Results from HCHS/SOL revealed an overall obesity prevalence of 36.5% for men and 42.6% for women. Puerto Ricans had the highest prevalence, followed by Dominicans, Mexicans, and Cubans [31, 41]. Central and South American participants had the lowest obesity prevalence.

As with other cardiovascular disease risk factors, research has found that several nutritional, metabolic, genetic, social, and environmental factors seem to play a role in the development of obesity. The major contributors, undeniably, are excess caloric intake and sedentarism. Even so, a lot of attention is being paid to proinflammatory adipokines (tumor necrosis factor-alpha, interleukin-1, interleukin-6, resistin, leptin, monocyte chemoattractant protein-1, angiotensin II, fibrinogen, plasminogen activator inhibitor-1, and adiponectin). Of these factors, adiponectin seems to be the only one that confers a protective anti-inflammatory role. Certain polymorphisms that promote the formation of dysfunctional adiponectin, which has been found to lead to metabolic syndrome, type 2 diabetes, and obesity, have been found to be more common in certain Hispanic/Latino populations [75–78].

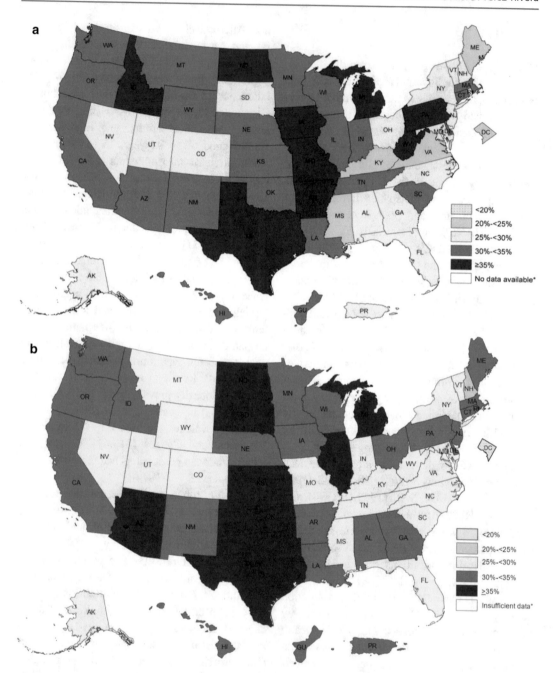

Fig. 11.2 Prevalence of self-reported obesity among Hispanic adults by states and territory, BRFSS, (**a**) 2012–2014 and (**b**) 2015–2017, respectively [72, 73]. (Source: Center for Disease Control and Prevention. USA)

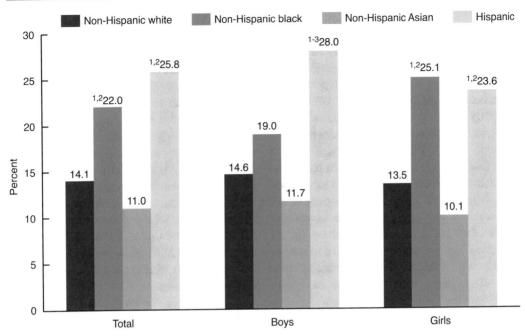

[1]Significantly different from non-Hispanic Asian persons.
[2]Significantly different from non-Hispanic white persons.
[3]Significantly different from non-Hispanic black persons.
NOTE: Access data table for figure 4 at: https://www.cdc.gov/nchs/data/databriefs/db288_table.pdf#4.
SOURCE: NCHS, National Health and Nutrition Examination Survey, 2015-2016

Fig. 11.3 Prevalence of obesity among youth aged 2-19 years, by sex and race and Hispanic origin, United States, 2015-2016. (Source: Center for Disease Control and Prevention. USA)

The causes of these obesity trends are likely related to an interplay between genetic/metabolic traits, environmental, and acculturation issues [79].

The Hispanic/Latino Paradox

For decades, epidemiologic studies have shown that health disparities among ethnic minorities lead to overall poorer outcomes. However, in 1986 Markides & Coreil provided evidence of a strange phenomenon among the Hispanic/Latino population that would be coined "The Hispanic/Latino Paradox." [1, 80] This paradox, although initially representative of Mexican Americans, suggested that despite having similar socioeconomic disadvantages as African Americans, the health outcomes of Hispanics/Latinos were closer to non-Hispanic Whites. Key indicators found in their study that supported these findings were related to infant mortality, life expectancy, mortal-

ity from cardiovascular disease, psychiatric issues, cancer, and general measures of functional health. These findings were in part supported by subsequent studies in the late 1990s and 2000s [81, 82, 85]. In general, it is thought that these outcomes are the result of healthier behaviors, better family and cultural support, less prevalence of smoking, and possible genetic factors, among others. Three recent systematic reviews and meta-analyses validated the existence of the Hispanic/Latino Paradox [83, 84, 86].

Hispanics/Latinos are the fastest growing minority group in the United States. From 2000 to 2010 the Hispanic/Latino population grew by 43%. Prior to the year 2000, most migrants came from Mexico. However, due to political turmoil, food insecurity, economic instability, and other reasons, the migratory landscape has greatly shifted from predominantly Mexican to a mixture of Mexican, Central American, South American, and Caribbean migrations.

The Final Deaths Data for 2016 published by the National Vital Statistics Reports [60] revealed that age-adjusted death rates for Hispanics/Latinos were lower than non-Hispanic Blacks and non-Hispanic Whites. It also reported that life expectancy for both males and females was higher by 3 years or more for Hispanics/Latinos as compared with non-Hispanic Blacks and non-Hispanic Whites [60]. Interestingly, since life expectancy data for Hispanics/Latinos have been available since 2006, the trend in life expectancy used to be increasing on a year-by-year basis. However, for the past 2 years life expectancy trends for Hispanics/Latinos have slightly decreased. This pattern has been also observed in non-Hispanic Blacks and non-Hispanic Whites. Life expectancy (years) for Hispanic/Latino females/males, non-Hispanic Black females/males, and non-Hispanic White females/males was 84.2/79.1, 77.9/71.5, and 81.0/76.1, respectively.

Opponents of this paradox were quick to analyze trends and establish several hypotheses for these outcomes [87]. Some simply stated that Hispanics/Latinos have lower prevalence of smoking than other ethnicities, resulting in a powerfully positive risk factor in their favor. The "Salmon Bias" establishes that many of the Hispanics/Latinos that once moved into the United States end up returning, and henceforth dying, in their country of origin. This migratory pattern would ultimately create an "immortal" statistic in the sense that the person will count as a migrant when he/she arrives in the United States, but there will be no record of them leaving. Hence, that migrant became permanently recorded as alive no matter of his/her actual outcome after returning to the country of origin. Some people challenging this theory state that Cubans are not allowed to return to their homeland due to political issues. Furthermore, Puerto Ricans who return to the island (commonwealth) are still considered in the US national statistics [88]. The "Healthy Migrant effect" states that most people who migrate from their country of origin tend to be healthier and have better socioeconomic support than those who do not migrate [81]. "Data Artifacts" could likely be the largest

contributor to the Hispanic/Latino Paradox, as explained by Palloni [89]. One example could be related to ethnic identification which is usually self-reported and occasionally found to be mislabeled on death certificates. Age identification has also been found to be mislabeled since some immigrants tended to overstate their age. This misreporting leads to lower mortality rates in falsely self-reported older age groups. Additionally, in some studies containing US-born Hispanics/Latinos, this population could classify themselves as non-Hispanic Whites rather than Hispanic/Latino Whites due to their belief that being born in the United States might eliminate their Hispanic/Latino ethnicity. Finally, undocumented migrants tend to use health services less than their counterparts. As a result, this population may be accounted for in census statistics but might not be well represented in health statistics [84, 90].

Does migrating from country of origin or being born in the United States confer any sort of cardiovascular advantage? Rodriguez et al. found that cardiovascular mortality rates were higher in foreign-born Hispanics/Latinos than in US-born Hispanics/Latinos [48–50].

Inojosa et al. provided further evidence about the existence of the Hispanic/Latino paradox and tabulated the most influential studies (Table 11.2) [88]. Whether this paradox is real or not, cardiovascular disease is still one of the top three leading causes of mortality and morbidity among Hispanics/Latinos in the United States and worldwide.

The Puerto Rican Disadvantage

Puerto Rican colonization by Spain ranged from 1493 until 1898 when the United States gained control of the island during the Spanish-American War. Since then, Puerto Ricans were granted US citizenship through the Jones Act of 1917, which granted the right to a US nationality, passport, and several federal benefits. Although Puerto Ricans have their own culture, traditions, geographic location, and speak Spanish as their main language, they also share many of the con-

Table 11.2 Influential studies on the Hispanic paradox

Study	Outcomes	Population	Results compared no NHW	Advantages	Limitations	Opinion
Corpus Christi [51]	CHD mortality	Mexican Americans Non-Hispanic Whites	Greater CHD mortality in Mexican Americans	Coded death certificates Coronary mortality blinded to ethnicity	Community base study	Against the paradox
San Antonio Study [48]	All-cause mortality	Diabetic Mexicans	Greater overall all-cause mortality for Mexican American non statistical significance	Ethnic classification algorithm reduces bias	Limits to diabetic patients	Against the paradox
	CVD mortality	Diabetic Mexican Americans	Greater cardiovascular mortality for Mexican American non statistical significance	Includes native and US born Mexicans		
		Diabetic non-Hispanic Whites	Similar risk on Mexicans			
Northern Manhattan study [8]	Nonfatal MI	Self-identified Hispanics	Increased prevalence of risk factors among Hispanics	Systematic follow-up	Insufficient demographic data	Supports the paradox on coronary mortality
	CHD mortality CVD mortality		Lower CHD mortality lower CVD mortality	Decreased risk of Salmon bias Multiple outcome analysis	Small quantity of nonfatal MI Hispanic health barriers remain present	Supports the paradox on cardiovascular mortality against the paradox on nonfatal MI
			No difference in nonfatal MI	Risk analysis that favored the paradox	Questionable external validity	
Frerichs, R [54]	All-cause mortality	Hispanics	Lower all-cause mortality	Includes multiple minority populations	Data gathered from U.S. Census	Supports the paradox
	CVD mortality	Non-Hispanic Whites AA Asians	Lower CVD mortality			
Friss, R [4]	All-cause mortality	Hispanics	Increased all-cause mortality	Coded death certificates	Data gathered from U.S. Census	Supports the paradox on cardiovascular mortality
	CVD mortality	Non-Hispanic Whites	Lower CVD mortality			

(continued)

Table 11.2 (continued)

Study	Outcomes	Population	Results compared no NHW	Advantages	Limitations	Opinion
Iribarren, C [5]	All-cause mortality CVD mortality	Hispanic Non-Hispanic Whites	Lower all-cause mortality Lower CVD mortality	Prospective cohort study	Community base study	Supports the paradox
Palaniappan, L [46]	All-cause mortality	Hispanics	Lower all-cause mortality	Includes multiple minority populations	Data gathered from U.S. Census	Supports the paradox
	CHD mortality	Non-Hispanic Whites AA Asians	Lower CHD mortality			
Sorlie, P [47]	All-cause mortality	Hispanic	Lower all-cause mortality	Includes multiple minority populations	Data gathered from U.S. Census	Supports the paradox
	CHD mortality	Non-Hispanic Whites	Lower CHD mortality			
Stern, M [55]	All-cause mortality	Mexican Americans	Lower all-cause mortality		Hispanic status established by surnames	Supports the paradox
	CHD mortality MI mortality	Non-Hispanic whites	Lower CHD mortality Lower MI mortality			
Wild, S [57]	CHD mortality Stroke mortality	Hispanic Non-Hispanic Whites AA Asians	Lower CHD mortality Lower stroke mortality	Coded death certificates	Data gathered from U S. Census and death certificates	Supports the paradox

Reproduced with permission from Medina-Inojosa et al. [88]

tinental US customs and lifestyles. Therefore, we should hypothesize that health outcomes should be comparable with either non-Hispanics/Latinos or Hispanics/Latinos in general. We can even speculate that access to care should not be a major issue in this Hispanic/Latino subgroup.

In 2015, the CDC published statistics from 2009 to 2013 showing that Puerto Ricans living in the continental United States had the overall worst health outcomes among Hispanics/Latinos and non-Hispanics/Latinos. They had moderate-to-higher rates of cancer, cardiovascular disease, diabetes, smoking, homicides, unintentional injuries, unemployment, living under the poverty line, cerebrovascular accidents, Alzheimer's disease, nephritic/nephrotic syndromes, septicemia, perinatal conditions, and high blood pressure [96]. Comparisons with Puerto Ricans living on the island were not done nor were there any comparisons between island-born and US-born Puerto Ricans. As evidenced by the data contained in this chapter, Puerto Ricans tend to have a higher overall prevalence of negative risk factors and outcomes.

A recent study investigating the quality of care provided to non-Hispanic Whites and Hispanics/Latinos enrolled in Medicare Advantage included Hispanics/Latinos living in the continental United States and Puerto Rico. They found that Hispanics/Latinos living in Puerto Rico had far worse care than non-Hispanic Whites and Hispanics/Latinos living in the continental

United States. Unadjusted data from Hispanics/Latinos in Puerto Rico showed significantly worse performance for 15 out of 17 Healthcare Effectiveness Data and Information Set (HEDIS) measures. When adjusting these data for age-sex and age-sex-poverty, Hispanics/Latinos living in Puerto Rico had significantly worse care for 12 and 10 measures, respectively [97].

Why are island and continental Puerto Ricans having worst cardiovascular outcomes than their Hispanic/Latino and non-Hispanic US counterparts? The response is likely multifactorial. We could speculate that the political status of Puerto Rico (i.e., US territory/commonwealth with partial US benefits) confers certain advantages and disadvantages, which will not be addressed in this book. From a public health perspective, several small studies have tried to investigate such reasons but no specific pattern can primarily explain these differences [91, 98, 99]. A recent systematic review identified plausible sociocultural factors that might play a role in diabetes mellitus outcomes among Puerto Ricans living in mainland United States: fatalistic views (when complications are unavoidable despite appropriate care); different treatment goals between clinicians and patients; negative attitudes towards insulin; lack of Puerto Rican specific dietary interventions and programs; a preference for Spanish-speaking clinicians despite fluency in English; higher rates of depression; among others [100]. However, all of these factors are important for and also affect all other Hispanic/Latino background groups with regard to cardiovascular health. A significant difference between Puerto Ricans and other Hispanic/Latino groups is their higher degree of acculturation with US culture given their inclusion history versus other groups [55, 56]. This deserves further exploration.

Finally, to what extent migration between Latin American countries and the United States impact on cardiovascular health by Hispanic/Latino subgroups in the United States remains understudied. However, what is evident is that each Hispanic/Latino subgroup is clearly unique and should be disaggregated from one another when analyzing trends between ethnic/racial groups [48–50, 100]. In summary, there is no one-size-fits-all for Hispanics/Latinos.

References

1. Keith C, Ferdinand AA. Cardiovascular disease in racial and ethnic minorities. 1st ed. Humana Press; 2010. 331 p
2. Hossain P, Kawar B, El Nahas M. Obesity and diabetes in the developing world–a growing challenge. N Engl J Med. 2007;356(3):213–5.
3. Heiss G, Snyder ML, Teng Y, Schneiderman N, Llabre MM, Cowie C, et al. Prevalence of metabolic syndrome among Hispanics/Latinos of diverse background: the Hispanic Community Health Study/Study of Latinos. Diabetes Care. 2014;37(8):2391–9.
4. Stančáková A, Laakso M. Genetics of metabolic syndrome. Rev Endocr Metab Disord. 2014;15(4):243–52.
5. Reaven GM. Banting Lecture 1988. Role of insulin resistance in human disease. 1988. Nutrition (Burbank, Los Angeles County, Calif). 1997;13(1):65; discussion 4, 6.
6. Eckel RH, Grundy SM, Zimmet PZ. The metabolic syndrome. Lancet. 2005;365(9468):1415–28.
7. Alberti KG, Zimmet PZ. Definition, diagnosis and classification of diabetes mellitus and its complications. Part 1: diagnosis and classification of diabetes mellitus provisional report of a WHO consultation. Diabet Med. 1998;15(7):539–53.
8. Grundy SM, Cleeman JI, Daniels SR, Donato KA, Eckel RH, Franklin BA, et al. Diagnosis and management of the metabolic syndrome: an American Heart Association/National Heart, Lung, and Blood Institute Scientific Statement. Circulation. 2005;112(17):2735–52.
9. Alberti KG, Zimmet P, Shaw J. The metabolic syndrome–a new worldwide definition. Lancet (London, England). 2005;366(9491):1059–62.
10. Meigs JB. Metabolic syndrome and risk for Type 2 diabetes. Expert Rev Endocrinol Metab. 2006;1(1):57–66.
11. McCracken E, Monaghan M, Sreenivasan S. Pathophysiology of the metabolic syndrome. Clin Dermatol. 2018;36(1):14–20.
12. Alberti KG, Eckel RH, Grundy SM, Zimmet PZ, Cleeman JI, Donato KA, et al. Harmonizing the metabolic syndrome: a joint interim statement of the International Diabetes Federation Task Force on Epidemiology and Prevention; National Heart, Lung, and Blood Institute; American Heart Association; World Heart Federation; International Atherosclerosis Society; and International Association for the Study of Obesity. Circulation. 2009;120(16):1640–5.
13. Wilson PW, D'Agostino RB, Parise H, Sullivan L, Meigs JB. Metabolic syndrome as a precursor of

cardiovascular disease and type 2 diabetes mellitus. Circulation. 2005;112(20):3066–72.

14. Cannon CP. Mixed dyslipidemia, metabolic syndrome, diabetes mellitus, and cardiovascular disease: clinical implications. Am J Cardiol. 2008;102(12, Supplement):5L–9L.

15. Lakka HM, Laaksonen DE, Lakka TA, Niskanen LK, Kumpusalo E, Tuomilehto J, et al. The metabolic syndrome and total and cardiovascular disease mortality in middle-aged men. JAMA. 2002;288(21):2709–16.

16. Costa LA, Canani LH, Lisboa HR, Tres GS, Gross JL. Aggregation of features of the metabolic syndrome is associated with increased prevalence of chronic complications in Type 2 diabetes. Diabet Med. 2004;21(3):252–5.

17. Alexander CM, Landsman PB, Teutsch SM, Haffner SM. NCEP-defined metabolic syndrome, diabetes, and prevalence of coronary heart disease among NHANES III participants age 50 years and older. Diabetes. 2003;52(5):1210–4.

18. Nwankwo T, Yoon SS, Burt V, Gu Q. Hypertension among adults in the United States: National Health and Nutrition Examination Survey, 2011–2012. NCHS Data Brief. 2013;133:1–8.

19. Maes HH, Neale MC, Eaves LJ. Genetic and environmental factors in relative body weight and human adiposity. Behav Genet. 1997;27(4):325–51.

20. Rankinen T, Zuberi A, Chagnon YC, Weisnagel SJ, Argyropoulos G, Walts B, et al. The human obesity gene map: the 2005 update. Obesity (Silver Spring, MD). 2006;14(4):529–644.

21. Lin HF, Boden-Albala B, Juo SH, Park N, Rundek T, Sacco RL. Heritabilities of the metabolic syndrome and its components in the Northern Manhattan Family Study. Diabetologia. 2005;48(10):2006–12.

22. Whitaker RC, Wright JA, Pepe MS, Seidel KD, Dietz WH. Predicting obesity in young adulthood from childhood and parental obesity. N Engl J Med. 1997;337(13):869–73.

23. Mitchell BD, Kammerer CM, Blangero J, Mahaney MC, Rainwater DL, Dyke B, et al. Genetic and environmental contributions to cardiovascular risk factors in Mexican Americans. The San Antonio Family Heart Study. Circulation. 1996;94(9):2159–70.

24. Aguilera CM, Olza J, Gil Á. Genetic susceptibility to obesity and metabolic syndrome in childhood (Susceptibilidad genética de obesidad y síndrome metabólico en la infancia). Nutr Hosp. 2013;28:44–55.

25. Friend A, Craig L, Turner S. The prevalence of metabolic syndrome in children: a systematic review of the literature. Metab Syndr Relat Disord. 2013;11(2):71–80.

26. Palmer ND, Goodarzi MO, Langefeld CD, Wang N, Guo X, Taylor KD, et al. Genetic variants associated with quantitative glucose homeostasis traits translate to type 2 diabetes in Mexican Americans: the GUARDIAN (genetics underlying diabetes in Hispanics) consortium. Diabetes. 2015;64(5):1853–66.

27. Schargrodsky H, Hernandez-Hernandez R, Champagne BM, Silva H, Vinueza R, Silva Aycaguer LC, et al. CARMELA: assessment of cardiovascular risk in seven Latin American cities. Am J Med. 2008;121(1):58–65.

28. Yala SM, Fleck EM, Sciacca R, Castro D, Joseph Z, Giardina EG. Metabolic syndrome and the burden of cardiovascular disease in Caribbean Hispanic women living in northern Manhattan: a red flag for education. Metab Syndr Relat Disord. 2009;7(4):315–22.

29. Gill R, Jackson RT, Duane M, Miner A, Khan SA. Comparison of metabolic syndrome indicators in two samples of Central and South Americans living in the Washington, D.C. area in 1993–1994 and 2008–2009: secular changes in metabolic syndrome in hispanics. Int J Environ Res Public Health. 2017;14(8):PMC5580585.

30. Moore JX, Chaudhary N, Akinyemiju T. Metabolic syndrome prevalence by race/ethnicity and sex in the United States, National Health and nutrition examination survey, 1988–2012. Prev Chronic Dis. 2017;14:E24.

31. Daviglus ML, Talavera GA, Aviles-Santa ML, Allison M, Cai J, Criqui MH, et al. Prevalence of major cardiovascular risk factors and cardiovascular diseases among Hispanic/Latino individuals of diverse backgrounds in the United States. JAMA. 2012;308(17):1775–84.

32. Ford ES. Prevalence of the metabolic syndrome defined by the International Diabetes Federation among adults in the U.S. Diabetes Care. 2005;28(11):2745–9.

33. Ford ES, Giles WH, Dietz WH. Prevalence of the metabolic syndrome among US adults: findings from the third National Health and Nutrition Examination Survey. JAMA. 2002;287(3):356–9.

34. Beltran-Sanchez H, Harhay MO, Harhay MM, McElligott S. Prevalence and trends of metabolic syndrome in the adult U.S. population, 1999–2010. J Am Coll Cardiol. 2013;62(8):697–703.

35. Whelton PK, Carey RM, Aronow WS, Casey DE, Jr., Collins KJ, Dennison Himmelfarb C, et al. 2017 ACC/AHA/AAPA/ABC/ACPM/AGS/APhA/ASH/ASPC/NMA/PCNA Guideline for the Prevention, Detection, Evaluation, and Management of High Blood Pressure in Adults: A Report of the American College of Cardiology/American Heart Association Task Force on Clinical Practice Guidelines. Hypertension (Dallas, Tex: 1979). 2018;71(6):e13–e115.

36. Shimamoto K, Ando K, Fujita T, Hasebe N, Higaki J, Horiuchi M, et al. The Japanese Society of Hypertension Guidelines for the Management of Hypertension (JSH 2014). Hypertens Res. 2014;37(4):253–390.

37. Qaseem A, Wilt TJ, Rich R, Humphrey LL, Frost J, Forciea MA, et al. Pharmacologic treatment of

hypertension in adults aged 60 years or older to higher versus lower blood pressure targets: a clinical practice guideline from the American College of Physicians and the American Academy of family PhysiciansPharmacologic treatment of hypertension in adults. Ann Intern Med. 2017;166(6):430–7.

38. Williams B, Mancia G, Spiering W, Agabiti Rosei E, Azizi M, Burnier M, et al. 2018 ESC/ESH guidelines for the management of arterial hypertension. Eur Heart J. 2018;39(33):3021–104.

39. Hertz RP, Unger AN, Cornell JA, Saunders E. Racial disparities in hypertension prevalence, awareness, and management. Arch Intern Med. 2005;165(18):2098–104.

40. Fryar CD, Ostchega Y, Hales CM, Zhang G, Kruszon-Moran D. Hypertension prevalence and control among adults: United States, 2015–2016. NCHS Data Brief. 2017;(289):1–8.

41. Daviglus ML, Pirzada A, Talavera GA. Cardiovascular disease risk factors in the Hispanic/Latino population: lessons from the Hispanic Community Health Study/Study of Latinos (HCHS/SOL). Prog Cardiovasc Dis. 2014;57(3):230–6.

42. Aviles-Santa ML, Colon-Ramos U, Lindberg NM, Mattei J, Pasquel FJ, Perez CM. From sea to shining sea and the great plains to Patagonia: a review on current knowledge of diabetes mellitus in Hispanics/Latinos in the US and Latin America. Front Endocrinol. 2017;8:298.

43. Yusuf S, Hawken S, Ounpuu S, Dans T, Avezum A, Lanas F, et al. Effect of potentially modifiable risk factors associated with myocardial infarction in 52 countries (the INTERHEART study): case-control study. Lancet (London, England). 2004;364(9438):937–52.

44. Lanas F, Avezum A, Bautista LE, Diaz R, Luna M, Islam S, et al. Risk factors for acute myocardial infarction in Latin America: the INTERHEART Latin American study. Circulation. 2007;115(9):1067–74.

45. Margolis KL, Piller LB, Ford CE, Henriquez MA, Cushman WC, Einhorn PT, et al. Blood pressure control in Hispanics in the antihypertensive and lipid-lowering treatment to prevent heart attack trial. Hypertension (Dallas, Tex : 1979). 2007;50(5):854–61.

46. Cooper-DeHoff RM, Aranda JM Jr, Gaxiola E, Cangiano JL, Garcia-Barreto D, Conti CR, et al. Blood pressure control and cardiovascular outcomes in high-risk Hispanic patients–findings from the International Verapamil SR/Trandolapril Study (INVEST). Am Heart J. 2006;151(5):1072–9.

47. Still CH, Rodriguez CJ, Wright JT Jr, Craven TE, Bress AP, Chertow GM, et al. Clinical outcomes by race and ethnicity in the Systolic Blood Pressure Intervention Trial (SPRINT): a randomized clinical trial. Am J Hypertens. 2018;31(1):97–107.

48. Rodriguez CJ, Still CH, Garcia KR, Wagenknecht L, White S, Bates JT, et al. Baseline blood pressure control in Hispanics: characteristics of Hispanics in

the Systolic Blood Pressure Intervention Trial. J Clin Hypertens (Greenwich, Conn). 2017a;19(2):116–25.

49. Rodriguez F, Hastings KG, Boothroyd DB, Echeverria S, Lopez L, Cullen M, et al. Disaggregation of cause-specific cardiovascular disease mortality among Hispanic subgroups. JAMA Cardiol. 2017b;2(3):240–7.

50. Rodriguez F, Hastings KG, Hu J, Lopez L, Cullen M, Harrington RA, et al. Nativity status and cardiovascular disease mortality among hispanic adults. J Am Heart Assoc. 2017c;6(12):e007207.

51. Dong C, Della-Morte D, Rundek T, Wright CB, Elkind MS, Sacco RL. Evidence to maintain the systolic blood pressure treatment threshold at 140 mm Hg for stroke prevention: The Northern Manhattan Study. Hypertension (Dallas, Tex : 1979). 2016;67(3):520–6.

52. Guzman NJ. Epidemiology and management of hypertension in the Hispanic population: a review of the available literature. Am J Cardiovas Drugs. 2012;12(3):165–78.

53. Thomas IC, Allison MA. Hypertension in Hispanics/Latinos: Epidemiology and Considerations for Management. Curr Hypertens Rep. 2019;21(6):43.

54. Pu J, Romanelli R, Zhao B, Azar KM, Hastings KG, Nimbal V, et al. Dyslipidemia in special ethnic populations. Cardiol Clin. 2015;33(2):325–33.

55. Rodriguez CJ, Daviglus ML, Swett K, González HM, Gallo LC, Wassertheil-Smoller S, et al. Dyslipidemia patterns among Hispanics/Latinos of diverse background in the United States. Am J Med. 2014a;127(12):1186–94.e1.

56. Rodriguez CJ, Allison M, Daviglus ML, Isasi CR, Keller C, Leira EC, et al. Status of cardiovascular disease and stroke in Hispanics/Latinos in the United States: a science advisory from the American Heart Association. Circulation. 2014b;130(7):593–625.

57. Lloret R, Ycas J, Stein M, Haffner S. Comparison of rosuvastatin versus atorvastatin in Hispanic-Americans with hypercholesterolemia (from the STARSHIP trial). Am J Cardiol. 2006;98(6):768–73.

58. Pencina MJ, Navar-Boggan AM, D'Agostino RB Sr, Williams K, Neely B, Sniderman AD, et al. Application of new cholesterol guidelines to a population-based sample. N Engl J Med. 2014;370(15):1422–31.

59. Grundy SM, et al. 2018 AHA/ACC/AACVPR/ AAPA/ABC/ACPM/ADA/AGS/APhA/ASPC/NLA/ PCNA Guideline on the Management of Blood Cholesterol: a report of the American College of Cardiology Foundation/American Heart Association Task Force on Clinical Practice Guidelines. J Am Coll Cardiol. 2018;73(24):3168–209.

60. Xu J, Murphy SL, Kochanek KD, Bastian B, Arias E. Deaths: final data for 2016. National vital statistics reports: from the Centers for Disease Control and Prevention, National Center for Health Statistics, National Vital Statistics System. 2018;67(5):1–76.

61. Prevention CDC. National Diabetes Statistics Report, 2017. US Department of Health and Human Services. 2017.

62. Vivo RP, Krim SR, Cevik C, Witteles RM. Heart failure in Hispanics. J Am Coll Cardiol. 2009;53(14):1167–75.

63. Bahrami H, Kronmal R, Bluemke DA, Olson J, Shea S, Liu K, et al. Differences in the incidence of congestive heart failure by ethnicity: the multiethnic study of atherosclerosis. Arch Intern Med. 2008;168(19):2138–45.

64. Casagrande SS, Aviles-Santa L, Corsino L, Daviglus ML, Gallo LC, Espinoza Giacinto RA, et al. Hemoglobin A1c, blood pressure, and LDL-Choelsetrol control among Hispanic/Latino adults with diabetes: results from the HCHS/SOL. Endocr Pract. 2017;23(10):1232–53.

65. Balfour PC Jr, Ruiz JM, Talavera GA, Allison MA, Rodriguez CJ. Cardiovascular disease in Hispanics/ Latinos in the United States. J Lat Psychol. 2016;4(2):98–113.

66. Kposowa AJ. Mortality from diabetes by Hispanic groups: evidence from the US National Longitudinal Mortality Study. Int J Populat Res. 2013;2013:12.

67. Pabon-Nau LP, Cohen A, Meigs JB, Grant RW. Hypertension and diabetes prevalence among U.S. Hispanics by country of origin: the National Health Interview Survey 2000–2005. J Gen Intern Med. 2010;25(8):847–52.

68. Hales CM, Carroll MD, Fryar CD, Ogden CL. Prevalence of obesity among adults and youth: United States, 2015–2016. NCHS Data Brief. 2017;288:1–8.

69. Petersen R, Pan L, Blanck HM. Racial and ethnic disparities in adult obesity in the United States: CDC's tracking to inform state and local action. Prev Chronic Dis. 2019;16:E46.

70. Flegal KM, Kruszon-Moran D, Carroll MD, Fryar CD, Ogden CL. Trends in obesity among adults in the United States, 2005 to 2014. JAMA. 2016;315(21):2284.

71. Bermudez OI, Tucker KL. Total and Central Obesity among Elderly Hispanics and the Association with Type 2 diabetes. Obes Res. 2001;9(8):443–51.

72. Prevalence of Self-Reported Obesity Among U.S. Adults by Race/Ethnicity, State and Territory, BRFSS, 2012–2014 [Internet]. Division of Nutrition, Physical Activity, and Obesity, National Center for Chronic Disease Prevention and Health Promotion. 2016. Available from: https://www.cdc.gov/obesity/downloads/data/2014-obesity-prevalence-map-by-raceethnicity-non-hispanic-508-compliant.pdf.

73. Prevalence of Self-Reported Obesity Among U.S. Adults by Race/Ethnicity, State and Territory, BRFSS, 2015-2017 [Internet]. Division of Nutrition, Physical Activity, and Obesity, National Center for Chronic Disease Prevention and Health Promotion. 2019. Available from: https://www.cdc.gov/obesity/data/prevalence-maps.html.

74. Goodpaster BH, Krishnaswami S, Harris TB, Katsiaras A, Kritchevsky SB, Simonsick EM, et al. Obesity, regional body fat distribution, and the metabolic syndrome in older men and women. Arch Intern Med. 2005;165(7):777.

75. Sutton BS, Weinert S, Langefeld CD, Williams AH, Campbell JK, Saad MF, et al. Genetic analysis of adiponectin and obesity in Hispanic families: the IRAS Family Study. Hum Genet. 2005;117(2–3):107–18.

76. Gilardini L, McTernan PG, Girola A, Da Silva NF, Alberti L, Kumar S, et al. Adiponectin is a candidate marker of metabolic syndrome in obese children and adolescents. Atherosclerosis. 2006;189(2):401–7.

77. Lastra-Gonzalez G, Manrique-Acevedo C, Lastra-Lastra G. Central obesity and the cardiometabolic syndrome in Hispanics. Therapy. 2007;4:609.

78. Shaibi GQ, Cruz ML, Weigensberg MJ, Toledo-Corral CM, Lane CJ, Kelly LA, et al. Adiponectin independently predicts metabolic syndrome in overweight Latino Youth. J Clin Endocrinol Metab. 2007;92(5):1809–13.

79. Isasi CR, Ayala GX, Sotres-Alvarez D, Madanat H, Penedo F, Loria CM, et al. Is acculturation related to obesity in Hispanic/Latino adults? Results from the Hispanic Community Health Study/Study of Latinos. J Obes. 2015;2015:186276.

80. Markides KS, Coreil J. The health of Hispanics in the southwestern United States: an epidemiologic paradox. Public Health Rep (Washington, DC: 1974). 1986;101(3):253–65.

81. Abraido-Lanza AF, Dohrenwend BP, Ng-Mak DS, Turner JB. The Latino mortality paradox: a test of the "salmon bias" and healthy migrant hypotheses. Am J Public Health. 1999;89(10):1543–8.

82. Forbang NI, Hughes-Austin JM, Allison MA, Criqui MH. Peripheral artery disease and non-coronary atherosclerosis in Hispanics: another paradox? Prog Cardiovasc Dis. 2014;57(3):237–43.

83. Ruiz JM, Steffen P, Smith TB. Hispanic mortality paradox: a systematic review and meta-analysis of the longitudinal literature. Am J Public Health. 2013;103(3):e52–60.

84. Shor E, Roelfs D, Vang ZM. The "Hispanic mortality paradox" revisited: meta-analysis and meta-regression of life-course differentials in Latin American and Caribbean immigrants' mortality. Soc Sci Med (1982). 2017;186:20–33.

85. Liao Y, Cooper RS, Cao G, Durazo-Arvizu R, Kaufman JS, Luke A, et al. Mortality patterns among adult Hispanics: findings from the NHIS, 1986 to 1990. Am J Public Health. 1998;88(2):227–32.

86. Cortes-Bergoderi M, Goel K, Murad MH, Allison T, Somers VK, Erwin PJ, et al. Cardiovascular mortality in Hispanics compared to non-Hispanic whites: a systematic review and meta-analysis of the Hispanic paradox. Eur J Intern Med. 2013;24(8):791–9.

87. Hunt KJ, Williams K, Resendez RG, Hazuda HP, Haffner SM, Stern MP. All-cause and cardiovascular mortality among diabetic participants in the San

Antonio Heart Study: evidence against the "Hispanic paradox". Diabetes Care. 2002;25(9):1557–63.

88. Medina-Inojosa J, Jean N, Cortes-Bergoderi M, Lopez-Jimenez F. The Hispanic paradox in cardiovascular disease and total mortality. Prog Cardiovasc Dis. 2014;57(3):286–92.

89. Palloni A, Arias E. A re-examination of the Hispanic mortality paradox. 2003.

90. Velasco-Mondragon E, Jimenez A, Palladino-Davis AG, Davis D, Escamilla-Cejudo JA. Hispanic health in the USA: a scoping review of the literature. Public Health Rev. 2016;37:31.

91. Ramos BM. Acculturation and depression among Puerto Ricans in the mainland. Soc Work Res. 2005;29:95.

92. Gerstein HC, Miller ME, Byington RP, Goff DC Jr, Bigger JT, Buse JB, et al. Effects of intensive glucose lowering in type 2 diabetes. N Engl J Med. 2008;358(24):2545–59.

93. Getaneh A, Light LS, Brillon DJ, Calles Escandon J, Felicetta J, Evans GW, et al. Diabetes control among Hispanics in the action to control cardiovascular risk in diabetes trial. J Gen Intern Med. 2012;27(11):1499–505.

94. Duckworth W, Abraira C, Moritz T, Reda D, Emanuele N, Reaven PD, et al. Glucose control and vascular complications in veterans with type 2 diabetes. N Engl J Med. 2009;360(2):129–39.

95. Saremi A, Schwenke DC, Bahn G, Ge L, Emanuele N, Reaven PD. The effect of intensive glucose lowering therapy among major racial/ethnic groups in the veterans affairs diabetes trial. Metabolism. 2015;64(2):218–25.

96. Dominguez K, Penman-Aguilar A, Chang MH, Moonesinghe R, Castellanos T, Rodriguez-Lainz A, et al. Vital signs: leading causes of death, prevalence of diseases and risk factors, and use of health services among Hispanics in the United States – 2009–2013. MMWR Morb Mortal Wkly Rep. 2015;64(17):469–78.

97. Rivera-Hernandez M, Leyva B, Keohane LM, Trivedi AN. Quality of Care for White and Hispanic Medicare Advantage Enrollees in the United States and Puerto Rico. JAMA Intern Med. 2016;176(6):787–94.

98. Torres JM, Wallace SP. Migration circumstances, psychological distress, and self-rated physical health for Latino immigrants in the United States. Am J Public Health. 2013;103(9):1619–27.

99. Capielo Rosario C, Lance CE, Delgado-Romero EA, Domenech Rodriguez MM. Acculturated and acultura'os: testing bidimensional acculturation across Central Florida and island Puerto Ricans. Cultur Divers Ethnic Minor Psychol. 2019;25(2):152–69.

100. Johnson JA, Cavanagh S, Jacelon CS, Chasan-Taber L. The diabetes disparity and Puerto Rican identified individuals. Diabetes Educ. 2017;43(2):153–62.

Progress in ASCVD Risk Assessment in African Americans and Hispanic Americans

12

Peter W. F. Wilson

Introduction

Atherosclerotic cardiovascular disease (ASCVD) is a major cause of death and disability in the United States. The key clinical outcome of interest for prediction and primary prevention in the 1980s was Hard Coronary Heart Disease (CHD), which included myocardial infarction (MI) and CHD death, and did not include angina pectoris. Over the past 30 years Hard ASCVD (first occurrence of MI, stroke, or cardiovascular disease (CVD) death has evolved to become the composite major adverse cardiovascular outcome of greatest interest. This chapter reviews information related to the prediction of Hard CHD and Hard ASCVD outcomes across African American (AA), Hispanic American (HA), and European American (EA) subgroups.

The prediction of vascular and heart disease outcomes such as angina pectoris, cardiac failure, and intermittent claudication will not be discussed. Population-based epidemiologic studies with baseline risk factor information and follow-up with adjudicated outcomes will provide the basis for most of this review. Data accrued from clinical trials will generally not be included as trial participants typically receive more clinical care, and closer follow-up in comparison to persons enrolled in observational studies. Such data are believed to provide biased estimates of ASCVD risk in populations.

Initial ASCVD Risk Estimation in Populations

Initial ASCVD risk estimates originated from the experience of population-based observational cardiovascular investigations such as the Framingham Heart Study (FHS), which focused on middle-aged participants with baseline measurements and periodic follow-up for the development of ASCVD events. Observational cohorts like Framingham and others that originated in the 1940s and 1950s were designed to investigate the role of blood pressure, smoking, and blood cholesterol level as determinants of risk for heart disease and stroke. Analyses in the 1960s first identified "factors of risk for the development of heart disease" in Framingham and other population studies [1]. Additionally, the Lipid Research Clinics Program and blood pressure intervention trial successes in the 1970s led to an awareness that simple assessments such as the presence or absence of a single risk factor did not adequately identify ASCVD risk for individuals. In fact, information for several variables could be combined. Statistical methods such as multivariable logistic regression, and later proportion hazards regression analyses, were used to estimate

P. W. F. Wilson (✉)
Atlanta VAMC and Emory Clinical Cardiovascular Research Institute, Atlanta, GA, USA
e-mail: pwwilso@emory.edu

© Springer Nature Switzerland AG 2021
K. C. Ferdinand et al. (eds.), *Cardiovascular Disease in Racial and Ethnic Minority Populations*,
Contemporary Cardiology, https://doi.org/10.1007/978-3-030-81034-4_12

absolute risk of developing an event such as an MI or CHD death over a specified follow up interval [2, 3]. To undertake such analyses, it generally meant following a cohort of at least several thousand persons for approximately 10 years or more to accrue the large number of outcomes that allowed investigators to undertake the statistical analyses needed to reliably estimate the effects of several risk factors on a CVD outcome [4].

With this backdrop Framingham investigators developed vascular disease risk estimating algorithms based on a suburban EA population sample. A 1998 publication reported effects for age, sex, systolic pressure, current smoking history, total cholesterol, HDL-C, and diabetes status to predict risk of CHD in 5345 middle-aged adults followed for approximately 12 years, an interval during which 610 persons developed a first ASCVD event. The major focus at the time was risk estimation for Hard CHD. Other algorithms were published for the prediction of several other ASCVD outcomes [5, 6].

Key Risk Factors for ASCVD Event Prediction

Age and Sex Greater age is an especially important ASCVD risk determinant, and men experience greater risk for CAD than women throughout most of adulthood. Clinical ASCVD is uncommon prior to age 40 in men and prior to the menopause in women. The absolute risk of developing clinical CAD in women increases greatly after the menopause, and by age 70–80 years the incidence of CAD is roughly similar in both sexes. Women more commonly experience angina pectoris as the first evidence of ASCVD. On the other hand, MI is the most common first ASCVD events in men [7]. Sudden cardiac death is much less common in women than in men [8].

Smoking Self-reported cigarette-smoking habit over the past year typically doubles the risk of CAD events [9]. Relative risks may be much higher for heavy smokers. Older research has shown that filter and non-filter cigarettes have similarly adverse effects on CHD risk [10].

Quitting smoking has been associated with improved long-term survival in persons with CHD, and the benefit of smoking cessation is typically evident within a few years of stopping, as shown in the Multiple Risk Factor Intervention Trial [11]. The prevalence of current smoking in the United States has declined over the last 50 years and is now in the 15–25% range for men and 5–25% range for women, which helps to account for a reduced impact of smoking on ASCVD risk at the population level [12].

Dyslipidemia Higher levels of total cholesterol, LDL-cholesterol (LDL-C), or non-HDL cholesterol (non-HDL-C), and apolipoprotein B are all associated with greater risk of CHD events. A large number of clinical trials have shown that lowering the concentration of atherogenic lipids such as LDL-C translates into reduced CAD risk [13]. In recent years researchers have extended this field to investigate atherogenic lipid measures such as apolipoprotein B levels and the LDL particle number in an effort to refine estimates of ASCVD risk [14, 15]. Higher levels of HDL-cholesterol (HDL-C) appear to be cardioprotective and lifestyle factors such as lower body mass index, greater alcohol intake, higher estrogen levels, avoidance of smoking, and greater physical activity are partially responsible for favorable HDL-C effects. Elevated triglyceride levels contribute to greater CHD risk and in multivariable models that include cholesterol, HDL-C, and triglycerides the effects of triglycerides are generally modest [16].

Blood Pressure Elevated blood pressure is a well-established risk factor for vascular disease. Population studies have shown that ASCVD risk increases in proportion to BP levels, even in the non-hypertensive range, as shown in 2007–2012 US NHANES data [12]. The prevalence of hypertension (>140/90 mmHg or on BP medication) increases inexorably with age, affecting approximately 8% of young adults and rising to 80% at age > 75 years, with little difference in the prevalence estimates for men and women. In analyses across AA, EA, and HA, the awareness of hypertension is generally in the 70–90% range,

BP treatment is in the 60–80% range, and BP control is in the 40–60% range [17], with considerable heterogeneity in these estimates across the different ethnic/racial groups [12].

The gradient of risk between CHD and BP is stronger for systolic pressure than for diastolic pressure. To avoid collinearity using both systolic and diastolic information in prediction models, systolic pressure is typically used to estimate risk for CHD events [9]. Pharmacotherapy is generally recommended for persons with elevated systolic or diastolic pressure, as published by expert committees [18]. Blood pressure management guidelines have become increasingly more aggressive, with initiation of therapy at lower arterial pressure levels than in the past [19]. Blood pressure treatment information, when available, has typically been included in multivariable risk models to predict ASCVD risk, but the hazard ratio for current BP therapy is typically greater than 1.00, which denotes increased ASCVD risk. This result has been interpreted to indicate that blood pressure intervention may have been initiated late in the natural history of ASCVD and did not provide cardioprotection [7].

Diabetes Mellitus For middle-aged adults the presence of type 2 diabetes mellitus typically doubles CHD risk for men and triples risk for women [7]. At older ages diabetes mellitus increases risk twofold in both sexes. The increased CHD risk in diabetic patients is attributable to higher BP levels, more dyslipidemia, elevated glucose levels, and increased levels of inflammatory markers [20].

ASCVD Risk Score Algorithms

Multivariable risk models, namely, ASCVD risk models were developed and published in the 1980s and early 1990s based on the experience of the Framingham Heart Study. The key variables were age, sex, smoking, systolic blood pressure, blood pressure treatment, total cholesterol (or LDL-C), HDL-C, and diabetes mellitus. The focus was on the experience of asymptomatic

adults without clinical vascular disease at baseline and the follow-up was typically 10 years or more. Clinical notes, inpatient and outpatient records, and death certificate information aided the adjudication of ASCVD events [5, 21]. Computers or specially programmed pocket calculators were used to estimate the risks, and an updated version that used categories of risk factor levels was published in 1998 [7]. Both the Original Cohort and the Offspring Cohort in Framingham were of European origin and the applicability of the ASCVD estimates to HA and AA groups was not known at the time.

In 2001, the utility of ASCVD risk prediction was assessed in a National Heart, Lung, and Blood Institute (NHLBI) ASCVD Risk Assessment Workshop. Results from Framingham were compared across several US cohorts [22]. Many of the comparison cohorts were predominantly EA adults from suburban adults such as from Rancho Bernardo, Physicians Health Study, Cardiovascular Health Study (older EA), and ARIC sites in North Carolina, Maryland, and Minnesota. Native American data were contributed from the Strong Heart Study and Japanese American data for men were contributed from the Honolulu Heart Program. The ARIC site in Jackson, Mississippi provided the only AA data and the Puerto Rico Heart Study supplied the only HA data evaluated in the 2001 NHLBI workshop. The analyses were largely based on baseline data from the 1970s and 1980s with 10 years of follow-up for ASCVD events up to the mid-1990s [22]. During this era aggressive blood pressure treatment became more prevalent, newer lipid medications such as statins were introduced, smaller heart attacks could be diagnosed, persons were more likely to survive a myocardial infarction, and coronary disease mortality was declining.

The 2001 NHLBI CVD Risk Workshop comparisons of Hard CHD relative risks for specific risk factors reported using variables without logarithmic transformation are shown in Table 12.1 (men) and Table 12.2 (women) for the FHS, ARIC, and Puerto Rican Heart Program Participants. The risk factors assessed included baseline age, blood pressure catego-

Table 12.1 Relative risks for CHD: Framingham, ARIC, and Puerto Rican men

Factor	Framingham Heart Study	Atherosclerosis risk in communities		Puerto Rico
	Euro American	Euro American	African American	Hispanic American
Age (years)	1.05 (1.04–1.07)	1.05 (1.02–1.07)	1.05 (1.01–1.10)	1.03 (1.00–1.05)
Blood pressure (mmHg)				
Optimal (BPs < 120, BPd < 80)	1.10 (0.67–1.82)	0.75 (0.53–1.06)	1.25 (0.48–3.23)	0.57 (0.35–0.91)
Normal (BPs < 140, BPd < 90)	Reference	Reference	Reference	
High normal (BPs < 140, BPd < 90)	1.53 (0.98–2.36)	0.93 (0.60–1.44)	2.67 (1.10–6.48)	1.22 (0.82–1.83)
Stage I Htn (BPs < 160, BPd < 100)	1.93 (1.28–2.92)	1.66 (1.11–2.47)	3.07 (1.31–7.18)	1.79 (1.25–2.57)
Stage II–IV (BPs ≥ 160, BPd ≥ 100)	2.45 (1.59–3.79)	1.72 (0.94–3.17)	1.55 (0.52–4.65)	3.26 (2.29–4.65)
Total cholesterol (mg/dL)				
<160	0.69 (0.31–1.52)	0.92 (0.51–1.67)	0.85 (0.31–2.31)	0.94 (0.59–1.49)
160–199	Reference	Reference	Reference	
200–239	1.77 (1.25–2.50)	1.40 (1.00–1.97)	1.32 (0.72–2.43)	1.21 (0.89–1.65)
240–279	2.10 (1.43–3.10)	1.93 (1.31–2.83)	1.10 (0.50–2.46)	1.36 (0.90–2.06)
≥280	2.29 (1.39–3.76)	2.23 (1.25–3.97)	2.23 (0.97–5.16)	2.08 (1.26–3.44)
HDL-C (mg/dL)				
<35	1.84 (1.17–2.88)	2.66 (1.55–4.56)	1.82 (0.76–4.37)	1.00 (1.00–1.00)
35–44	1.45 (0.94–2.21)	1.97 (1.16–3.36)	1.16 (0.51–2.65)	0.73 (0.50–1.07)
45–49	Reference	Reference	Reference	
50–59	1.00 (0.62–1.60)	1.40 (0.76–2.59)	0.71 (0.28–1.78)	1.00 (1.00–1.00)
≥60	0.63 (0.34–1.18)	0.55 (0.21–1.40)	0.71 (0.28–1.78)	1.00 (1.00–1.00)
Diabetes	1.69 (1.11–2.57)	2.42 (1.69–3.46)	1.40 (0.75–2.62)	2.07 (1.50–2.85)
Current smoking	2.07 (1.60–2.68)	1.94 (1.47–2.56)	1.65 (1.00–2.71)	1.74 (1.38–2.20)

Table adapted from D'Agostino [22]

ries, blood pressure treatment, total cholesterol categories, HDL-C categories, diabetes status, and current smoking status. Many risk factor effects were similar across the different ethnic and racial groups but some striking differences were noted. The impact of high normal and stage I hypertension on ASCVD risk was especially elevated in both AA men and AA women, and diabetes mellitus exerted a smaller effect on risk in AA men than in EA men or HA men. The consensus following the 2001 NHLBI Workshop was that the FHS risk estimators could be used to predict CHD risk in Americans and that validity of the FHS prediction models was greatest in EA. The report noted the relative paucity of data for AA and HA population groups, and it was hoped that more data would become available in the future to provide data for race and ethnic specific CHD risk estimation in the future.

Following the 2001 NHLBI Workshop, an Expert Committee published the Adult Treatment

Table 12.2 Relative risks for CHD: Framingham and ARIC women

Factor	Framingham Heart Study Euro American	Atherosclerosis risk in communities Euro American	African American
Age (years)	1.19 (0.97–1.45)	1.67 (0.73–3.83)	0.88 (0.33–2.33)
Blood pressure (mmHg)			
Optimal (BPs < 120, BPd < 80)	0.48 (0.22–1.05)	0.42 (0.24–0.73)	0.71 (0.24–2.130)
Normal (BPs < 140, BPd < 90)	Reference	Reference	Reference
High normal (BPs < 140, BPd < 90)	0.69 (0.34–1.42)	1.12 (0.61–2.08)	2.82 (1.10–7.23)
Stage I Htn (BPs < 160, BPd < 100)	1.24 (0.69–2.24)	1.17 (0.59–2.28)	1.94 (0.75–5.020)
Stage II-IV (BPs ≥ 160, BPd ≥ 100)	1.84 (1.00–3.39)	2.80 (1.24–6.36)	8.86 (3.81–20.63)
Total cholesterol (mg/dL)			
<160	1.23 (0.27–5.64)	0	1.46 (0.51–4.17)
160–199	Reference	Reference	Reference
200–239	1.55 (0.81–2.96)	0.90 (0.52–1.56)	1.17 (0.56–2.48)
240–279	1.74 (0.90–3.40)	1.16 (0.64–2.10)	1.36 (0.61–2.99)
≥280	2.44 (1.21–4.93)	1.48 (0.75–2.93)	2.98 (1.35–6.58)
HDL-C (mg/dL)			
<35	2.08 (1.00–4.31)	2.34 (1.21–4.52)	3.08 (1.20–7.86)
35–44	1.82 (1.05–3.16)	0.84 (0.44–1.61)	1.80 (0.88–3.71)
45–49	1.82 (1.05–3.14)	1.80 (0.99–3.28)	1.08 (0.44–2.63)
50–59	Reference	Reference	Reference
≥60	0.58 (0.33–1.02)	0.47 (0.23–0.93)	0.87 (0.41–1.86)
Diabetes	2.38 (1.40–4.06)	3.62 (2.21–5.94)	2.01 (1.16–3.48)
Current smoking	2.65 (1.77–3.97)	3.92 (2.56–5.99)	2.78 (1.64–4.73)

Table adapted from D'Agostino [22]

Cholesterol Adult Treatment Panel III Guidelines in 2001 and the algorithm adopted to guide care for the prevention of first coronary disease events was a categorical approach to CHD risk estimation that was based on the 1998 Framingham publication and the 2001 Workshop validation analyses. The prevention outcome of interest was the composite event of first major CHD event (MI or Coronary Heart Disease death) [23].

The next major update for ASCVD prediction took place in 2014 when an American Heart Association/American College of Cardiology (AHA/ACC) Expert Committee published Pooled Cohort Equations (PCE) to estimate the risk of first Hard ASCVD events (MI, stroke, or CVD death). The EA estimates were derived from the experience of the FHS, ARIC, CARDIA, and CHS White cohorts and the AA estimates were developed from Jackson Heart Study data. The variables used to develop the risk estimates were the same as for the 2001 algorithm, but the variables were logarithmically transformed prior to model fitting. The effects of various combinations of risk factor levels on estimates of Hard ASCVD risk for EA and AA men and women are shown in Fig. 12.1. In general, women experience much lower ASCVD risk than men, and ASCVD risk in AA is greater than for EA, even with the same risk factor burden.

External validation, largely based on the experience of EA adults in other US studies, was provided from the experience of the REasons for Geographic And Racial Differences in Stroke (REGARDS) and the Multiethnic Study of Atherosclerosis (MESA) [24]. Concomitant to the 2013 PCE publication, other investigators reported that the 2018 equations estimated absolute Hard ASCVD risk at twice the incidence rate that was actually observed [25]. Unfortunately, data were not available to make comparisons across HA and AA groups. A later analysis from REGARDS and the Kaiser Permanente Southern California (KPSC) experience with baseline lipid

measurements in 2003–2007 compared results to ARIC findings that had baseline measurements obtained in 1987–1989. The authors showed that CHD rates declined in recent years and the association between lipids and CHD in contemporary studies may be attenuated by the preferential use of statins by high-risk individuals [26].

Lifetime risk of CAD and other vascular events, largely confined to analysis of EA data, has been possible since the turn of century using methods that censored for competing causes of death and had follow-up periods of long duration. A recent report that included information from 18 cohorts and more than 200,000 adults showed that the lifetime risk of ASCVD was 15% for persons without risk factors at age 55 years and absolute risk rose to approximately 40% for those with two or more of the traditional risk factors [27].

Several electrocardiogram (ECG) abnormalities have been associated with greater ASCVD

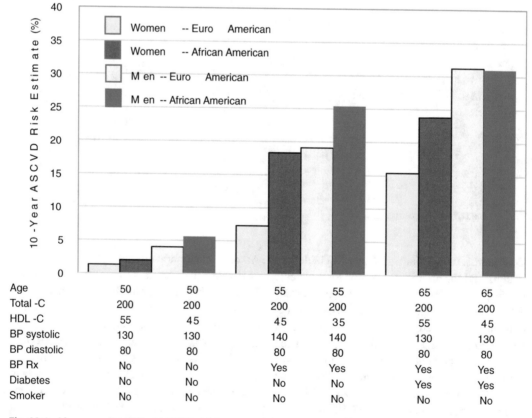

Fig. 12.1 10-year predicted Hard ASCVD risk by race and for US adults 2013. (Adapted from Table by Goff, based on Pooled Cohort Equations [24])

risk but they are not included in ASCVD prediction algorithms because the ECG is typically not included in ASCVD screening programs and the abnormalities are relatively uncommon. Examples of such ECG abnormalities in asymptomatic persons include ST depression, T wave inversion, left ventricular hypertrophy (LVH) or strain, and premature ventricular contractions, which can have a two-to tenfold increased risk of CHD compared to those with a normal ECG [28]. Some early ASCVD prediction algorithms included LVH, which is highly associated with hypertension, older age, and obesity and historically more prevalent in AA populations. Among >15,000 patients in ARIC who were followed for 15 years, both women and men with baseline ECG-identified LVH were significantly more likely to die from ASCVD than from non-ASCVD causes (HR in women 8.4, 95% CI 4.5–15.6, HR in men 4.9, 95% CI 3.0–7.8) [29]. The prevalence of ECG in recent times is only a few percent and is lower than in the past. It is impor-

tant to recognize that the presence of LVH does help to identify persons at greater risk to develop ASCVD events.

Since the 2013 PCE publication the Jackson Heart Study investigators reported that the 2013 ACC/AHA CVD Pooled Cohort Equations "work well in Black individuals and are not easily improved upon." [30] A second report, based on an analysis of electronic health records from Kaiser Healthcare enrollees in Northern California, included 19,760 HA and 4117 AA, and 151,615 EA age 40–79 years at baseline with an average of 3.9 years of follow-up for first Hard ASCVD events. They concluded that the 2013 ACC/AHA PCE generally overestimated risk 20% in HA, 60% in AA, and 50% in EA, and there was a fair degree of heterogeneity in the risk estimation across ASCVD quantiles, as shown in Fig. 12.2 [31].

The distribution of 10-year predicted Hard ASCVD risk by race and ethnicity for US men aged 40–79 years is shown in Fig. 12.3, and simi-

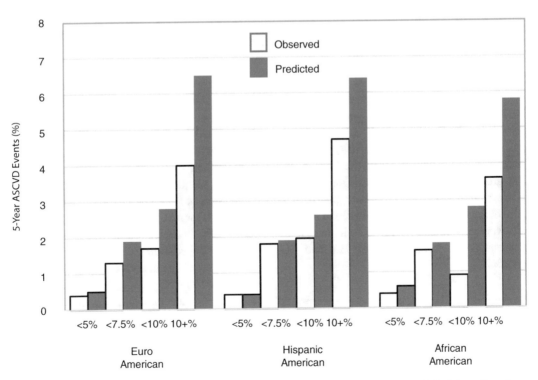

Fig. 12.2 A 5-year observed versus predicted Hard ASCVD risk by race and ethnicity for Kaiser Healthcare North California enrollees. Risk estimates were made with the 2013 ACC/AHA Pooled Cohort Equations. (Adapted from Rodriguez [31])

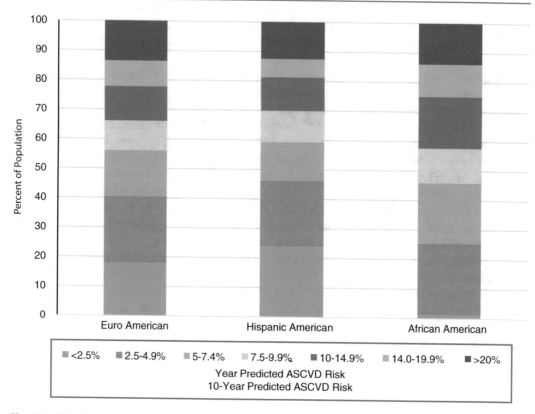

Fig. 12.3 Distribution of 10-year predicted Hard ASCVD risk by race and ethnicity for US adult men aged 40–79 years. (After Goff [24])

lar information for women is displayed in Fig. 12.4. These figures were developed from the 2013 ACC/AHA Guideline report on the Assessment of Cardiovascular Risk [24]. Lower risk (<2.5% 10-year predicted risk) was especially common in women across the AA, EA, and HA groups. The highest risk categories (>10% 10-year predicted risk) comprise approximately 30% of the men and 20% of women, and AA men and women were more likely to be in these high-risk categories compared with EA and HA groups.

Beyond Traditional Risk Factors for ASCVD

The factor that was emphasized the most in the 2018 ACC/AHA Cholesterol Guideline to help guide risk decisions is coronary artery calcification (CAC) detected by electron beam computed tomography or multidetector computed tomography [32]. After age 40 coronary calcium is frequently seen in the coronary arteries, an aggregate coronary calcium score can be developed from the images, and ASCVD risk is greater in persons in proportion to the quantity of calcium [33]. Coronary plaque volume, calcium density, and progression of the calcification are all related to greater risk for ASCVD events [34, 35]. Analyses from MESA investigators showed that CAC was especially effective in reclassifying the ASCVD risk for persons estimated to be at intermediate risk across all racial groups. High CAC was associated with greater risk [36, 37], and a low CAC score, especially a score of zero, was associated with very low ASCVD risk [38].

Many factors can be considered beyond the common ASCVD risk factors and were categorized as Risk-Enhancing Factors for Clinician-Patient Discussion in the 2018 ACC/AHA Cholesterol Guideline [32]. They include a posi-

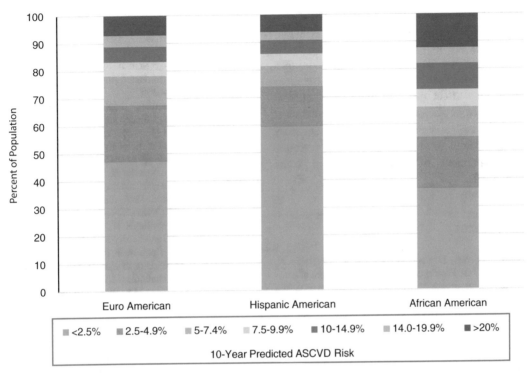

Fig. 12.4 Distribution of 10-year predicted Hard ASCVD risk by race and ethnicity for US adult women aged 40–79 years. (After Goff [24])

tive family history of ASCVD, hypercholesterolemia, metabolic syndrome, chronic kidney disease, chronic inflammatory conditions, premature menopause, high-risk race or ethnicity such as South Asian, and a variety of biomarkers. The list of candidate ASCVD biomarkers in the blood highlighted C-reactive protein, lipoprotein (a), and apolipoprotein B, but the list is long and constantly growing. Information related to subclinical atherosclerotic disease such as an abnormal ankle brachial index was also included. Not emphasized in the 2018 ACC/AHA Cholesterol guideline but considered important is that disadvantaged socioeconomic status has been consistently associated with higher ASCVD risk in many studies and has also been utilized in some British ASCVD risk estimates [39–42].

Although individual genetic markers are associated with ASCVD, their aggregate effect beyond traditional factors has not been well established and at this point not integrated into ASCVD risk assessment. For example, a genetic risk score created from 101 SNPs associated with

ASCVD did not improve discrimination or reclassification of risk after adjustment for traditional factors in a cohort of over 19,000 White women [43]. Peripheral blood cell gene expression has also been investigated as a means of estimating the risk of ASCVD, specifically obstructive CAD, and based on limited data the technique may be comparable to stress testing with myocardial perfusion imaging in terms of accuracy of diagnosing CHD [44–46].

Summary

The epidemiology of ASCVD has evolved to the point where clinical Hard ASCVD events—myocardial infarction, ischemic stroke, and cardiovascular disease death—are extremely common on a worldwide basis, and antecedent prediction of such events is a key focus for ASCVD prevention. Traditional factors such as age, male sex, recent smoking habit, diabetes mellitus, hypertension, hypertension therapy, and lipid measures are important determinants of risk. Newer biomarkers continue to be studied and are complemented by research findings concerning genetic variants that augment ASCVD risk. In addition, a variety of other situations, conditions, and diagnoses may affect risk development of clinical ischemic heart disease. Finally, use of subclinical heart disease assessments, especially coronary artery calcium scoring, holds promise to refine the assessment of ASCVD risk in some individuals.

References

1. Kannel WB, Dawber TR, Kagan A, Revotskie N, Stokes J III. Factors of risk in the development of coronary heart disease–six year follow-up experience. The Framingham Study. Ann Intern Med. 1961;55:33–50.
2. Castelli WP, Garrison RJ, Wilson PWF, Abbott RD, Kalousdian S, Kannel WB. Coronary heart disease incidence and lipoprotein cholesterol levels: the Framingham Study. JAMA. 1986;256:2835–8.
3. Abbott RD, Wilson PW, Kannel WB, Castelli WP. High density lipoprotein cholesterol, total cholesterol screening, and myocardial infarction. The Framingham Study. Arteriosclerosis. 1988;8(3):207–11.
4. Harrell FE Jr. Regression modeling strategies: with applications to linear models, logistic regression, and survival analysis. New York: Springer; 2001.
5. Anderson KM, Odell PM, Wilson PWF, Kannel WB. Cardiovascular disease risk profiles. Am Heart J. 1991;121:293–8.
6. Anderson KM, Wilson PWF, Odell PM, Kannel WB. An updated coronary risk profile. A statement for health professionals. Circulation. 1991;83:357–63.
7. Wilson PW, D'Agostino RB, Levy D, Belanger AM, Silbershatz H, Kannel WB. Prediction of coronary heart disease using risk factor categories. Circulation. 1998;97(18):1837–47.
8. Kannel WB, Wilson PW, D'Agostino RB, Cobb J. Sudden coronary death in women. Am Heart J. 1998;136(2):205–12.
9. Goff DC Jr, Lloyd-Jones DM, Bennett G, et al. 2013 ACC/AHA guideline on the assessment of cardiovascular risk: a report of the American College of Cardiology/American Heart Association Task Force on Practice Guidelines. Circulation. 2014;129(25 Suppl 2):S49–73.
10. Castelli WP, Garrison RJ, Dawber TR, McNamara PM, Feinleib M, Kannel WB. The filter cigarette and coronary heart disease: the Framingham study. Lancet. 1981;2(8238):109–13.
11. Hammal F, Ezekowitz JA, Norris CM, Wild TC, Finegan BA, Investigators A. Smoking status and survival: impact on mortality of continuing to smoke
one year after the angiographic diagnosis of coronary artery disease, a prospective cohort study. BMC Cardiovasc Disord. 2014;14:133.
12. Mozaffarian D, Benjamin EJ, Go AS, et al. Heart Disease and Stroke Statistics-2016 update: a report from the American Heart Association. Circulation. 2016;133(4):e38–e360.
13. Cholesterol Treatment Trialists C, Baigent C, Blackwell L, et al. Efficacy and safety of more intensive lowering of LDL cholesterol: a meta-analysis of data from 170,000 participants in 26 randomised trials. Lancet. 2010;376(9753):1670–81.
14. Sniderman AD, Lamarche B, Contois JH, de Graaf J. Discordance analysis and the Gordian Knot of LDL and non-HDL cholesterol versus apoB. Curr Opin Lipidol. 2014;25(6):461–7.
15. Sniderman AD, Williams K, Contois JH, et al. A meta-analysis of low-density lipoprotein cholesterol, non-high-density lipoprotein cholesterol, and apolipoprotein B as markers of cardiovascular risk. Circ Cardiovasc Qual Outcomes. 2011;4(3):337–45.
16. Hokanson JE, Austin MA. Plasma triglyceride level is a risk factor for cardiovascular disease independent of high-density lipoprotein cholesterol level: a meta-analysis of population-based prospective studies. J Cardiov Risk. 1996;3:213–9.
17. Benjamin EJ, Muntner P, Alonso A, et al. Heart disease and stroke statistics-2019 update: a report from the American Heart Association. Circulation. 2019;139(10):e56–66.
18. James PA, Oparil S, Carter BL, et al. 2014 evidence-based guideline for the management of high blood pressure in adults: report from the panel members appointed to the Eighth Joint National Committee (JNC 8). JAMA. 2014;311(5):507–20.
19. Whelton PK, Carey RM, Aronow WS, et al. 2017 ACC/AHA/AAPA/ABC/ACPM/AGS/APhA/ASH/ASPC/NMA/PCNA guideline for the Prevention, Detection, Evaluation, and Management of High Blood Pressure in adults: a report of the American College of Cardiology/American Heart Association Task Force on Clinical Practice Guidelines. Circulation. 2018;138(17):e484–594.
20. Regensteiner JG, Golden S, Huebschmann AG, et al. Sex differences in the cardiovascular consequences of diabetes mellitus: a scientific statement from the American Heart Association. Circulation. 2015;132(25):2424–47.
21. Wilson PWF, Castelli WP, Kannel WB. Coronary risk prediction in adults: the Framingham Heart Study. Am J Cardiol. 1987;59(G):91–4.
22. D'Agostino RB Sr, Grundy S, Sullivan LM, Wilson P. Validation of the Framingham coronary heart disease prediction scores: results of a multiple ethnic groups investigation. JAMA. 2001;286(2):180–7.
23. Executive Summary of the Third Report of The National Cholesterol Education Program (NCEP) Expert Panel on Detection, Evaluation, and Treatment of High Blood Cholesterol In Adults (Adult Treatment Panel III). JAMA. 2001;285(19):2486–2497.

24. Goff DC Jr, Lloyd-Jones DM, Bennett G, et al. ACC/ AHA guideline on the assessment of cardiovascular risk: a report of the American College of Cardiology/ American Heart Association Task Force on Practice guidelines. Circulation. 2014; 129 (25 suppl): S49–73
25. Ridker PM, Cook NR. Statins: new American guidelines for prevention of cardiovascular disease. Lancet. 2013;382(9907):1762–5.
26. Colantonio LD, Bittner V, Reynolds K, et al. Association of Serum Lipids and Coronary Heart Disease in contemporary observational studies. Circulation. 2016;133(3):256–64.
27. Berry JD, Dyer A, Cai X, et al. Lifetime risks of cardiovascular disease. N Engl J Med. 2012;366(4):321–9.
28. Auer R, Bauer DC, Marques-Vidal P, et al. Association of major and minor ECG abnormalities with coronary heart disease events. JAMA. 2012;307(14):1497–505.
29. Desai CS, Ning H, Lloyd-Jones DM. Competing cardiovascular outcomes associated with electrocardiographic left ventricular hypertrophy: the Atherosclerosis Risk in Communities Study. Heart. 2012;98(4):330–4.
30. Fox ER, Samdarshi TE, Musani SK, et al. Development and validation of risk prediction models for cardiovascular events in black adults: the Jackson Heart Study Cohort. JAMA Cardiol. 2016;1(1):15–25.
31. Rodriguez F, Chung S, Blum MR, Coulet A, Basu S, Palaniappan LP. Atherosclerotic cardiovascular disease risk prediction in disaggregated Asian and Hispanic subgroups using electronic health records. J Am Heart Assoc. 2019;8(14):e011874.
32. Grundy SM, Stone NJ, Bailey AL, et al. AHA/ACC/ AACVPR/AAPA/ABC/ACPM/ADA/AGS/APhA/ ASPC/NLA/PCNA guideline on the Management of Blood Cholesterol: a report of the American College of Cardiology/American Heart Association Task Force on clinical practice guidelines. J Am Coll Cardiol. 2018;2018
33. Detrano R, Guerci AD, Carr JJ, et al. Coronary calcium as a predictor of coronary events in four racial or ethnic groups. N Engl J Med. 2008;358(13):1336–45.
34. Budoff MJ, Young R, Lopez VA, et al. Progression of coronary calcium and incident coronary heart disease events: MESA (Multi-Ethnic Study of Atherosclerosis). J Am Coll Cardiol. 2013;61(12):1231–9.
35. Criqui MH, Denenberg JO, Ix JH, et al. Calcium density of coronary artery plaque and risk of incident cardiovascular events. JAMA. 2014;311(3):271–8.
36. Polonsky TS, McClelland RL, Jorgensen NW, et al. Coronary artery calcium score and risk classification for coronary heart disease prediction. JAMA. 2010;303(16):1610–6.
37. Nasir K, Shaw LJ, Liu ST, et al. Ethnic differences in the prognostic value of coronary artery calcification for all-cause mortality. J Am Coll Cardiol. 2007;50(10):953–60.
38. Nasir K. Message for 2018 cholesterol management guidelines update: time to accept the power of zero. J Am Coll Cardiol. 2018;72(25):3243–5.
39. Virtanen M, Nyberg ST, Batty GD, et al. Perceived job insecurity as a risk factor for incident coronary heart disease: systematic review and meta-analysis. BMJ. 2013;347:f4746.
40. Kivimaki M, Nyberg ST, Batty GD, et al. Job strain as a risk factor for coronary heart disease: a collaborative meta-analysis of individual participant data. Lancet. 2012;380(9852):1491–7.
41. Kivimaki M, Jokela M, Nyberg ST, et al. Long working hours and risk of coronary heart disease and stroke: a systematic review and meta-analysis of published and unpublished data for 603,838 individuals. Lancet. 2015;386(10005):1739–46.
42. Hippisley-Cox J, Coupland C, Robson J, Brindle P. QRISK2 validation by ethnic group. Heart. 2014;100(5):436.
43. Paynter NP, Chasman DI, Pare G, et al. Association between a literature-based genetic risk score and cardiovascular events in women. JAMA. 2010;303(7):631–7.
44. Elashoff MR, Wingrove JA, Beineke P, et al. Development of a blood-based gene expression algorithm for assessment of obstructive coronary artery disease in non-diabetic patients. BMC Med Genet. 2011;4:26.
45. Rosenberg S, Elashoff MR, Beineke P, et al. Multicenter validation of the diagnostic accuracy of a blood-based gene expression test for assessing obstructive coronary artery disease in nondiabetic patients. Ann Intern Med. 2010;153(7):425–34.
46. Thomas GS, Voros S, McPherson JA, et al. A blood-based gene expression test for obstructive coronary artery disease tested in symptomatic nondiabetic patients referred for myocardial perfusion imaging the COMPASS study. Circ Cardiovasc Genet. 2013;6(2):154–62.

Cardiovascular Disease in Minorities: Unique Considerations: Hypertension in African and Hispanic Americans

13

Kenneth A. Jamerson, Samar A. Nasser, and Keith C. Ferdinand

Introduction

Hypertension (HTN) is one of the most common chronic diseases in adults and a leading cause of morbidity and mortality affecting approximately 30% of adults in the United States [1]. Although hypertension is a leading cause of preventable disease, only 48% of hypertensive adults have blood pressure (BP) lower than 140/90 mmHg [2]. Not only does the prevalence of hypertension increase with age, it is higher among African Americans (AA), and BP control has not substantially improved in the last decade [3]. Data from the 2014 National Health Interview Survey (NHIS) showed that AA adults $\geq$18 years of age were more likely (33.0%) to have been told on $\geq$2 occasions that they had hypertension than American Indian/Alaska Native adults (26.4%), White adults (23.5%), Hispanic or Latino adults (22.9%), or Asian adults (19.5%) [4]. Additionally, among adults with hypertension, AAs were more likely to have resistant hypertension (19.0%) than Whites (13.5%) or Hispanics (11.2%) [5].

Among more than four million adults who were overweight or obese in ten healthcare systems, the prevalence of hypertension was 47.3% among Blacks, 39.6% among Whites, 38.6% among Native Hawaiians/ Pacific Islanders, 38.3% among American Indians/Native Americans, 34.8% among Asians, and 24.8% among Hispanics [6]. Although HTN treatment and control have been improving overall during the past several decades, AA patients still have poorer HTN control than their non-Hispanic White (NHW) counterparts. Additionally, even though the prevalence of controlled HTN increased from 31.6% in 1999–2000 to 53.1% in 2009–2010, no significant changes in control were observed from 2009–2010 through 2015–2016 [2]. Furthermore, age-standardized hypertension prevalence decreased among non-Hispanic White Americans, but not among AA or Mexican Americans [7].

For adults 45 years of age without HTN, the 40-year risk for developing HTN was 93% for AAs, 92% for Hispanics, 86% for Whites, and 84% for Chinese adults [1]. According to the National Health and Nutrition Examination Survey (2015–2016), the prevalence of HTN among non-Hispanic Black (NHB) adults

K. A. Jamerson
University of Michigan Health System, Division of Cardiovascular Medicine, Ann Arbor, MI, USA
e-mail: jamerson@umich.edu

S. A. Nasser (✉)
School of Medicine and Health Sciences, The George Washington University, Washington, DC, USA
e-mail: snasser@gwu.edu

K. C. Ferdinand
Tulane University School of Medicine,
New Orleans, LA, USA
e-mail: kferdina@tulane.edu

© Springer Nature Switzerland AG 2021
K. C. Ferdinand et al. (eds.), *Cardiovascular Disease in Racial and Ethnic Minority Populations*,
Contemporary Cardiology, https://doi.org/10.1007/978-3-030-81034-4_13

(40.3%) was higher than among NHW (27.8%), Hispanic (27.8%), and non-Hispanic Asian (25.0%) adults [2]. Furthermore, the prevalence of HTN was higher among NHB men (40.6%) than among NHW (29.7%), Hispanic men (27.3%), and non-Hispanic Asian (28.7%). Likewise, in women, the prevalence of HTN was higher among NHB (39.9%) adults than among NHW (25.6%), Hispanic adults (28.0%), and non-Hispanic Asian (21.9%).

Hispanic Americans

The Hispanic American population is among the fastest growing, and minority population in the United States, contributing to more than 17% of the US population [8], a number that is expected to reach 30% by 2050. Hypertension is a leading cause of CVD for Hispanic individuals. Although the prevalence of hypertension is highest among non-Hispanic Black individuals, the prevalence of antihypertensive medication use is lowest among Hispanic individuals [9]. Poor adherence to prescribed medication for HTN is a major contributor to disparities in effective blood pressure control among Hispanics. From 2013 to 2016, among Hispanics age 20 and older, 47.4% of males and 40.8% of females had HTN [10].

For US Hispanic or Latino males, the age-standardized prevalence of hypertension in 2008–2011 varied from a low of 19.9% among individuals of South American background to a high of 32.6% among individuals of Dominican background. For US Hispanic or Latino females, the age-standardized prevalence of hypertension was lowest for individuals of South American background (15.9%) and highest for individuals of Puerto Rican background (29.1%) [11].

Hispanic Americans experience a disproportionate burden of CVD risk factors, including obesity, HTN, and type 2 diabetes. Overall, Hispanic subjects demonstrated lower cardiovascular death rates when compared with non-Hispanic White subjects (244.8 vs. 189.0 per 100,000) [12]. However, when evaluating varying densities of Hispanic populations at the county level, higher Hispanic population was associated with greater mortality from CVD for both Hispanics and non-Hispanic White individuals. Thus, Hispanics living in the United States endure more cardiovascular-related death in counties heavily populated by Hispanics than those living in more diverse areas.

To evaluate the relationship between Hispanic population density and CVD mortality, Rodriguez and colleagues analyzed data from 715 counties across the United States and reviewed records for a total of 4,769,040 deaths, including 382,416 Hispanic adults and 4,386,624 non-Hispanic White adults [12]. Overall, the data demonstrated that counties with higher Hispanic populations faced more economic disadvantages, a lack of access to quality healthcare, and language barriers. Compared with counties that had the lowest Hispanic populations, those with the highest had 60% more Hispanic deaths from CVD (215.3 vs. 134.2 per 100,000). Notably, socioeconomic factors impact these statistics demonstrating that counties with higher Hispanic populations were more likely to be lower-income, lacking education, living below the poverty level, fewer primary care physicians, increased rates of uninsured, and more residents with limited English proficiency. The higher county Hispanic populations were also more likely to be rural, and mostly located in the Southwestern United States, South Florida, and in a few regions in the Northeast—thus demonstrating the critical impact of Hispanic population density, or residential segregation, at the county level on CVD deaths. Rodriguez and colleagues advocate future interventions focusing upon areas of high-proportion Hispanic density, as well as exploring the adverse health consequences of residential segregation.

Evidence demonstrates that poor adherence to prescribed antihypertensive medication is a major contributor to disparities in the Hispanic community. In a recent study, Lor and colleagues [13] investigated the association between health literacy level and adherence to antihypertensive medications in Hispanic adults who self-reported hypertension in a cross-sectional survey of 1355 Hispanics, primarily Dominicans.

The results demonstrated that 88.4% (n = 1026) had low adherence to their antihypertensive medications and 84.9% (n = 1151) exhibited inadequate health literacy— thus, leading the investigators to conclude that tailored interventions regarding health literacy are needed to support medication adherence to improve hypertension outcomes in Hispanics.

Pathophysiology

Hypertension is one of the most important modifiable risk factors for CVD; however, essential hypertension is categorized as primary hypertension, in view of the lack of a clear identifiable etiology or single pathogenesis. More than 90% of patients commonly treated for hypertension are essential or primary in origin, likely due to the results of multiple, poorly characterized genetic and environmental factors [14]. Although there are several modifiable lifestyle risk factors for essential hypertension (i.e., obesity, high sodium intake, insufficient physical activity, excessive alcohol consumption), non-modifiable factors also play important contributing roles (i.e., age, race/ethnicity, family history). The modifiable risk factors for essential primary hypertension are strongly and independently associated with its development, despite the lack of a clear etiology for most cases of elevated BP. Overweight and obesity have a precipitous racial gradient with the highest prevalence rate among Black and Hispanic adults and the lowest prevalence among Asians [6]. For instance, African American women have the highest rates (approximately four out of five) of being overweight or obese compared to other groups in the United States [15]. Obesity may additionally increase rates of heart disease and stroke events, and is strongly associated with higher rates of diabetes, which is more prevalent in AAs and Hispanics than in White groups [16]. Additionally, there are several potential determinants of hypertension that especially affect AAs. These include and stem from obesity (>50% of AA women have a body mass index ≥40), higher salt sensitivity, low levels of plasma renin, sympathetic over

activity, attenuated nocturnal fall in BP, and an increased risk for diabetes mellitus, physical inactivity, and a positive family history [14, 17]. Clearly, implementation of therapeutic lifestyle changes lies at the heart of hypertension care, especially in patients with milder forms of hypertension.

Hypertension Categorization

The 2017 American College of Cardiology/ American Heart Association guideline for the prevention, detection, evaluation, and management of high blood pressure (BP) (2017 ACC/ AHA HBP Guideline) in adults now defines HTN in stages (1 and 2). Stage 1 HTN entails a systolic BP of 130–139 mmHg or diastolic BP of 80–89 mmHg, while stage 2 HTN is a systolic BP ≥140 or diastolic BP ≥ 90 mmHg [1]. This paradigm shift recognizes the linear, consistent cardiovascular risk with elevated BP. Hypertension is the leading cause of death and disability worldwide and causes more CVD deaths than any other modifiable CVD risk factor and is a critical contributor to a myriad of cardiovascular and renal diseases [1].

Impact of Hypertension Prevalence and Management

Using data from the National Health and Nutrition Examination Survey 2013–2016, Bundy and colleagues estimated the risk reductions of CVD and all-cause mortality assuming the entire US adult population achieved guideline-recommended BP treatment goals of the 2017 high blood pressure guideline versus the 2014 guidelines [18]. According to the 2017 guideline, they determined that 45.4% of US adults, or 105.3 million people, had hypertension as compared to estimates under the 2014 guideline where 32% of Americans, or 74.1 million people, were classified as having hypertension—thus reflecting a significant increase in HTN estimates with the greatest difference evident in men aged 40–50 years. Furthermore, under the 2017 guideline, 35.9% of

US adults, or 83.2 million people, would be eligible for antihypertensive treatment versus 31.1%, or 72.2 million people, under the 2014 guideline.

Importantly, among those for whom treatment was recommended under the 2017 guideline, 12.1% (27.9 million) people were untreated, 12.9% (29.9 million) were treated but had not achieved their BP goal, and 10.9% (25.3 million) were treated and had achieved their BP goal. When compared to the 2014 version, the 2017 guideline was estimated to recommend more men than women for treatment with a 5.4% (6.0 million) increase in men and a 4.1% (5.0 million) increase in women. This may also be potentially due to the recommended treatment to more people over 60 years of age (a 10.5% increase or 6.6 million people) than people under age 60 (a 2.6% increase or 4.4 million people). As per race and ethnicity, there were consistent increases in the proportions of people recommended for treatment as well.

Accordingly, Bundy and colleagues mentioned with achievement of the 2017 guidelines, an estimated 610,000 CVD events and 334,000 total deaths would be prevented each year in those aged 40 or older versus 270,000 and 170,000, respectively, under the 2014 guideline. Therefore, implementation could potentially prevent 340,000 CVD events and 156,000 deaths each year.

Treatment for Hypertension

According to the National Health and Nutrition Examination Survey (2003–2012), incorporating 8796 hypertensive individuals ≥18 years of age among three racial groups (NHW, NHB or AAs, and Hispanics), AAs were more likely to receive combination therapy and had the highest average number of antihypertensive medications (NHW: 1.78; 95% CI, 1.73–1.82; AAs: 1.91; 95% CI, 1.84–1.97; Hispanics: 1.69; 95% CI, 1.61–1.77). Yet, AAs were less likely to achieve HTN control (adjusted OR, 0.73; 95% CI, 0.63–0.83) [19]. Although there are posi-

tive trends in both antihypertensive therapy utilization and HTN control in all racial groups during the 10-year study period, AAs continue to experience disparities in BP control. The 2017 ACC/AHA HBP Guideline recommends two or more antihypertensive medications to achieve a BP target of <130/80 mmHg in most adults and especially in AA adults with HTN [1].

Moreover, Gu and colleagues detected a difference in BP responsiveness to various antihypertensive drug classes in AA patients. Not only did AA patients receive more intensive antihypertensive therapy compared with White patients, they also utilized higher rates of combination therapy. In regard to the various classes of antihypertensive drugs, AAs were more likely to receive calcium channel blockers (CCBs) and diuretics in favor of angiotensin-converting enzyme inhibitors (ACEIs). Besides these observations, AA hypertensive patients were still less likely to achieve hypertension control. Several lifestyle differences may have contributed to the observed racial disparities. When compared to White patients, AA patients had an increased prevalence of obesity, a lower physical activity level, and a higher caloric, lower potassium intake [19]. Accordingly, in a previous study, compared with monotherapy, single-pill combination and multiple-pill combinations were associated with 55% and 26% greater likelihood of BP control, respectively [20].

Moreover, the Study of Women's Health Across the Nation (SWAN), a prospective cohort of women (n = 3,302, aged 42–52), evaluated antihypertensive medications grouped by class and examined by race/ethnicity. After adjusting for potential confounders, 1707 (51.7%) women (mean age 50.6 years) reported hypertension or used antihypertensive medications at baseline or during follow-up (mean 9.1 years). Compared with White patients, AAs were almost three times as likely to receive a CCB (odds ratio, 2.92; 95% CI, 2.24–3.82) and twice as likely to receive a thiazide diuretic (odds ratio, 2.38; 95% CI, 1.93–2.94). Additionally, AA women also had a higher probability of reporting use of ≥2 antihypertensive medications (odds ratio, 1.95; 95% CI, 1.55–2.45) compared with White women. ACEI/angiotensin receptor blocker use increased over time among all groups with the exception of Chinese women who reported thiazide diuretics as the most commonly used antihypertensive medication class [21].

Hypertension Guidelines: Comparison of the American College of Cardiology/American Heart Association (ACC/AHA) guideline for the Prevention, Detection, Evaluation, and Management of High Blood Pressure (BP) in Adults and European Guidelines (2018 European Society of Hypertension [ESH]/ European Society of Cardiology [ESC] Guidelines).

There are some key differences in the recently published US and European guidelines recommendations that modify the diagnostic and therapeutic approach to hypertension [1, 22] (Table 13.1). Some differences include a lower BP threshold for drug treatment in the adult and the elderly hypertensive population, lower BP goals to achieve with treatment, emphasis on utilization of home. and ambulatory BP measurements for the confirmation of hypertension. The ACC/AHA guideline uses the atherosclerotic CVD risk calculator for individualized cardiovascular risk assessment before defining treatment options. Thus, those patients with greater than a 10%, ten-year cardiovascular risk require more aggressive management to achieve levels below 130/80 mmHg and in concert with lifestyle modification will require antihypertensive drug therapy.

One of the largest differences between the ACC/AHA and ESH/ESC BP guidelines is the BP goal and definition of hypertension. Per ACC/AHA, threshold for hypertension diagnosis begins at >130/80 mmHg and threshold for initiation of drug therapy begins at >140/90 mmHg if low risk and at >130/80 mmHg if age >65, high risk, CV history, or diabetes. Accordingly, goal is to treat all patients to <130/80 mmHg as tolerated regardless of age. The ESH/ESC guideline maintains the diagnostic threshold of HTN at 140/90 mmHg.

Table 13.1 Similarities and differences between ACC/AHA and ESH/ESC guidelines

Similarities	
ACC/AHA	ESH/ESC
More emphasis on home BP and patient empowerment	Wider use of home BP monitoring to confirm diagnosis
Single-pill combination if >20/10 mmHg above goal	Initial single-pill combination as initial therapy
More attention to detail of BP measurement	More attention to detail of BP measurement
Focus on improving adherence	Detection of poor adherence
Differences	
	Does not have Specific focus on >10% 10-year absolute CV risk—Rather focuses on cardiovascular risk estimator, identified as SCORE system, to consider in timing and intensity of therapy
	Specific attention to prevention as BP approaches 130/80 mmHg
	Much attention to specific ethnic/racial groups
Retained definition of hypertension >140/90 mmHg and encouraged patient discussion and education to get <130/80 mmHg in those who require it by the evidence	
Limits on BP reduction—Not below 120/70 mmHg	

Table adapted from: Bakris [23]
ACC/AHA American College of Cardiology/American Heart Association, *BP* blood pressure, *ESC/ESH* European Society of Cardiology/European Society of Hypertension, *SCORE* Systematic Coronary Risk Evaluation

Public Health Perspectives and Future Considerations

Despite public health initiatives such as Healthy People 2020 and the Million Hearts initiative goals for 2017, the rates of HTN prevalence and control have not been attained. These national health initiatives help address the public health burden associated with health disparities through primary and secondary prevention efforts targeting HTN at the individual, community, health systems, and population levels. The Million Hearts campaign was sponsored by the US Department of Health and Human Services and consisted of comprehensive evidence-based interventions and strategies to prevent one million heart attacks and strokes over the period from 2012 to 2016 [24, 25]. Community-based interventions sponsored by the Association of Black Cardiologists, local programs such as the Healthy Heart Community Prevention Project (HHCPP) in New Orleans, and the International Society of Hypertension in Blacks outreach in Baltimore were early proponents of utilizing barbershops and churches as centers to provide education and screening specifically for HTN [26, 27]. More recently, Victor and colleagues completed a study funded by the National Heart, Lung, and Blood Institute in Los Angeles comparing two types of barber-based, patient-centered BP programs to evaluate which type was more effective in improving the customers' high blood pressure [28]. The author's approach linked the barber-based intervention to team-based care delivery, and demonstrated an effective intervention among AA male barbershop patrons with uncontrolled hypertension. By incorporating health promotion by barbers, there was a larger blood pressure reduction when coupled with medication management in barbershops by specialty trained clinical pharmacists [28].

As a measure of impacting disparities in the near future, health information technology (HIT) holds the potential to improve the quality, safety, and equity of healthcare. Internet-enabled electronic health (eHealth) applications, such as patient portals, help patients with chronic diseases communicate with providers, enable family caregivers to be better healthcare advocates, and provide a vehicle for individuals to receive ongoing self-management support. Moreover, clinicians who use electronic health records have the capability to electronically prescribe and utilize clinical decision support tools to enhance patient health and safety. Thus, HIT facilitates communication between patients "at-risk" for health disparities and their healthcare providers, and it provides patients online access to test results, immunization records, prescription refills, and patient education information.

On the other hand, the benefits of these technologies may disproportionately accrue to patients and providers with the physical access to eHealth and the resources and skills needed to use them. For instance, digital disparities persist among older adults, racial and ethnic minorities, physically disabled, lower-income and those with limited English proficiency. Thus, there is emerging evidence of pervasive racial/ethnic and educational disparities in use of patient portals [29, 30].

However, a considerable effort is in place to help bridge the technology gap between well-resourced and under-resourced providers to provide the tools necessary for all patients to successfully utilize and navigate HIT. Technological health interventions may deliver positive effects on reducing disparities at both the patient and provider levels, however; this will require cultural competence, language support, and cost-conscious pricing to avoid alienating minorities [31, 32]. In a recent effort to address the impact of HIT and health disparities, the National Institute on Minority Health and Health Disparities, in partnership with the National Science Foundation and the National Health IT Collaborative for the Underserved, convened a scientific workshop which proposed innovative strategies on the role of health IT in addressing health disparities. Using a comprehensive perspective at multiple levels of care, they found that community engagement, cultural competency, and patient-centered care were key to improving health equity as well as promoting scalable, sustainable, and effective health IT interventions. In addition, expanding public–private partnerships was emphasized as well. Collaboration between clinicians and IT developers may lead to innovative methods to improve upon healthcare decision-making [33]. Ultimately, if applied properly, HIT may improve health outcomes for minority populations, reduce disparities, and promote health equity.

Conclusion

Over recent decades, dramatic improvements in US CVD mortality, life expectancy, and overall healthcare have not occurred equally across

African American and Hispanic communities. Better targeting of interventions to reduce CV morbidity and mortality, specifically hypertension, not only by race/ethnicity, but also by risk factors and social determinants, must be addressed. Hypertension prevalence among AAs is among the highest in the world, and the Hispanic American population is among the fastest growing minority population in the United States. Collectively, these two disparate populations contribute to a disproportionate burden of CVD risk factors in the United States . Therefore, implementing interventions within the community will lead to greater reduction and impact in CV morbidity and mortality. In addition to preventative programs or lifestyle changes or medication adherence, interventions may help offset the negative effects of uncontrolled HTN as a long-term approach to management and control.

References

1. Whelton PK, Carey RM, Aronow WS, et al. 2017 ACC/AHA/AAPA/ABC/ACPM/AGS/APhA/ASH/ASPC/NMA/PCNA guideline for the prevention, detection, evaluation, and management of high blood pressure in adults: a report of the American College of Cardiology/American Heart Association Task Force on Clinical Practice Guidelines. Circulation. 2018;138(17):e426–81.
2. Fryar CD, Ostchega Y, Hales CM, Zhang G, Kruszon-Moran D. Hypertension prevalence and control among adults: United States, 2015–2016. NCHS Data Brief, No 289. Hyattsville: National Center for Health Statistics; 2017.
3. Egan BM, Li J, Small J, Nietert PJ, Sinopoli A. The growing gap in hypertension control between insured and uninsured adults: National Health and Nutrition Examination Survey 1988 to 2010. Hypertension. 2014;64:997–1004.
4. National Health Interview Survey: 2014 data release. Public-use data file and documentation. http://www.cdc.gov/nchs/nhis/nhis_2014_data_release.htm. Accessed Feb 10, 2019.
5. Sim JJ, Bhandari SK, Shi J, Liu IL, Calhoun DA, McGlynn EA, Kalantar-Zadeh K, Jacobsen SJ. Characteristics of resistant hypertension in a large, ethnically diverse hypertension population of an integrated health system. Mayo Clin Proc. 2013;88:1099–107. https://doi.org/10.1016/j.mayocp.2013.06.017.
6. Young DR, Fischer H, Arterburn D, Bessesen D, Cromwell L, Daley MF, Desai J, Ferrara A, Fitzpatrick SL, Horberg MA, Koebnick C, Nau CL, Oshiro C, Waitzfelder B, Yamamoto A. Associations of overweight/obesity and socioeconomic status with hypertension prevalence across racial and ethnic groups. J Clin Hypertens (Greenwich). 2018a;20:532–40. https://doi.org/10.1111/jch.13217.
7. Dorans KS, Mills KT, Liu Y, He J. Trends in prevalence and control of hypertension according to the 2017 American College of Cardiology/American Heart Association (ACC/AHA) guideline. J Am Heart Assoc. 2018;7(11):e008888. Published 2018 Jun 1. https://doi.org/10.1161/JAHA.118.008888.
8. Nittle NK. Interesting Facts about Racial Minorities in America. ThoughtCo. https://www.thoughtco.com/racial-minority-groups-in-the-us-2834984. Accessed February 11, 2019.
9. Fang J, Gillespie C, Ayala C, Loustalot F. Prevalence of self-reported hypertension and antihypertensive medication use among adults aged ≥18 years – United States, 2011–2015. MMWR Morb Mortal Wkly Rep. 2018;67(7):219–224. Published 2018 Feb 23. https://doi.org/10.15585/mmwr.mm6707a4.
10. Benjamin EJ, Muntner P, Alonso A, Bittencourt MS, Callaway CW, Carson AP, Chamberlain AM, Chang AR, Cheng S, Das SR, Delling FN, Djousse L, Elkind MSV, Ferguson JF, Fornage M, Jordan LC, Khan SS, Kissela BM, Knutson KL, Kwan TW, Lackland DT, Lewis TT, Lichtman JH, Longenecker CT, Loop MS, Lutsey PL, Martin SS, Matsushita K, Moran AE, Mussolino ME, O'Flaherty M, Pandey A, Perak AM, Rosamond WD, Roth GA, Sampson UKA, Satou GM, Schroeder EB, Shah SH, Spartano NL, Stokes A, Tirschwell DL, Tsao CW, Turakhia MP, VanWagner LB, Wilkins JT, Wong SS, Virani SS; on behalf of the American Heart Association Council on Epidemiology and Prevention Statistics Committee and Stroke Statistics Subcommittee. Heart disease and stroke statistics – 2019 update: a report from the American Heart Association [published online ahead of print January 31, 2019]. Circulation. https://doi.org/10.1161/CIR.0000000000000659.
11. Daviglus ML, Talavera GA, Avilés-Santa ML, Allison M, Cai J, Criqui MH, Gellman M, Giachello AL, Gouskova N, Kaplan RC, LaVange L, Penedo F, Perreira K, Pirzada A, Schneiderman N, Wassertheil-Smoller S, Sorlie PD, Stamler J. Prevalence of major cardiovascular risk factors and cardiovascular diseases among Hispanic/Latino individuals of diverse backgrounds in the United States. JAMA. 2012;308:1775–84. https://doi.org/10.1001/jama.2012.14517.
12. Rodriguez F, Hu J, Kershaw K, Hastings KG, López L, Cullen MR, Harrington RA, Palaniappan LP. County-level Hispanic ethnic density and cardiovascular disease mortality. J Am Heart Assoc. 2018;7(19):e009107.
13. Lor M, Koleck TA, Bakken S, Yoon S, Navarra AM. Association between health literacy and medication adherence among Hispanics with hypertension. J Racial Ethn Health Disparities. 2019;6:517–24.
14. Ferdinand KC, Nasser SA. Managing essential hypertension. Cardiol Clin. 2017;35(2):231–46.

15. US Dept of Health and Human Services. Office of Minority Health Website: https://minorityhealth.hhs.gov/omh/browse.aspx?lvl=4&lvlid=25. Accessed: February 16, 2019.

16. Goutham R, Powell-Wiley TM, Ancheta I, Hairston K, Kirley K, Lear SA, Palaniappan L, Rosal MC, et al. Identification of obesity and cardiovascular risk in ethnically and racially diverse populations: a scientific statement from the American Heart Association. Circulation. 2015;132(5):457–72.

17. Jiang SZ, Lu W, Zong XF, Ruan HY, Liu Y. Obesity and hypertension. Exp Ther Med. 2016;12(4):2395–9.

18. Bundy JD, Mills KT, Chen J, Li C, Greenland P, He J. Estimating the association of the 2017 and 2014 hypertension guidelines with cardiovascular events and deaths in US adults: an analysis of national data. JAMA Cardiol. 2018;3(7):572–81.

19. Gu A, Yu Y, Desai RP, Argulian E. Racial and ethnic differences in antihypertensive medication use and blood pressure control among US adults with hypertension. Circ Cardiovasc Qual Outcomes. 2017a;10:e003166.

20. Gu Q, Burt VL, Dillon CF, Yoon S. Trends in antihypertensive medication use and blood pressure control among United States adults with hypertension: the National Health and Nutrition Examination Survey, 2001 to 2010. Circulation. 2012;126:2105–14.

21. Jackson EA, Ruppert K, Derby CA, et al. Effect of race and ethnicity on antihypertensive medication utilization among women in the United States: Study of Women's Health Across the Nation (SWAN). J Am Heart Assoc. 2017;6(3):e004758. Published 2017 Feb 23. https://doi.org/10.1161/JAHA.116.004758.

22. Williams B, Mancia G, Spiering W, Authors/Task Force Members, et al. 2018 ESC/ESH guidelines for the management of arterial hypertension: the task force for the management of arterial hypertension of the European Society of Cardiology and the European Society of Hypertension:the task force for the management of arterial hypertension of the European Society of Cardiology and the European Society of Hypertension. J Hypertens. 2018;36:1953–2041.

23. Bakris G. Similarities and differences between the ACC/AHA and ESH/ESC guidelines for the prevention, detection, evaluation, and management of high blood pressure in adults: a perspective. Circ Res. 2019;124(7):969–71.

24. Ritchey MD, Wall HK, Gillespie C, George MG, Jamal A. Division for Heart Disease and Stroke Prevention, CDC. Million hearts: prevalence of leading cardiovascular disease risk factors—United States, 2005–2012. MMWR Morb Mortal Wkly Rep. 2014;63(21): 462–7.

25. Centers for Disease Control and Prevention (CDC). Million hearts: strategies to reduce the prevalence of leading cardiovascular disease risk factors—United States, 2011. MMWR Morb Mortal Wkly Rep. 2011;60(36):1248–51.

26. Ferdinand KC, Patterson KP, Taylor C, Fergus IV, Nasser SA, Ferdinand DP. Community-based approaches to prevention and management of hypertension and cardiovascular disease. J Clin Hypertens (Greenwich). 2012;14(5):336–43.

27. Victor RG, Ravenell JE, Freeman A, Leonard D, Bhat DG, Shafiq M, et al. Effectiveness of a barber-based intervention for improving hypertension control in black men: the BARBER-1 study: a cluster randomized trial. Arch Intern Med. 2011;171(4):342–50.

28. Victor RG, Lynch K, Li N, Blyler C, Muhammad E, Handler J, Brettler J, Rashid M, Hsu B, Foxx-Drew D, Moy N, Reid AE, Elashoff RM. A cluster-randomized trial of blood-pressure reduction in black barbershops. N Engl J Med. 2018;378:1291–301.

29. Sarkar U, Karter AJ, Liu JY, Adler NE, Nguyen R, López A, Schillinger D. Social disparities in internet patient portal use in diabetes: evidence that the digital divide extends beyond access. J Am Med Inform Assoc. 2011;18(3):318–21.

30. Roblin DW, et al. Disparities in use of a personal health record in a managed care organization. JAMIA. 2009;16:683–9. https://doi.org/10.1197/jamia.M3169.

31. Palmer MJ, Barnard S, Perel P, Free C. Mobile phone-based interventions for improving adherence to medication prescribed for the primary prevention of cardiovascular disease in adults. Cochrane Database Syst Rev. 2018;6:CD012675.

32. Lyles CR, Sarkar U, Schillinger D, Ralston JD, Allen JY, Nguyen R, et al. Refilling medications through an online patient portal: consistent improvements in adherence across racial/ethnic groups. J Am Med Inform Assoc. 2016;23:e28–33.

33. Zhang X, Hailu B, Tabor DC, Gold R, Sayre MH, Sim I, et al. Role of health information technology in addressing health disparities: patient, clinician, and system perspectives. Med Care. 2019;57(Suppl 6 Suppl 2):S115–20.

Weight Loss, Lifestyle, and Dietary Factors in Cardiovascular Disease in African Americans and Hispanics

14

Nia S. Mitchell and Jamy D. Ard

Abbreviations

BP	Blood pressure
BRS	Baroreflex sensitivity
CAD	Coronary artery disease
CHD	Coronary heart disease
CHF	Congestive heart failure
CVD	Cardiovascular disease
DASH	Dietary Approaches to Stop Hypertension
DASH-A	Dietary Approaches to Stop Hypertension with weekly session with nutritionist
DASH-WM	Dietary Approaches to Stop Hypertension—weight management
DBP	Diastolic blood pressure
ENCORE	Exercise and Nutrition interventions for CardiOvasculaR hEalth
FMD	Flow mediated dilation
HDL	High-density lipoprotein
HTN	Hypertension
LDL	Low-density lipoprotein
MESA	Multi-Ethnic Study of Atherosclerosis
MVPA	Moderately vigorous physical activity
OMNI	Optimal Macronutrient Intake Trial
OMNI-Carb	Optimal Macronutrient Intake—carbohydrate
OMNI-MUFA	Optimal Macronutrient Intake—monounsaturated fat
OMNI-Protein	Optimal Macronutrient Intake—protein
PA	Physical activity
PWV	Pulse wave velocity
SBP	Systolic blood pressure
TGs	Triglycerides
UC	Usual control diet

N. S. Mitchell
Division of General Internal Medicine, Department of Medicine, Duke University School of Medicine, Durham, NC, USA
e-mail: nia.s.mitchell@duke.edu

J. D. Ard (✉)
Department of Epidemiology and Prevention, Wake Forest School of Medicine, Winston-Salem, NC, USA
e-mail: jard@wakehealth.edu

Introduction

It has been estimated that a large fraction of cardiovascular disease (CVD) in the United States is preventable [16]. CVD is largely preventable because many of the contributors to the risk of CVD are lifestyle related. A variety of lifestyle behaviors can have direct and indirect influences on CVD risk including, but not limited to, physical activity and intake of energy, dietary pattern,

© Springer Nature Switzerland AG 2021
K. C. Ferdinand et al. (eds.), *Cardiovascular Disease in Racial and Ethnic Minority Populations*,
Contemporary Cardiology, https://doi.org/10.1007/978-3-030-81034-4_14

and alcohol. More recent work has begun to focus on the importance of other lifestyle factors like sedentary behaviors and sleep duration and quality in promoting CVD risk. To the extent that individuals can make choices to actively engage in healthful behaviors and avoid or limit engagement in less healthful behaviors, these actions account for the fraction of disease risk that is preventable.

Association of Lifestyle Behaviors with CVD Risk

The contributions of traditional lifestyle behaviors to CVD risk have been well defined, with some recent evidence expanding our thinking. Physical activity provides a clear example of this relationship. Individuals who report higher levels of leisure time physical activity have lower risk of CVD and CVD-related mortality [8]. There are nuances within this broad category of physical activity to consider more closely. For example, sedentary behavior, or physical inactivity, is increasingly being recognized as an independent risk factor for CVD. It is important to note that one can meet goals for leisure time physical activity but still have a high amount of sedentary time. Sedentary has been defined as "waking behavior characterized by an energy expenditure ≤ 1.5 metabolic equivalents while in a sitting or reclining posture" [43]. One metabolic equivalent is the amount of energy expended at rest in a sitting position; by contrast, three metabolic equivalents define moderate intensity physical activity [1]. Individuals who have a high amount of sedentary time appear to be at increased risk of CVD even when considering their overall activity levels [50]. The recommended amount of leisure time physical activity is 150 minutes per week of moderate intensity activity [36]. Despite a growing body of evidence suggesting a relationship between sedentary behavior and increased risk of CVD, there are no quantitative guidelines for what an acceptable amount of sedentary time may be. Experts note that it is still prudent advice to "sit less and move more" [50].

There are several dietary variables that can improve or worsen CVD risk. Dietary patterns that are high in added sugar, sodium, and saturated fat are associated with higher risk of CVD [16]. Conversely, individuals who consume diets that are low in refined grains and processed red meat and high in fruits, vegetables, and whole grains have lower rates of CVD [17]. Dietary intakes that are lower in sodium are associated with lower blood pressure and reduced rates of heart disease and stroke [17]. Maintaining energy balance and a healthy body weight is also an important CVD risk factor influenced by dietary intake [47]. Universally, poor-quality dietary patterns are associated with higher body mass index (BMI), elevated waist circumference, and insulin resistance—all of which contribute to metabolic syndrome and increased CVD risk [47]. Unfortunately, based on surveys of American dietary habits, fewer than 10% of the population currently meets goals for fruit and vegetable intake, while approximately 90% of the US population exceeds recommended intakes for solid fats and added sugar—primary sources of high energy-dense, low nutrient-rich calories [47].

In an effort to promote healthful dietary intake and reduce risk of CVD in the American population, current dietary guidelines include several dietary patterns such as the DASH (Dietary Approaches to Stop Hypertension) or Mediterranean dietary pattern that are associated with a reduced risk of CVD [46]. Both of these dietary patterns are characterized by high intakes of fruits and vegetables and limited amounts of red meat, added sugar, and refined grains. In addition to being high in nutrient-dense foods, these types of dietary patterns tend to be low-energy dense and associated with lower overall energy intake and energy balance [47]. Current sodium intake recommendations are for adults to consume <2400 mg sodium per day with evidence that even more reduction in blood pressure can be achieved by reducing sodium further to 1500 mg per day. However, for those who find it difficult to reach those levels of sodium intake, reducing one's current sodium intake by 1000 mg per day from current levels is also associated with significant reductions in blood pressure [17].

Differences in Lifestyle Behaviors by Race/Ethnicity

As noted previously, most Americans are falling short of recommended levels of physical activity and key dietary intakes. While the challenge to achieve healthy behaviors affects all Americans, some groups seem to be experiencing even greater difficulty in meeting some key goals. For example, the average American adult spends 6–8 hours daily in sedentary behavior [50]. Sedentary behavior has been shown to be higher in ethnic minority groups in some studies, noting that television watching is significantly higher in these populations, with one report noting that Black adults spent an average of 7 hours and 13 minutes per day watching television. Use of smartphones is also higher among African American and Hispanic adults, likely further contributing to sedentary time [8]. In this general context, African Americans have lower levels of physical activity on average compared to non-Hispanic White and Hispanic Americans. The proportion of people meeting the weekly goal of ≥150 minutes of moderate or ≥75 minutes of vigorous leisure time physical activity based on self-report was lowest for African American women (39.1%), followed closely by Hispanic women (41.8%) compared to non-Hispanic White women (53.6%) [8].

Dietary intake patterns show similar differences by race/ethnicity that would be expected to contribute to higher risk in African Americans and Hispanic Americans. African Americans and Hispanic Americans tend to have lower intakes of fruits and vegetables. African Americans have higher intakes of fish and shellfish, but at least one study suggests that a large proportion of that fish intake is fried fish, which has been associated with increased risk of cardiovascular disease events [32, 33]. Only one in six African Americans and one in eight Mexican Americans meet recommendations for servings of nuts and seeds (≥4 servings per week) [47]. Compared to 7–10% of non-Hispanic White Americans, only 4–5% of African Americans consumed the recommended 28 g of dietary fiber on a daily basis. However, 13–14% of Mexican Americans consume at least

the recommended amount of fiber [47]. Racial and ethnic minorities are more likely to exceed recommended guidelines for sugar intake, with only 32% of African Americans being below the target for sugar intake, compared to 43% of non-Hispanic White Americans and 41% of Hispanic Americans [12].

Many of the differences in lifestyle behaviors by race/ethnicity are notable, especially in the setting of significant disparities in CVD. When considering the etiology of the differences in lifestyle behaviors, it is important to note that the ability to engage in healthful lifestyle behaviors may not be consistent across various populations. Certainly, there are social determinants that influence one's ability to engage in some lifestyle behaviors. For example, limited space for safe exercise will have an influence on one's ability to engage in certain types of physical activity. While some circumstances create barriers to actively engaging in healthful lifestyle behaviors, there may be an equal or increasing number of factors that actively facilitate engagement in less healthful behaviors. The confluence of fewer options for healthy foods and the presence of highly marketed fast-food outlets in poor neighborhoods has been associated with lower-quality dietary intakes [11, 28, 31]. Discussion of the social determinants or influences of some behaviors is beyond the scope of this chapter, but it is discussed elsewhere. However, it is worth mentioning in this context to remind the reader that accessibility to healthful lifestyle behaviors is not equitable and may contribute to observed disparities in CVD risk and outcomes.

Changes in Lifestyle Behaviors Can Improve Risk and Prevent CVD

Preventing CVD using lifestyle behaviors is often considered a long-term process, because a CVD event is typically the culmination of years of persistent insults, like the rupture of a plaque that began many years prior as a fatty streak. However, prevention can also come in the form of reversing abnormal CVD risk factors by improving lifestyle behaviors, even when there has been prior long-term exposure to poor lifestyle behaviors. Individuals can improve risk factors like blood pressure, blood glucose, and body weight by focusing on improving a variety of lifestyle behaviors. Many of the lifestyle behaviors will have pleiotropic effects, leading to a wide range of risk factor improvements. For example, reducing body weight is associated with improvements in blood pressure, blood glucose, and lipids. In many instances, combining several lifestyle interventions can have additive or complementary effects for the individual. One example of this would be combining a lower sodium intake with a high-quality dietary pattern like the DASH diet.

The benefit to individuals from racial/ethnic minority groups for improving CVD risk by engaging in healthful lifestyle interventions has been demonstrated in several clinical trials. This chapter will review that evidence base and highlight the impact that healthful lifestyle behaviors can have in addressing CVD risk disparities. We will review the physiologic links between lifestyle and the risk factors that impact CV health. This will be followed by a discussion of the primary lifestyle interventions (aside from smoking cessation) that have evidence for modifying CVD risk, including weight reduction, improving diet pattern, and physical activity.

Evidence That Key Dietary Patterns Are Associated with Lower Risk of CVD

Food Groups and Risk of CVD

A large systematic review and meta-analysis published in 2019 examined the association of food groups and the risk of coronary heart disease, heart failure, and stroke [7]. This analysis found that consumption of whole grains, fruits and vegetables, nuts, and fish was associated with decreased risk of cardiovascular disease, including CHD, stroke, and heart failure, to varying degrees. However, eggs, red meat, processed meat, and sugar-sweetened beverages are associated with increased risk for CVD [7]. Outcomes were not reported by race or ethnicity.

Dietary Patterns

Compared to food groups, dietary patterns are defined by the combinations of various food groups. The dietary pattern is therefore defined by the specific combinations of food groups, denoting the inclusion of key food groups and the omission or limited intake of other food groups. A dietary pattern is typically analyzed as a unit, rather than reducing the effect down to the component food groups that make up the pattern. To derive the intended effect, the combination of food groups would need to be consumed consistently. Most assessments of dietary patterns typically include a scoring system or quantitative assessment of how closely an individual is to consuming all of the required component food groups while avoiding those that are excluded from the dietary pattern. Below, we will review the literature about the effects of several dietary patterns, including the vegetarian, Dietary Approached to Stop Hypertension (DASH), Mediterranean, and Optimal Macronutrient Intake Trial to Prevent Heart Disease (OMNI-Heart) on cardiovascular outcomes.

Vegetarian Dietary Patterns and CVD

Another systematic review and meta-analysis published in 2019 examined the association of vegetarian dietary pattern and CHD mortality and incidence, CVD mortality, and stroke mortality [20]. Vegetarian dietary patterns included lacto-ovo vegetarian diets, which include fruit, vegetables, grains, dairy and egg products, and vegan diets, which exclude dairy and egg products. These vegetarian patterns were compared with omnivorous dietary patterns, which include meat. Compared to omnivorous dietary pattern, the lacto-ovo-vegetarian or vegan dietary pattern did not affect either CVD mortality (0.92 [0.84, 1.02], $p = 0.13$) or stroke mortality (0.92 [0.77, 1.10], $p = 0.36$). However, there was a 22% reduction in CHD mortality (0.78 [0.69, 0.88], $p = <0.001$) and 28% reduction in CHD incidence (0.72 [0.61, 0.85], no p value reported). Although the authors noted the quality of the evidence was "very low" for all outcomes, outcomes were not reported by race or ethnicity.

Dietary Approaches to Stop Hypertension (DASH) Diet

Results from the Dietary Approaches to Stop Hypertension (DASH) diet were originally published in 1997 [2]. This study showed that compared to the "typical US diet," a diet "rich in fruits, vegetables, and low-fat dairy with reduced saturated and total fat" significantly lowered both systolic and diastolic blood pressure. Compared to individuals without hypertension, the effects of the diet were larger among individuals with hypertension. Regardless of hypertension status, compared to White Americans, African Americans had greater lowering of blood pressure [45].

Based on the Framingham risk equations, compared to the control diet, the DASH diet reduced the 10-year CHD risk by 18% for all participants [13]. However, the 10-year CHD risk among African Americans on the DASH diet compared to control diet was 22% lower ($p < 0.001$), whereas among White Americans the difference was 8% lower ($p = 0.296$). No outcomes were reported for Hispanic Americans.

Dietary Approaches to Stop Hypertension—Sodium

The DASH diet was also studied with different levels of sodium. DASH—Sodium was a two-arm trial where participants were randomized to either the DASH or control diet. For 30 consecutive days, in random order, participants ate foods with varying levels of sodium—high (150 mmol/day), intermediate (100 mmol/day), or low (50 mmol/day) [42]. On both the DASH and control diets, lower sodium lowered blood pressure. Compared to lowering sodium, the DASH diet was better at lowering blood pressure. Combining the DASH and low-sodium diets lowered blood pressure more than either diet alone, but the cumulative effects were sub-additive. For both the DASH and control diets, decreased sodium

had a greater effect on blood pressure for individuals with hypertension. A subgroup analysis confirmed these results in African Americans as well. No outcomes were reported for Hispanic Americans.

DASH Dietary Patterns and Cardiovascular Outcomes

A review published in 2019 analyzed DASH dietary patterns and cardiometabolic outcomes, including cardiovascular disease, coronary heart disease, and stroke [14]. This review of DASH and cardiometabolic outcomes included three systematic reviews and meta-analyses of prospective cohort studies and four systematic reviews and meta-analyses of prospective RCTs. In the prospective cohort studies, the DASH diet decreased the relative risk of cardiovascular disease by 20% (RR = 0.80 [0.76–0.85], $p < 0.001$); lowered the incidence coronary heart disease incidence by 21% (RR = 0.79 [0.71–0.88], $p < 0.001$); and lowered the incidence of stroke by 19% (RR = 0.81 [0.72–0.92], $p < 0.001$). Authors described the strength of evidence for these outcomes as either "low" or "very low." Outcomes were not reported by race or ethnicity.

In the prospective RCTs, the DASH diet lowered SBP (weighted mean difference [WMD] = -5.20 mmHg [-7.00 to -3.40 mmHg], $p < 0.001$) (moderate evidence) and DBP (WMD = -2.60 mmHg [-3.50 to -1.70 mmHg], $p < 0.001$) (low evidence). The DASH diet lowered total cholesterol (WMD = -0.20 mmol/L [-0.31 to -0.10 mmol/L], $p < 0.001$) (low evidence) and LDL cholesterol (WMD = -0.10 mmol/L [-0.20 to -0.01 mmol/L], $p = 0.03$) (moderate evidence), but did not change HDL cholesterol (low evidence) or triglycerides (low evidence) significantly.

DASH Dietary Patterns and Left Ventricular Function

One study examined how the DASH eating pattern affects left ventricular function [34]. The MESA

(Multi-Ethnic Study of Atherosclerosis) cohort was recruited between 2000 and 2002, and it includes 6814 women and men who were 28% African American, 12% Asian (predominantly Chinese), 22% Hispanic, and 38% White. At the time of enrollment, participants were aged 45–84 without evidence of cardiovascular disease. The current study included 4506 men and women from the MESA Study, which consists of individuals who were 40% White, 24% African American, 22% Hispanic American, and 14% Chinese American. MRI was used to measure left ventricular end-diastolic volume, stroke volume, and ejection fraction. DASH eating patterns were measured by a food frequency questionnaire that ranked eight food groups: (1) fruits; (2) vegetables; (3) whole grains; (4) nuts and legumes; (5) low-fat dairy products; (6) red meat and processed meats; (7) sweetened beverages; and (8) sodium. Scores for each group were divided into quintiles.

For food groups that were positively associated with the DASH eating pattern, a score of 1 was given to the lowest quintile and 5 was given to the highest quintile. For food groups that were negatively associated with the DASH eating pattern, a score of 1 was given to the highest quintile and 5 was given to the lowest quintile. The total scores ranged from 8 to 40—8 was minimally aligned with DASH eating patterns and 40 was strongly aligned with DASH eating pattern. After adjustment, for every one-unit increase in the score, there was a 0.26 mL increase in end-diastolic volume ($p < 0.01$) and 0.10 mL/m^2 increase in stroke volume ($p < 0.001$). The change in ejection fraction was not significant. Outcomes were adjusted for race, but not reported by race.

DASH Adaptations in African Americans and Hispanic Americans

DASH interventions are clearly efficacious in well-controlled academic settings. However, it is important to understand how the intervention works in real-world community settings. In several small studies, the DASH diet has been modified and tested in African American and Latino communities.

DASH Adaptations in African American Communities

One of the adaptations of the DASH diet among African Americans occurred in a neighborhood healthcare center [37]. The study included 82 African American patients aged 45–65 with a diagnosis of hypertension, an average BP above 140/90 for three previous clinic visits, and who were prescribed antihypertensive medications. Patients were divided into six groups of 12–15 patients, and patients were allowed to bring a guest to their sessions. Each group met weekly for 2 hours over eight consecutive weeks. Meetings included blood pressure and weight measurement; a presentation about nutritional information; a meal and discussion; and recipe demonstrations. Blood pressure and serum folate were the primary and secondary outcomes, respectively. Results were reported based on the number of sessions missed. Over 8 weeks, the SBP/DBP of 32 individuals who missed ≤2 sessions decreased by 8.4/4.3 mmHg ($p < 0.01$ and 0.05, respectively). Additionally, for the 18 individuals with data, the serum folate levels increased significantly ($p < 0.05$). The BP for the other groups who missed either three or four sessions; five to seven sessions; or all eight sessions was not significantly different, and there were not enough folate data for significant comparisons. Therefore, those who completed the intervention had significant changes in their blood pressure.

This same group conducted another community-based participatory research study where women were recruited from a neighborhood health center for a two-part study [38]. In the first part of the study, eight women, who participated in a previous DASH intervention, modified traditional African American ("soul food") recipes over 10 weeks with the help of nutrition students. Thirty-nine modified recipes were included in a cookbook and recorded on VHS and DVD. In the second part of the study, the neighborhood health center hosted eight dinner sessions where modified recipes were introduced. Based on nutritional analyses, the modified recipes successfully met DASH principles. Based on focus groups and surveys, participants found the recipes appealing.

Another group tested a culturally modified version of DASH among African Americans in urban communities with lower income, higher unemployment, and less availability of healthy food in North Carolina in a 12-week pilot randomized controlled trial [49]. The intervention group received two individual and nine group DASH sessions with a dietician and professional chef. The control group received one individual session with the study physician and dietician; they also received handouts about lowering blood pressure and the DASH diet. Fourteen individuals were assigned to the intervention group and 11 were assigned to the control group. The study was not powered to show differences in blood pressure, but outcomes included changes in behavior and dietary intake. Compared to the control group, the intervention group increased its consumption of fruits and vegetables, but neither group reached the daily targets of fruit, vegetable, low-fat dairy, saturated fat, or sodium intake.

One multiyear community-based participatory research project produced culturally appropriate nutrition information based on DASH-Sodium study, distributed the information through community health workers, and increased access to healthier foods through community gardens, and partnerships with farmers' markets, community organizations, and grocery stores [5]. Baseline data were collected in 2008 and follow-up data were collected in 2013. Compared to the county that did not get the intervention, the county that received the intervention had a decrease in the prevalence of hypertension and overweight/obesity. In the intervention county, the prevalence of hypertension decreased from 61.0% to 43.5% ($p < 0.01$), whereas in the control county it was essentially unchanged, 46.7% to 49.1% ($p = 0.48$). The trends in the prevalence of overweight and obesity were similar. In the intervention county, the prevalence of overweight and obesity decreased from 69.8% to 62.8% ($p < 0.01$), whereas in the control county it was not significantly different, 65.2% vs. 66% ($p = 0.39$). Individuals in the intervention county who had "high" participation in the intervention activities were more likely to report both higher

consumption of fruits and vegetables (OR 1.46, 95% CI 1.00, 21.12) and greater diversity of fruit and vegetable intake (OR 1.75, 95% CI 1.14, 2.71).

The Five Plus Nuts and Beans was an 8-week trial that randomized 123 African Americans who were recruited from urban primary care clinic to either a control group or the DASH-Plus group [30]. The control group received a handout about the DASH diet and a debit account with $30/week. The DASH-Plus group received an individual 1-hour coaching session about the DASH diet, weekly 15-minute phone coaching sessions, $30/week in a debit account for participants to buy high-potassium foods that would be delivered to a library near the clinic from which patients were recruited. Food purchases were tracked through the debit card. The primary outcome was change in blood pressure. Although the DASH-Plus group increased their consumption of fruits and vegetables, there was no difference in the change in BP between the two groups ($p = 0.48$).

DASH Adaptations in Latino Communities

The Hypertension Improvement Project (HIP) Latino Pilot Study tested the feasibility of a Spanish-language, culturally adapted intervention, delivered by a Latina facilitator in a community setting [41]. Its goals were to help pre-hypertensive and hypertensive adult participants lose weight (if they were overweight or obese), adopt DASH dietary eating patterns, and increase physical activity. Most participants were recruited through a community health center and a Hispanic-serving community organization. Six weekly sessions were held at both the community health center and the community organization. Sessions lasted between 90 and 120 minutes. Follow-up data were available for 17 participants. The mean (SD) weight change was −1.5 (3.2) lbs, change in systolic blood pressure was −10.4 (10.6) mmHg, and change in diastolic BP was −9.0 (13.0) mmHg. The median (IQR) difference in number of minutes of exercise per week was

+40 (115). Authors reported that the change in SBP as a "large effect size" and changes in weight and exercise as "medium-large effect sizes."

The same group expanded their intervention to 20 weeks, and it was held at the same community organization as the previous intervention [15]. Outcomes included changes in weight, blood pressure, eating patterns, and physical activity. In this study, 56 individuals were included in the final analysis. Average weight change was −5.1 lbs ($p = 0.006$). Average change in BP was −2.6/−0.5 mmHg ($p = 0.013$ for SBP, $p = 0.596$ for DBP). On average, participants consumed 0.6 fewer servings of meat per day ($p = 0.03$). However, there was no difference in the number of servings of vegetables, fruit, grains, dairy, or fats. Authors were unable to calculate changes in physical activity due to missing data.

Mediterranean Diet

The Mediterranean dietary pattern includes plant-based foods, including fruits, vegetables, whole grains, nuts, and seeds; olive oil; dairy products, usually yogurt or cheese; select animal protein, twice weekly fish and poultry and limiting red meat to a few times per month; red wine; and herbs and spices, in place of salt and fat [44]. It has been associated with improvement in numerous cardiovascular risk factors, including decreased hypertension and improved lipid profiles.

Mediterranean Dietary Patterns and Cardiovascular Outcomes

A Cochrane review published in 2019 in 30 RCTs examined four comparisons: (1) Mediterranean diet to no/minimal intervention to prevent onset of CVD; (2) Mediterranean diet to another diet to prevent onset of CVD; (3) Mediterranean diet to usual care to prevent CVD recurrence; and (4) Mediterranean diet to another diet to prevent CVD recurrence [39]. The primary outcomes were cardiovascular mortality; all-cause mortality; and non-fatal cardiovascular events—myo-

cardial infarction; coronary artery bypass grafting; percutaneous transluminal coronary angioplasty; angina or angiographically defined CHD; stroke; carotid endarterectomy; or peripheral artery disease. For primary prevention, the review cited the PREDIMED Diet (Prevención con Diets Mediterránea) [Prevention with Mediterranean Diet], which compared the Mediterranean diet with olive oil or nuts with a low-fat diet in Spain. It had a significant effect on composite clinical endpoints—MI, stroke, and death from cardiovascular causes (HR 0.70, 95% CI 0.58–0.85), but "little or no effect … on total mortality, CVD mortality, or MI." For secondary prevention, the review cited the Lyon Diet Heart Study, which compared a Mediterranean diet with a control diet in individuals with a previous MI over 46 months. The Mediterranean diet lowered the composite endpoint—CVD deaths and non-fatal MI (HR 0.28 [0.15–0.52]), CVD mortality (HR 0.35 [0.15–0.82]), and total mortality (HR 0.44 [0.21–0.92]). In terms of primary prevention of secondary outcomes, when compared to no/minimal intervention, the Mediterranean diet lowered total cholesterol (−0.16 mmol/L [−0.32–0.00]), systolic BP (−2.99 mmHg [−3.45 to −2.53]) and diastolic BP (−2.0 Hg [−2.29 to −1.71]). When compared to another diet intervention, the Mediterranean diet lowered LDL cholesterol (−0.15 mmol/L [−0.27 to −0.02]) and triglycerides (−0.09 mmol/L [−0.16 to −0.01]). There was "little or no effect" on lipids or BP for individuals with previous CVD. The PREDIMED intervention lowered the incidence of diabetes (HR 0.71 [0.52–0.96]).

Mediterranean Dietary Patterns and Left Ventricular Function

One study examined how the Mediterranean eating pattern affects left ventricular function in the MESA cohort [29]. The MESA cohort was recruited between 2000 and 2002, and it includes 6814 women and men who were African American, Chinese, Hispanic, and White. At the time of enrollment, participants were aged 45–84 without evidence of cardiovascular disease. The current study included 4497 men and women from all of the represented ethnic groups (although race data were presented within the results by quartile, it was not described for the entire cohort). MRI was used to measure left ventricular end-diastolic volume, stroke volume, and ejection fraction. The Mediterranean diet score was measured by a food frequency questionnaire that ranked nine food groups: (1) fruit; (2) vegetables; (3) nuts; (4) legumes; (5) whole grains; (6) fish; (7) ratio of monounsaturated to saturated fat; (8) red and processed meats; and (9) alcohol.

For food groups that were positively associated with the Mediterranean eating pattern, a score of 1 was given to those above the sex-specific medians for the sample. For foods groups that were negatively associated with the Mediterranean eating pattern, a score of 1 was given to those below the sex-specific medians for the sample. Total scores could range from 0 to 9—0 was minimally aligned with Mediterranean eating patterns and 9 was strongly aligned with Mediterranean eating patterns. Scores for each group were divided into quartiles. The Mediterranean Diet Score was positively associated with LV stroke volume ($p < 0.001$) and ejection fraction ($p = 0.004$). There was a U-shaped association for LV mass and Mediterranean diet score (p quad $= 0.04$). There was no significant association between the Mediterranean Diet Score and end-diastolic volume ($p = 0.055$). Outcomes were adjusted for race, but not reported by race.

DASH and Mediterranean Dietary Patterns and CVD Mortality

The Dietary Patterns Methods Project examined the relationship between several diet quality indices, including the DASH and Mediterranean patterns, with mortality [22]. Authors calculated hazard ratios for quintile 1 versus quintile 5 for each dietary pattern—quintile 1 was minimally aligned with the dietary pattern and quintile 5 was strongly aligned with the dietary pattern. For African Americans, the hazard ratios (95% CI)

for CVD mortality for the DASH and Mediterranean dietary patterns were 0.65 (0.54, 0.77) and 0.82 (0.70, 0.97) [women] and 0.73 (0.60, 0.89) and 0.75 (0.62, 0.90) [men], respectively. For Latinos, the hazard ratios (95% CI) for CVD mortality for the DASH and Mediterranean dietary patterns ranged were 0.91 (0.73, 1.14) and 0.89 (0.71, 1.11) [women] and 1.12 (0.93, 1.36) and 0.90 (0.75, 1.08) [men].

Optimal Macronutrient Intake Trial to Prevent Heart Disease (OMNI-Heart)

The OMNI-Heart trial examined how the effects of the DASH dietary pattern might change with substitution of protein or unsaturated fat for some of the carbohydrates in the original DASH dietary pattern (55% of calories from carbohydrate). Three different macronutrient diets—OMNI-Carb (i.e., original DASH), OMNI-Protein, and OMNI-MUFA (monounsaturated fat)—were compared to determine the effects on blood pressure and lipids [4]. Table 14.1 details the macronutrient content of the diets. The study included 164 individuals (55% were African American, 40% non-Hispanic White, and 5% other race). The primary outcomes were systolic blood pressure and LDL. Secondary outcomes were diastolic blood pressure, HDL, and triglycerides. SBP, DBP, LDL, and total cholesterol were significantly lower on all diets. HDL was significantly lower on OMNI-Carb and OMNI-Protein, but there was no significant difference on OMNI-MUFA. The 10-year CVD risk score decreased by 16.1%, 21.0%, and 19.6% in the OMNI-Carb, OMNI-Protein, and OMNI-MUFA diets, respectively. For African Americans, SBP was

Table 14.1 Macronutrient content of the dietary patterns in the OMNI-Heart Trial

Macronutrient	OMNI-carbohydrate (%)	OMNI-protein (%)	OMNI-MUFA (%)
Carbohydrate	58	48	48
Protein	15	25	15
Fat	27	27	37

1.5 mmHg lower on OMNI-Protein than OMNI-Carb ($p = 0.009$), but there was no significant difference in SBP between the OMNI-MUFA and OMNI-Carb. For African Americans, there was also no significant difference between LDL on any of the diets. The authors concluded that within DASH dietary patterns, exchanging some of the carbohydrates with protein or monounsaturated fat can further decrease the risk for cardiovascular disease with additional reductions of blood pressure and improvements in lipids.

Barriers to Healthy Eating Patterns in African American and Latino Communities

Although there is a substantial amount of evidence about healthy dietary patterns to prevent and treat cardiovascular disease, African American and Latino populations are less likely to consume these foods.[8, 10–12] Several qualitative studies examined the environmental barriers to healthy eating in underprivileged African American and Latino communities. These barriers included the following: (1) lack of access to fresh produce, including decreased local access and lack of transportation to get to areas where it is available [48, 51]; (2) high cost of healthier food [6, 19, 40, 48, 51]; (3) easy access to fast foods [19, 40]; (4) lack of time to prepare health foods [19, 40, 48]; (5) lack of social support [6, 19]; and (6) lack of knowledge about foods [6].

Physical Activity

The 2018 Physical Activity Guidelines recommend that individuals get 150–300 minutes of moderate-to-vigorous physical activity (MVPA) per week, which is unchanged from the 2008 guidelines [35]. However, the 2018 guidelines no longer stipulate that the exercise must occur in sessions of at least 10 minutes. A subcommittee of that group published a systematic umbrella review that included physical activity and cardiovascular disease and mortality [26]. The authors reported an inverse dose response relationship between physical activity and CVD mortality, CHD, ischemic stroke, and heart failure, that is, increasing amounts of physical activity led to decreased incidence of cardiovascular outcomes. The authors observed that outcomes among subgroups were difficult to assess, but noted that because of the large size and diversity of the populations included, the results could be generalized across sex, race, age, and BMI.

Barriers to Physical Activity in African Americans

An integrative review of the barriers to physical activity encountered by African American women was published in 2015 [25]. Intrapersonal barriers included lack of time; lack of motivation; tiredness/fatigue; lack of knowledge; health conditions and physical activity-related health concerns; concerns about physical appearance; and cost of facilities. Interpersonal barriers included role of family and gender; lack of social support; and lack of a physical activity partner. Community/environmental barriers included lack of physically active role models; neighborhood/community safety concerns; lack of sidewalks; lack of facilities; and weather conditions.

The authors note that the intrapersonal barriers have been documented among all genders and races, but they also mention that concerns about hair and the desire to maintain a "full-figured body shape" might be unique to African American women. However, the full-figured body shape is also preferred among some Latina women as well [27]. Because some in the African American and Latino cultures prefer the full-figured body shape, it may lead to decreased social support for physical activity among family and friends.

Barriers to Physical Activity in Latinos

A review of the social and environmental influence on physical activity among Latinas was published in 2013 [27]. Social influences included family, friends, and social networks. The social barriers to physical activity included lack of time due to family obligations and household responsibilities; fatigue; lack of childcare; jealousy of male partners; lack of a physical activity partner; view that physical activity is "unfeminine"; and the preference for larger body types among some in the Latino culture. The environmental barriers were similar to those in the African American community [25], including unsafe neighborhoods with less "walk-ability," few exercise facilities, and weather. The authors noted one potential barrier that may be unique to some of the Latino population is "fear of immigration enforcement."

It is important to note that one study of semi-structured interviews with Hispanic men echoed the concern about the lack of safe places to engage in physical activity [19].

In both African Americans and Latinos, environmental barriers seem to be related to socioeconomic status. If individuals do not feel safe exercising in their neighborhoods or if they cannot afford exercise facilities, then it is unclear how or where they can exercise.

Physical Activity Interventions in African American Women

A systematic review of articles published from 2009 to 2015 about physical activity interventions in African American women included 13 interventions [9]. The interventions occurred in both urban and rural locations in a variety of settings, such as community health centers, a medical center, churches, beauty salons, and a college university. Many types of physical activities were included—walking, running, dancing, yoga, kickboxing, aerobic, and housework. The interventions lasted between 5 weeks and 24 months. Since there was so much variation in the intervention and methods, it is not surprising that the results from the studies were mixed. At the end of the interventions, 7 of the 13 studies showed an increase in physical activity, while others showed little change. Some studies were not designed to show definitive differences in physical activity, but to provide information about feasibility of certain interventions and understand barriers to

physical activity that African American women face. The authors concluded it is possible to increase physical activity among African American women and that the data collected from the studies could be used to improve future interventions.

An integrative review of articles published from 2000 to 2015 including interventions promoting physical activity in African American women was published in 2017, and it contained 32 studies [24]. Half of the studies focused only on physical activity, the other half included physical activity and nutrition. As in the systematic review, the interventions ran the gamut in terms of sites, duration, types of physical activity, facilitators, and methodology. Some of the interventions were in-person, over the phone, or a combination. Some non-faith-based interventions occurred in faith-based settings, but there were some faith-based interventions as well. The authors did not give a specific summary about how many of the studies had significant results, but noted that the results were "mixed" in almost all categories.

Both reviews recommended more randomized controlled trials and larger sample sizes to find definitive evidence about which interventions are successful.

A systematic review of physical activity interventions with African American or Latino men was published in 2018, and it included nine articles about seven studies [21]. Of the seven studies, six included African American men and two included Latino men. The number of African American participants ranged from 31 to 101, and the number of Latino male participants ranged from 6 to 49. Studies were conducted in several different settings, including churches, a gym, a community wellness center, a community outreach center, and an academic medical center. The interventions lasted from 7 days to 12 months. Only two of the seven studies reported improvements in physical activity, but the authors were encouraged that physical activity interventions are including African American and Latino men and suggest that interventions be specifically developed for them in the future.

One review that analyzed physical activity interventions in Hispanic adults was published in

2012 [23], and it included 20 studies of interventions that included at least 35% Hispanic adult participants. Interventions were held in community, clinical, faith-based, and family/home-based settings. The interventions lasted from one session to 12 months. According to the authors, 19 of the 20 studies indicated an improvement in either physical activity, knowledge, fitness, or psychological well-being. Authors recommended interventions include cultural components, social support, and self-management along with environmental and policy changes to have lasting effect on physical activity among Hispanic adults.

Diet and Exercise Interventions

PREMIER

The PREMIER Trial examined the effects of a comprehensive lifestyle intervention on blood pressure [3]. This was an 18-month trial where 810 women and men with prehypertension or hypertension were randomized to one of three groups. The "advice only" group received information about ways to treat elevated blood pressure including weight management, sodium intake, physical activity, and the DASH diet. The "established" group was given the following goals: (1) lose 15 pounds in 6 months; (2) 180 minutes of moderately vigorous physical activity weekly; (3) less than 100 mEq of sodium daily; and (4) less than 0.5 ounces and 1 ounce of alcohol daily for women and men, respectively. The "established plus DASH" group was given all the goals in the established group as well as instruction about meeting the dietary goals of the DASH diet. Individuals in the established and established plus DASH groups were expected to attend 14 group meetings and four individual counseling sessions. The primary outcome was change in SBP at 6 months. Blood pressure declined in all groups. Compared to the participants without hypertension, those with hypertension experienced a larger decline in their BP (Table 14.2). There was a significant difference between the change in SBP in the advice only

Table 14.2 Mean changes in SBP in the PREMIER Trial

	Advice only	Established	Established plus DASH
SBP (mmHg)			
All	6.6 (9.2)	10.5 (10.1)	11.1 (9.9)
Hypertensive	7.8 (10.3)	12.5 (11.5)	14.2 (10.1)
Non-hypertensive	5.8 (8.4)	9.4 (9.1)	9.2 (9.3)

group and both the established and established plus DASH groups ($p < 0.001$ for both). The difference between the change in SBP between the established and established plus DASH was not significant ($p = 0.30$). Individuals in the established and established plus DASH groups who attended more intervention sessions experienced greater declines in SBP.

The PREMEIR Trial group also examined the outcomes by race, sex, hypertension status, and age. Authors divided the population into African American women (26%) and men (9%) and non-African American women (36%) and men (29%). Although SBP decreased in all populations in all intervention groups, the difference between the advice-only group and the established and established plus DASH groups was not statistically significant for African American females ($p = 0.4028$ and 0.1851, respectively). These same numbers were statistically significant for African American men ($p = 0.0076$ and 0.0045, respectively), non-African American women ($p = 0.0005$ and 0.0013, respectively), and non-African American men ($p = 0.0004$ and <0.0001, respectively). The only population for which established plus DASH group was better than established group was participants aged 50 and older.

Exercise and Nutrition Interventions for CardiOvasculaR hEalth (ENCORE)

The Exercise and Nutrition interventions for CardiOvasculaR hEalth (ENCORE) study [10] was a 16-week intervention that included 144 men and women with pre-HTN or stage 1

HTN. Participants were randomized to either a control diet (UC); DASH diet with weekly sessions with a nutritionist (DASH-A); or reduced calorie-DASH diet with weekly session with nutritionist and cognitive behavioral therapy strategies, and thrice weekly supervised 45-minute exercise sessions (DASH-WM [weight management]). The primary outcome was changed in blood pressure. Secondary outcomes included changes in cardiovascular biomarkers including pulse wave velocity (PWV); baroreflex sensitivity (BRS); brachial artery flow-mediated dilation (FMD); and left ventricular mass index. Post-treatment blood pressure was lower in all three groups; the reduction in SBP/DBP was 16.1/9.9, 11.2/7.5, and 3.4/3.8 in DASH-WM, DASH-A, and UC, respectively. When compared to the UC group, the change in blood pressure was significantly lower in the DASH-WM and DASH-A groups ($p < 0.001$ for both comparisons). For both SBP and DBP, the change in blood pressure was significantly lower in DASH-WM group than the DASH-A ($p = 0.02$ and $p < 0.048$, respectively). For the cardiovascular biomarkers, DASH-A and DASH-WM were combined and compared with UC; then DASH-A and DASH-WM were compared to each other. Compared to the UC group, PWV was significantly lower in the DASH groups ($p = 0.001$); compared to the DASH-A group, PWV was significantly lower in the DASH-WM ($p = 0.045$). While FMD improved more in the DASH groups than UC group ($p = 0.06$), the difference was not statistically significant, and there was no difference in FMD between DASH-A and DASH-WM ($p = 0.99$). For BRS, there was no difference between the DASH groups and UC ($p = 0.38$), but DASH-WM showed greater improvements than DASH-A ($p = 0.01$). The left ventricular mass index was lower in the DASH groups than in the UC group, but it was not significant ($p = 0.26$); however, DASH-WM had lower LV mass index than DASH-A ($p = 0.02$). The authors concluded that adding weight loss and exercise to the DASH diet improved blood pressure and cardiovascular biomarkers than the DASH diet alone.

For the ENCORE trial, this same group examined how adherence and blood pressure outcomes varied by race [18]. The primary outcomes were composite index of adherence to the DASH diet and clinic BP. Even when adjusting for lower income and age, African Americans had lower pre-intervention DASH adherence largely due to less consumption of low-fat dairy and increased consumption of sweets. Although post-treatment DASH adherence increased in both White Americans and African Americans, it was still lower in African Americans ($p < 0.001$), who consumed more meat, fat, sweets, and less fruit. Overall, participants with higher DASH adherence had lower BP. Authors recommend modifying traditional African American recipes and using principle of community-based participatory research to increase dietary adherence.

References

1. Ainsworth BE, Haskell WL, Herrmann SD, Meckes N, Bassett DR Jr, Tudor-Locke C, Greer JL, Vezina J, Whitt-Glover MC, Leon AS. 2011 Compendium of Physical Activities: a second update of codes and MET values. Med Sci Sports Exerc. 2011;43:1575–81.
2. Appel LJ, Moore TJ, Obarzanek E, Vollmer WM, Svetkey LP, Sacks FM, Bray GA, Vogt TM, Cutler JA, Windhauser MM, Lin PH, Karanja N. A clinical trial of the effects of dietary patterns on blood pressure. DASH Collaborative Research Group. N Engl J Med. 1997;336:1117–24.
3. Appel LJ, Champagne CM, Harsha DW, Cooper LS, Obarzanek E, Elmer PJ, Stevens VJ, Vollmer WM, Lin PH, Svetkey LP, Stedman SW, Young DR, Writing Group of the PREMIER Collaborative Research Group. Effects of comprehensive lifestyle modification on blood pressure control: main results of the PREMIER clinical trial. JAMA. 2003;289:2083–93.
4. Appel LJ, Sacks FM, Carey VJ, Obarzanek E, Swain JF, Miller ER, Conlin PR, Erlinger TP, Rosner BA, Laranjo NM, Charleston J, McCarron P, Bishop LM, OmniHeart Collaborative Research Group. Effects of protein, monounsaturated fat, and carbohydrate intake on blood pressure and serum lipids: results of the OmniHeart randomized trial. JAMA. 2005;294:2455–64.
5. Baker EA, Barnidge EK, Schootman M, Sawicki M, Motton-Kershaw FL. Adaptation of a modified DASH diet to a rural African American community setting. Am J Prev Med. 2016;51:967–74.

6. Baruth M, Sharpe PA, Parra-Medina D, Wilcox S. Perceived barriers to exercise and healthy eating among women from disadvantaged neighborhoods: results from a focus groups assessment. Women Health. 2014;54:336–53.

7. Bechthold A, Boeing H, Schwedhelm C, Hoffmann G, Knüppel S, Iqbal K, De Henauw S, Michels N, Devleesschauwer B, Schlesinger S, Schwingshackl L. Food groups and risk of coronary heart disease, stroke and heart failure: a systematic review and dose-response meta-analysis of prospective studies. Crit Rev Food Sci Nutr. 2019;59:1071–90.

8. Benjamin EJ, Muntner P, Alonso A, Bittencourt MS, Callaway CW, Carson AP, Chamberlain AM, Chang AR, Cheng S, Das SR, Delling FN, Djousse L, Elkind MSV, Ferguson JF, Fornage M, Jordan LC, Khan SS, Kissela BM, Knutson KL, Kwan TW, Lackland DT, Lewis TT, Lichtman JH, Longenecker CT, Loop MS, Lutsey PL, Martin SS, Matsushita K, Moran AE, Mussolino ME, O'Flaherty M, Pandey A, Perak AM, Rosamond WD, Roth GA, Sampson UKA, Satou GM, Schroeder EB, Shah SH, Spartano NL, Stokes A, Tirschwell DL, Tsao CW, Turakhia MP, VanWagner LB, Wilkins JT, Wong SS, Virani SS, Epidemiology American Heart Association Council on, Committee Prevention Statistics, and Subcommittee Stroke Statistics. Heart disease and stroke statistics-2019 update: a report from the American Heart Association. Circulation. 2019;139:e56–e528.

9. Bland V, Sharma M. Physical activity interventions in African American women: a systematic review. Health Promot Perspect. 2017;7:52–9.

10. Blumenthal JA, Babyak MA, Hinderliter A, Watkins LL, Craighead L, Lin PH, Caccia C, Johnson J, Waugh R, Sherwood A. Effects of the DASH diet alone and in combination with exercise and weight loss on blood pressure and cardiovascular biomarkers in men and women with high blood pressure: the ENCORE study. Arch Intern Med. 2010;170:126–35.

11. Boone-Heinonen J, Gordon-Larsen P, Kiefe CI, Shikany JM, Lewis CE, Popkin BM. Fast food restaurants and food stores: longitudinal associations with diet in young to middle-aged adults: the CARDIA study. Arch Intern Med. 2011;171:1162–70.

12. Bowman SA, Clemens JC, Martin CL, Anand J, Steinfeldt LC, Moshfegh AJ. Added sugars intake of Americans: what we eat in America, NHANES 2013–2014. Edited by Food Surveys Research Group. Dietary Data Brief, No. 18. 2017.

13. Chen ST, Maruthur NM, Appel LJ. The effect of dietary patterns on estimated coronary heart disease risk: results from the Dietary Approaches to Stop Hypertension (DASH) trial. Circ Cardiovasc Qual Outcomes. 2010;3:484–9.

14. Chiavaroli L, Viguiliouk E, Nishi SK, Blanco Mejia S, Rahelić D, Kahleová H, Salas-Salvadó J, Kendall CW, Sievenpiper JL. DASH dietary pattern and cardiometabolic outcomes: an umbrella review of systematic reviews and meta-analyses. Nutrients. 2019;11(2):338.

15. Corsino L, Rocha-Goldberg MP, Batch BC, Ortiz-Melo DI, Bosworth HB, Svetkey LP. The Latino Health Project: pilot testing a culturally adapted behavioral weight loss intervention in obese and overweight Latino adults. Ethn Dis. 2012;22:51–7.

16. Danaei G, Ding EL, Mozaffarian D, Taylor B, Rehm J, Murray CJ, Ezzati M. The preventable causes of death in the United States: comparative risk assessment of dietary, lifestyle, and metabolic risk factors. PLoS Med. 2009;6:e1000058.

17. Eckel RH, Jakicic JM, Ard JD, de Jesus JM, Houston Miller N, Hubbard VS, Lee IM, Lichtenstein AH, Loria CM, Millen BE, Nonas CA, Sacks FM, Smith SC Jr, Svetkey LP, Wadden TA, Yanovski SZ. 2013 AHA/ACC guideline on lifestyle management to reduce cardiovascular risk: a report of the American College of Cardiology/American Heart Association Task Force on Practice Guidelines. J Am Coll Cardiol. 2014;63:2960–84.

18. Epstein DE, Sherwood A, Smith PJ, Craighead L, Caccia C, Lin PH, Babyak MA, Johnson JJ, Hinderliter A, Blumenthal JA. Determinants and consequences of adherence to the dietary approaches to stop hypertension diet in African-American and white adults with high blood pressure: results from the ENCORE trial. J Acad Nutr Diet. 2012;112:1763–73.

19. Garcia DO, Valdez LA, Hooker SP. Hispanic male's perspectives of health behaviors related to weight management. Am J Mens Health. 2017;11:1547–59.

20. Glenn AJ, Viguiliouk E, Seider M, Boucher BA, Khan TA, Blanco Mejia S, Jenkins DJA, Kahleová H, Rahelić D, Salas-Salvadó J, Kendall CWC, Sievenpiper JL. Relation of vegetarian dietary patterns with major cardiovascular outcomes: a systematic review and meta-analysis of prospective cohort studies. Front Nutr. 2019;6:80.

21. Griffith DM, Bergner EM, Cornish EK, McQueen CM. Physical activity interventions with African American or Latino men: a systematic review. Am J Mens Health. 2018;12:1102–17.

22. Harmon BE, Boushey CJ, Shvetsov YB, Ettienne R, Reedy J, Wilkens LR, Le Marchand L, Henderson BE, Kolonel LN. Associations of key diet-quality indexes with mortality in the Multiethnic Cohort: the Dietary Patterns Methods Project. Am J Clin Nutr. 2015;101:587–97.

23. Ickes MJ, Sharma M. A systematic review of physical activity interventions in Hispanic adults. J Environ Public Health. 2012;2012:156435.

24. Jenkins F, Jenkins C, Gregoski MJ, Magwood GS. Interventions promoting physical activity in African American women: an integrative review. J Cardiovasc Nurs. 2017;32:22–9.

25. Joseph RP, Ainsworth BE, Keller C, Dodgson JE. Barriers to physical activity among African American women: an integrative review of the literature. Women Health. 2015;55:679–99.

26. Kraus WE, Powell KE, Haskell WL, Janz KF, Campbell WW, Jakicic JM, Troiano RP, Sprow K, Torres A, Piercy KL, 2018 Physical Activity Guidelines

Advisory Committee*. Physical activity, all-cause and cardiovascular mortality, and cardiovascular disease. Med Sci Sports Exerc. 2019;51:1270–81.

27. Larsen BA, Pekmezi D, Marquez B, Benitez TJ, Marcus BH. Physical activity in Latinas: social and environmental influences. Womens Health (Lond). 2013;9:201–10.

28. Larson NI, Story MT, Nelson MC. Neighborhood environments: disparities in access to healthy foods in the U.S. Am J Prev Med. 2009;36:74–81.

29. Levitan EB, Ahmed A, Arnett DK, Polak JF, Hundley WG, Bluemke DA, Heckbert SR, Jacobs DR, Nettleton JA. Mediterranean diet score and left ventricular structure and function: the Multi-Ethnic Study of Atherosclerosis. Am J Clin Nutr. 2016;104:595–602.

30. Miller ER, Cooper LA, Carson KA, Wang NY, Appel LJ, Gayles D, Charleston J, White K, You N, Weng Y, Martin-Daniels M, Bates-Hopkins B, Robb I, Franz WK, Brown EL, Halbert JP, Albert MC, Dalcin AT, Yeh HC. A dietary intervention in urban African Americans: results of the "five plus nuts and beans" randomized trial. Am J Prev Med. 2016;50:87–95.

31. Morland K, Wing S, Diez Roux A. The contextual effect of the local food environment on residents' diets: the atherosclerosis risk in communities study. Am J Public Health. 2002;92:1761–7.

32. Nahab F, Le A, Judd S, Frankel MR, Ard J, Newby PK, Howard VJ. Racial and geographic differences in fish consumption: the REGARDS study. Neurology. 2011;76:154–8.

33. Nahab F, Pearson K, Frankel MR, Ard J, Safford MM, Kleindorfer D, Howard VJ, Judd S. Dietary fried fish intake increases risk of CVD: the REasons for Geographic And Racial Differences in Stroke (REGARDS) study. Public Health Nutr. 2016;19:3327–36.

34. Nguyen HT, Bertoni AG, Nettleton JA, Bluemke DA, Levitan EB, Burke GL. DASH eating pattern is associated with favorable left ventricular function in the multi-ethnic study of atherosclerosis. J Am Coll Nutr. 2012;31:401–7.

35. Physical Activity Guidelines Advisory Committee. 2018 Physical Activity Guidelines Advisory Committee scientific report. Washington, DC: US Department of Health and Human Services; 2018.

36. Piercy KL, Troiano RP, Ballard RM, Carlson SA, Fulton JE, Galuska DA, George SM, Olson RD. The physical activity guidelines for Americans. JAMA. 2018;320:2020–8.

37. Rankins J, Sampson W, Brown B, Jenkins-Salley T. Dietary Approaches to Stop Hypertension (DASH) intervention reduces blood pressure among hypertensive African American patients in a neighborhood health care center. J Nutr Educ Behav. 2005;37:259–64.

38. Rankins J, Wortham J, Brown LL. Modifying soul food for the Dietary Approaches to Stop Hypertension diet (DASH) plan: implications for metabolic syndrome (DASH of Soul). Ethn Dis. 2007;17:S4-7–12.

39. Rees K, Takeda A, Martin N, Ellis L, Wijesekara D, Vepa A, Das A, Hartley L, Stranges S. Mediterranean-style diet for the primary and secondary prevention of cardiovascular disease. Cochrane Database Syst Rev. 2019;3:CD009825.

40. Richards Adams IK, Figueroa W, Hatsu I, Odei JB, Sotos-Prieto M, Leson S, Huling J, Joseph JJ. An examination of demographic and psychosocial factors, barriers to healthy eating, and diet quality among African American adults. Nutrients. 2019;11(3):519.

41. Rocha-Goldberg MDP, Corsino L, Batch B, Voils CI, Thorpe CT, Bosworth HB, Svetkey LP. Hypertension Improvement Project (HIP) Latino: results of a pilot study of lifestyle intervention for lowering blood pressure in Latino adults. Ethn Health. 2010;15:269–82.

42. Sacks FM, Svetkey LP, Vollmer WM, Appel LJ, Bray GA, Harsha D, Obarzanek E, Conlin PR, Miller ER, Simons-Morton DG, Karanja N, Lin PH, DASH-Sodium Collaborative Research Group. Effects on blood pressure of reduced dietary sodium and the Dietary Approaches to Stop Hypertension (DASH) diet. DASH-Sodium Collaborative Research Group. N Engl J Med. 2001;344:3–10.

43. Sedentary Behaviour Research Network. Letter to the editor: standardized use of the terms "sedentary" and "sedentary behaviours". Appl Physiol Nutr Metab. 2012;37:540–2.

44. Shen J, Wilmot KA, Ghasemzadeh N, Molloy DL, Burkman G, Mekonnen G, Gongora MC, Quyyumi AA, Sperling LS. Mediterranean dietary patterns and cardiovascular health. Annu Rev Nutr. 2015;35:425–49.

45. Svetkey LP, Simons-Morton D, Vollmer WM, Appel LJ, Conlin PR, Ryan DH, Ard J, Kennedy BM. Effects of dietary patterns on blood pressure: subgroup analysis of the Dietary Approaches to Stop Hypertension (DASH) randomized clinical trial. Arch Intern Med. 1999;159:285–93.

46. US Department of Health and Human Services and US Department of Agriculture. Dietary guidelines for Americans, 2015–2020. Washington, DC: U.S. Government Printing Office; 2015.

47. US Dietary Guidelines Advisory Committee. Scientific report of the 2015 Dietary Guidelines Advisory Committee: advisory report to the Secretary of Health and Human Services and the Secretary of Agriculture. Washington, DC: United States Department of Agriculture; 2015.

48. White M, Addison C, Jenkins BWC, Henderson F, McGill D, Payton M, Antoine-LaVigne D. Factors affecting dietary practices in a Mississippi African American community. Int J Environ Res Public Health. 2017;14:718.

49. Whitt-Glover MC, Hunter JC, Foy CG, Quandt SA, Vitolins MZ, Leng I, Hornbuckle LM, Sanya KA, Bertoni AG. Translating the Dietary Approaches to Stop Hypertension (DASH) diet for use in underresourced, urban African American communities, 2010. Prev Chronic Dis. 2013;10:120088.

50. Young DR, Hivert MF, Alhassan S, Camhi SM, Ferguson JF, Katzmarzyk PT, Lewis CE, Owen N, Perry CK, Siddique J, Yong CM, Lifestyle Physical Activity Committee of the Council on, Health Cardiometabolic, Cardiology Council on Clinical, Epidemiology Council on, Prevention, Genomics Council on Functional, Biology Translational, and Council Stroke. Sedentary behavior and cardiovascular morbidity and mortality: a science advisory from the American Heart Association. Circulation. 2016;134:e262–79.

51. Zenk SN, Odoms-Young AM, Dallas C, Hardy E, Watkins A, Hoskins-Wroten J, Holland L. "You have to hunt for the fruits, the vegetables": environmental barriers and adaptive strategies to acquire food in a low-income African American neighborhood. Health Educ Behav. 2011;38:282–92.

Coronary Calcium Scoring in African American and Hispanic Patients

15

Robert Gillespie and Matthew Budoff

Summary

During our training at Harbor UCLA over 30 years ago, we learned from our mentors Bruce Brundage, Robert Detrano, and others the value of coronary calcium scoring. Yet 30 years later, the debate has continued on its role in risk stratifying patients.

This chapter is intended to present some of the data strongly supportive of its use in all patient populations, including AA and Hispanics. This chapter is also intended to highlight the integration of this modality into many of our guidelines.

This again emphasizes the advance in our knowledge and acceptance of this power tool.

Coronary calcification and its association with atherosclerotic disease are well known. Studies of ancient Egyptian mummies dating prior to 1500 BCE have demonstrated the presence of calcium in vascular beds consistent with atherosclerosis [2]. The initial detection of coronary calcium by fluoroscopic imaging was described in 1959 [6]. Coronary calcium scoring (CAC) has subsequently emerged as a powerful tool used to

assess future cardiac risk [27]. It is not a marker for coronary artery disease. Instead, it is a definitive evidence for the presence of coronary artery disease [33, 42]. CAC assessment with basic fluoroscopy has evolved to more advanced technologies that allow us to quantify plaque burden. Electron beam computed tomography utilizing the Agatston score [1] provided the framework and extensive data for the use of this technique in the 1980s, followed by expansion with widely utilized multidetector computed tomography (MDCT). Both Agatston and volume score have been shown to be reproducible when used with EBCT and MDCT [26]. While there are many potential confounding variables including obesity, motion, heart rate, and scanner type, reproducibility of this technique is very good with intraobserver and interobserver agreement exceeding 90% [13].

In 2007, an observational study of over 25,000 patients by Budoff and colleagues demonstrated significant added value of using calcium scoring to risk stratify patients. In this study, after adjusting for risk factors, a CAC of 0 denoted a 10-year survival of 99.4% compared to 87.8% with a score >1000 [1]. Other imaging modalities including carotid intimal thickening and ankle brachial index have not been as effective in determining risk for future cardiac events [16].

CAC can be accomplished without the need for contrast agents at low radiation doses typically in the range of 1 mSv and has been supported in

R. Gillespie (✉)
Sharp Rees-Stealy Medical Group,
San Diego, CA, USA

M. Budoff
David Geffen School of Medicine at UCLA, Division of Cardiology, Harbor-UCLA Medical Center, Torrance, CA, USA
e-mail: mbudoff@lunquist.org

© Springer Nature Switzerland AG 2021
K. C. Ferdinand et al. (eds.), *Cardiovascular Disease in Racial and Ethnic Minority Populations*,
Contemporary Cardiology, https://doi.org/10.1007/978-3-030-81034-4_15

the cardiology guidelines for screening low to intermediate risk patients [18]. A review of the St. Francis Heart Study suggested the guidelines for the use of statins might over-treat those with low calcium scores and undertreat those with high calcium scores [41]. This article as well as others brought attention to the potential utility of coronary calcium assessment to help determine the institution of medical therapy.

Additionally, CAC can also be used to risk-stratify those most appropriate for aspirin use, which may prove useful as our guidelines move away from the routine use of aspirin in primary prevention. A recent systematic review and meta-analysis of 13 trials with 14,225 participants without known cardiovascular disease showed an absolute risk reduction of cardiovascular events of 0.38% with an absolute risk increase of 0.47% [46]. This would suggest net harm in the general population despite some reduction in cardiovascular events. However, the Multi-Ethnic Study of Atherosclerosis (MESA) trial showed that CAC can better risk-stratify those patients who may benefit from aspirin. In this study, participants with CAC ≥ 100 had favorable risk/benefit outcome estimates for aspirin use while participants with zero CAC were estimated to have net harm [28]. Both statins and aspirin are widely used drugs. and statins have a particularly large group of patients who are very concerned about taking these drugs. CAC can allow for a more informed decision-making discussion with our patients. Additionally, the preponderance of data suggests CAC improves medical management in those patients with abnormal scores. In these studies, it is not entirely clear if this improvement is patient driven by a change in lifestyle or physician driven by more aggressive medical therapy. The data would suggest both are likely, though the effect on behavior has not been fully delineated [35].

Other populations that CAC may provide valuable risk stratification include the very low risk of events in diabetics with low CAC, such as that seen in a meta-analysis by Budoff [10] and colleagues showing a significantly lower myocardial infarction rate which correlated with CAC. The lower the score, the lower the risk.

Generally, calcium scoring is best applied to patients over the age of 45. Younger patients tend to have a higher percentage of non-calcified plaque, and use of CAC scoring may underestimate plaque burden. Also, the prevalence of disease is low in younger patients and the test is best used only in the highest-risk patients in this group.

In patients with multiple risk factors, such as family history of very early onset of CAD or documented atherosclerosis in other vascular beds, the test may be of some benefit to further risk-stratify patients.

Nasir et al. [32] evaluated the interaction of CAC and family history in 5347 asymptomatic individuals (47% men; mean age 62 +/− 10 years) in the Multi-Ethnic Study of Atherosclerosis (MESA). The age-, gender-, and race-adjusted prevalence of CAC 0 was significantly higher with the presence of family history of premature CHD than for those with no family history at low risk (35% vs. 23%, $P < 0.0001$) and among those at intermediate risk (70% vs. 60%, $P < 0.01$). The strongest predictor of CAC were participants reporting + family history in both a parent and a sibling (odds ratio, 2.74; 95% CI, 1.64–4.59), followed by those reporting a family history in a sibling only (odds ratio, 2.06; 95% CI, 1.64–2.58), and still significant were those reporting a family history of premature CHD only in a parent (odds ratio, 1.52; 95% CI, 1.19–1.93).

Reclassification

It has been long sought to identify ways of improving risk classification beyond risk calculators, as many individuals are left at intermediate risk, which makes recommendations for further testing and treatment unclear. Of all the tests studied (including biomarkers, genetics and atherosclerosis, and vascular testing), CAC scoring results in the highest reclassification rates among those found to be at intermediate risk. This has been confirmed in multiple large epidemiologic cohorts, demonstrating the benefit of imaging subclinical coronary atherosclerosis with CT. Coronary artery calcium provided superior discrimination and risk reclassification compared with other risk markers in the NIH Sponsored Multi-Ethnic Study of Atherosclerosis (MESA) study. CAC demonstrated a net 25.5% of the events group was reclassified to high risk appropriately, while a net 40.4% of the nonevents group was appropriately reclassified into the low-risk group by the addition of CAC to the Framingham Risk Score. Yeboah et al. [45] studied multiple different mechanisms to reclassify risk and CAC had the highest improvement in both appropriate use criteria (AUC) and net reclassification index (NRI) when added to the Framingham Risk Score as compared to carotid imaging, C-reactive protein, family history, endothelial function testing, and ankle–brachial index. This has subsequently been validated in multiple cohort studies, including Rotterdam heart, Heinz Nixdorff Recall (HNR) study, Dallas heart study and Framingham heart study, among others [19].

Compliance

Multiple studies have demonstrated that the visualization of coronary artery calcification stimulates better health behaviors including statin and aspirin use, increasing cardiovascular exercise, improving diet, and weight reduction [19]. A meta-analysis reported six studies (11,256 participants, mean follow-up time: 1.6–6.0 years). Pooled estimates of the odds of aspirin initiation (OR: 2.6; 95% confidence interval [CI]: 1.8–3.8), lipid-lowering medication initiation (OR: 2.9; 95% CI: 1.9–4.4), blood pressure-lowering medication initiation (OR: 1.9; 95% CI: 1.6–2.3), lipid-lowering medication continuation (OR: 2.3; 95% CI: 1.6–3.3), increase in exercise (OR: 1.8; 95% CI: 1.4–2.4), and dietary change (OR: 1.9; 95% CI: 1.5–2.5) were higher in individuals with nonzero CAC versus zero CAC scores [3].

The Eisner study is the most notable of these studies, as it represents a prospective, randomized trial of CAC visualization versus none. This trial demonstrated, as compared with the no-scan group, the CAC group showed a net favorable change in systolic blood pressure ($p = 0.02$), low-density lipoprotein cholesterol ($p = 0.04$), and waist circumference ($p = 0.01$), and a tendency of weight loss among overweight subjects ($p = 0.07$). Patients with CAC were more likely to comply with statins, and initiate and maintain higher levels of aspirin, blood pressure lowering, and statin use over the 4 years of the randomized trial. Costs were neutral for obtaining a CAC as compared to those who did not get the test, as those with zero scores used less resources (medications, testing) and those with higher CAC scores had increased resource utilization. This was found to match intensity of therapy with increasing cardiovascular risk [35, 36].

The Impact of Zero CAC Score

Research to date has found a very low cardiovascular event rate among those with zero CAC [37]. Approximately 50% of the MESA sample had CAC scores of zero and had event rates that were less than 5% over the 10-year follow-up. This demonstrates an excellent opportunity for this risk marker to accurately "de-risk" certain subjects [9, 32]. This is concordant with other prospective longitudinal studies demonstrating that coronary artery calcium score of 0 results in the most accurate downward risk reclassification [5, 23]. In MESA, the 10 + −year average event rates for those participants with zero CAC remain well under 6%, signifying a low risk state [11].

A CAC score of zero has proven to be quite reassuring for both clinicians and patients for risk stratification. The long-term prognostic value of a CAC score of zero for asymptomatic individuals has been described in several studies. Valenti et al. [40] reported that a CAC score of zero conferred a 15-year warranty period against mortality for individuals at low to intermediate risk by the Framingham Risk Score (FRS) that was unaffected by gender or age. A CAC score of zero showed the lowest rates of mortality among the low-risk categories such as FRS < 10% or no cardiovascular risk factors. CAC zero afforded lower-risk than no-risk factors, even if those with CAC zero had multiple risk factors for heart disease. The risk of all-cause mortality was greater in individuals with a CAC score > 0 plus low FRS or low ATP III cardiovascular risk categories (CAC > 0+ low FRS, HR 3.3, 95% CI: 2.49–4.32, CAC > 0+ low ATP III, HR 3.09, 95% CI: 2.45–3.90) compared with those with a CAC score of zero plus high FRS or high ATP III cardiovascular risk categories.

In older adults, a CAC score of zero was associated with a vascular age that was 30 years lower than their chronological age [40]. Similarly, mortality risk in patients without evidence of CAC was significantly lower compared to that in the general US population across various age groups regardless of gender [31]. A CAC score of zero was shown to be a stronger negative risk predictor for all CAD and CVD events after a mean follow-up of 10.3 years among protective atherosclerotic risk factors such as carotid intima-media thickness <25th percentile or absence of carotid plaque, ankle-brachial index between 0.9 and 1.3, high-sensitivity C-reactive protein <2 mg/L, and no family history of CHD and healthy lifestyle [5]. A CAC score of zero resulted in the greatest reduction in posttest risk among all risk markers. Of the available options, a CAC score of zero is most strongly warranted as a rationale to downgrade risk and reconsider lifelong statin therapy when the patient or clinician is otherwise uncertain.

CAC in 2018 ACC/AHA Guidelines

The 2018 Cholesterol guidelines recommend that if the CAC score is zero, treatment with statin therapy may be withheld or delayed for 5–10 years, except in cigarette smokers, those with diabetes mellitus, and those with a strong family history of premature ASCVD. "If the coronary calcium score is zero, it is reasonable to withhold statin therapy and reassess in 5 to 10 years." The guidelines cite that the most important recent observation has been the finding that a CAC score of zero indicates a low ASCVD risk for the subsequent 10 years.

For those with CAC, the 2018 ACC/AHA Guidelines on the Management of Blood Cholesterol states: In adults 40–75 years of age without diabetes mellitus and with LDL-C levels ≥70 mg/dL-89 mg/dL (≥1.8–4.9 mmol/L), at a 10-year ASCVD risk of ≥7.5–19.9%, if a decision about statin therapy is uncertain, consider measuring CAC. A CAC score of 1–99 favors statin therapy, especially in those >55 years of age. For any patient, if the CAC score is ≥100 Agatston units or ≥75th percentile, statin therapy is indicated unless otherwise deferred by the outcome of clinician–patient risk discussion (Class IIa) [20, 21].

Diabetes

Individuals with diabetes have greater extent and prevalence of subclinical atherosclerosis. Several studies have demonstrated the prognostic value of CAC in reclassifying asymptomatic patients with diabetes [25, 39]. Unlike the general population, women and men with type 2 DM have a similar extent CAC, confirming the clinical evidence that diabetes negates the well-known advantage of women over men in prevalence and extent of atherosclerosis [24, 29]. Khaleeli et al. [24] reported that there was no significant difference in coronary calcification between men and women with diabetes. In another study, Mielke et al. [29] performed EBCT in 3389 patients with diabetes. They showed that women with diabetes had greater plaque burden when compared to men with a history of diabetes.

A CAC score of zero was associated with very low short-term and long-term CVD and all-cause mortality in non-diabetic and diabetic males and females. Large population-based studies have shown that a significant proportion of adults with diabetes have CAC scores of zero [25, 34, 39]. Raggi et al. [34] demonstrated that 39% of individuals with diabetes had a CAC score of zero.

In the Multi-Ethnic Study of Atherosclerosis (MESA) [25], 38% of DM patients were reported to have a CAC score of 0, and in the Heinz Nixdorf Recall (HNR) study, 39.3% of women with diabetes and 13.4% of men with diabetes had a CAC score of 0 [30]. Importantly, the absence of CAC predicted a low short-term risk of death (~1% at 5 years) for diabetic patients, which was slightly higher but statistically similar to that of non-diabetic patients in both studies.

In summary, CAC provides strong risk stratification of patients with diabetes. The mortality risk is higher in patients with diabetes than in patients without diabetes. However, about 40% of adult diabetics have a CAC score of zero or <10, and a very low mortality rate. The overall evidence would support the use of CAC scanning for risk stratification and to guide management in the asymptomatic DM patient, as recommended by a Class IIa indication in the 2010 AHA/ACC guidelines [17, 18].

Combining Calcium Score with Stress Testing

Normal stress tests of all modalities are associated with low short-term risks. A normal stress nuclear test both with exercise or with pharmacologic agents confers a low short-term risk, though inability to exercise in itself increases risks for CV events. This holds true for stress echocardiography with exercise and with dobutamine also. As a result, patients requiring pharmacologic stress because of inability to exercise are intrinsically at higher risk. Adding calcium scoring to stress testing further risk-stratifies these patients and allows for better long-term risk classification. Additionally, patients with suboptimal endurance with a Ca score of 0 are at lower risk than patients with Ca in their coronary arteries particularly with CAC >400 as noted in combination with SPECT imaging. The addition of CAC to stress testing provides another way to further risk-stratify our patients and can also assist in being more definitive in borderline cases. If the CAC is 0 and the stress test is equivocal, the likelihood is that the patient does not have high-risk disease. Conversely, the presence of Ca and a borderline stress test confers a higher risk and likely deserves additional assessment.

Calcium Scoring in African American and Hispanic Patients

African Americans (AA) die of heart disease at a higher rate than any other ethnic groups in the United States. Recent data from the 2018 Center for Disease Control (CDC) show that there is an over 40% increased risk of cardiovascular death for AA compared to White and Hispanic Americans that have a lower incidence of cardiovascular death.

The causes for these differences for these outcomes in large part can be attributed to increased risk factors for AA with the impact of hypertension markedly higher. Racial disparity in systolic blood pressure control plays a major role in nearly 8000 excess deaths annually from heart disease and stroke [15]. The incidence of diabetics, physical inactivity, and obesity also play a major role in these outcomes with the prevalence of overweight and obese AA much higher than all other race or ethnic group, particularly in AA women [44].

With this increased burden of cardiovascular disease comes a potentially even greater role for CAC. In a group of those considered at high risk, a tool to better identify those truly at high risk is very useful and can help identify those who would benefit from more aggressive intervention. Use of the Framingham Risk Score and other models are less precise and may in some cases significantly miscalculate risk.

By the early 2000s, the data was clear that CAC in White populations provided a substantial improvement in risk assessment when calcium scoring was added to traditional risk factor assessment. But it had not been clear if the large accumulating data on the utility of CAC applied to AA. This was of particular concern because of the known differences in extent of coronary calcification in different ethnic groups. Previous studies had shown that there were highly variable differences in the prevalence and extent of calcification in different ethnic groups, generally with less calcification in AA and Hispanic patients. A study published by Doherty [14] appeared to be paradoxical. AA had lower CAC with clearly having higher event rates, despite having similar risk factor profiles. The hazard ratio for cardiovascular events after 70 months was 2.16. In this study, while overall risk factor profiles were similar, there were some important differences. AA had significantly higher systolic blood pressures, higher incidence of diabetes, and higher BMI, all of which may have played a role in the differences in outcomes.

Bild et al. [4] showed in a review of the MESA data, after adjustment for risk factors, that the prevalence of detectable coronary calcification was 22% and 15% lower among AA and Hispanic individuals. Those with a CAC > 0 was greatest among White individuals. This was seen in a number of other studies as well with the one notable exception [22]. In 2008, a review by Detrano et al. in 6722 asymptomatic men and women from the MESA cohort with 27.6% AA and 21% Hispanic and 11.9% Chinese showed that doubling of the CAC increased the risk of MI or death from CAD by 15–35% leading the authors to correctly conclude that coronary calcium is a strong predictor of incident coronary heart disease providing predictive data beyond traditional risk factor assessment in all patients, not only White individuals. There was no significant difference in predictive value for any of these groups [13]. The largest risk was in those with calcium scores of over 100, as seen in many studies as outlined previously. This was further supported by additional assessment of the MESA database which supported using absolute CAC instead of age–sex–race indices [7, 9]. Progressive increased cardiovascular risk was seen as the score increased to above 400. The 2013 multimodality AUC cited the threshold of Agatston Score >100 as appropriate for exercise ECG, stress RNI, and stress echo in asymptomatic patients and noted CTA may be appropriate [43].

The ethnic variation in the extent of calcium in coronary arteries has long been known. Tang et al. [38] looked at 1461 asymptomatic high-risk subjects using digital subtraction fluoroscopy and cinefluoroscopy. In this high-risk population, only 36% of AA had coronary calcium compared to 60% in White and Asian Americans despite using logistic regression algorithms to take into account variation in risk factors. As in other studies, AA still had poorer outcomes, when followed for 20 months. Budoff et al. [8] used EBCT to assess the correlation between ethnic differences and symptomatic patients with coronary obstruction. The incidence of coronary calcium and obstructive disease in symptomatic AA and Hispanic patients was lower than White patients independent of risk factor profiles. The burden of atherosclerosis is higher in White patients despite an overall better prognosis. The reasons for the variation in the extent of coronary calcium in both asymptomatic and symptomatic patients are not known. Possible etiologies include variation in calcium intake, vitamin D metabolism, or other genetic differences.

NHLBI's Multi-Ethnic Atherosclerosis Study (MESA) [4] measured CAC in participants including White, Black, Hispanic, and Chinese participants. Significant ethnic differences were noted in the prevalence of CAC after adjustment for risk factors, with a relative risk of CAC being 15% less in Hispanic individuals, 22% less in Black individuals, and 8% less in Chinese individuals than in White Individuals. Budoff et al. [12] published a report on 16,560 asymptomatic individuals from multiple ethnicities, demonstrating similar results.

Conclusively, racial differences do exist in the prevalence and severity of CAC. These differences are more prominent in men. White patients and South Asian patients have been noted to have a higher prevalence of CAC as compared to other ethnic groups, even after the adjustment of risk factors. In light of these findings, studies, and statements mentioned above, the prevalence and extent of coronary calcification differ considerably among ethnic groups. From current data, mostly from MESA and HNR, these differences do not seem to reduce the predictive value of this subclinical marker in US minority groups. Regardless of the prevalence of calcification across different ages, race/ethnicity and gender, a CAC score of >100 imparts a high-risk patient. Budoff demonstrated in MESA that all participants, regardless of demographics, had a 10-year ASCVD event rate of >7.5%, imparting similar high-risk status [11].

In conclusion, CAC score is a robust imaging modality that allows for accurate assessment of cardiac risks in asymptomatic patients. It is more accurate in predicting events than any technique available in asymptomatic patients. CAC scoring provides incremental improvement in classification of risk beyond our traditional modalities such as the Framingham Risk Score or other algorithms. Finally, CAC score has been shown to help direct appropriate medical therapy with aspirin and statins in the appropriate risk populations. These findings also apply to all patients including Hispanic and African American populations.

References

1. Agatston AS, et al. Quantification of coronary calcium score using ultrafast computed tomography. JACC. 1990;15(4):827–8332.
2. Allam AH, et al. Atherosclerosis in ancient Egyptian mummies. JACC Cardiovasc Imaging. 2011;4(4):315–27. https://doi.org/10.1016/j.jcmg.2011.02.002.
3. Ankur G, et al. The identification of calcified coronary plaque is associated with initiation and continuation of pharmacological and lifestyle preventive therapies: a systematic review and meta-analysis. JACC Cardiovasc Imaging. 2017;10(8):833–42.
4. Bild DE, et al. Ethnic differences in coronary calcification: the multi-ethnic study of atherosclerosis (MESA). Circulation. 2005;111(10):1313–20.
5. Blaha MJ, Cainzos-Achirica M, Greenland P, McEvoy JW, Blankstein R, Budoff MJ, Dardari Z, Sibley CT, Burke GL, Kronmal RA, Szklo M, Blumenthal RS, Nasir K. Role of coronary artery calcium score of zero and other negative risk markers for cardiovascular disease: the Multi-Ethnic Study of Atherosclerosis (MESA). Circulation. 2016;133:849–58.
6. Blankenhorn DH, Stern D. Calcification of the coronary arteries. Am J Roentgenol Radium Therapy, Nucl Med. 1959;81(5):772.
7. Budoff MJ, et al. Coronary calcium predicts events better with absolute calcium scores than age-sex-race/ethnicity percentiles. JACC. 2009a;53(4):345–52.
8. Budoff MJ, et al. Ethnic differences in coronary atherosclerosis. J Am Coll Cardiol. 2002;39:408–12.
9. Budoff MJ, McClelland RL, Nasir K, Greenland P, Kronmal RA, Kondos GT, Shea S, Lima JA, Blumenthal RS. Cardiovascular events with absent or minimal coronary calcification: the Multi-Ethnic Study of Atherosclerosis (MESA). Am Heart J. 2009b;158:554–61.
10. Budoff MJ, Raggi P, Beller GA. Noninvasive cardiovascular risk assessment of the asymptomatic diabetic patient: the Imaging Council of the American College of Cardiology. JACC Cardiovasc Imaging. 2016;9(2):176–92.
11. Budoff MJ, Young R, Burke G, Jeffrey Carr J, Detrano RC, Folsom AR, Kronmal R, Lima JAC, Liu KJ, McClelland RL, Michos E, Post WS, Shea S, Watson KE, Wong ND. Ten-year association of coronary artery calcium with atherosclerotic cardiovascular disease (ASCVD) events: the multi-

12. ethnic study of atherosclerosis (MESA). Eur Heart J. 2018;39(25):2401–8.
12. Budoff MJ, et al. Ethnic differences of the presence and severity of coronary atherosclerosis. Atherosclerosis. 2006;187(2):343–50.
13. Detrano R, Guerci AD, Carr JJ, et al. Coronary calcium as a predictor of coronary events in four racial or ethnic groups. N Engl J Med. 2008;358:1336–45.
14. Doherty TM, et al. Racial differences in the significance of coronary calcium in asymptomatic black and white subjects with coronary risk factors. JACC. 1999;34(3):789–94.
15. Fiscella K. Racial disparity on hypertension control: tallying the death toll. Ann Fam Med. 2008;6(6):497–502.
16. Gepner AD, et al. Comparison of carotid plaque score and coronary artery calcium score for predicting cardiovascular disease events: the multi-EthnicStudy of atherosclerosis. J Am Heart Assoc. 2017;6:e005179. https://doi.org/10.1161/JAHA.116.005179.
17. Greenland P, et al. 2010 ACCF/AHA guideline for assessment of cardiovascular disease in asymptomatic adults: a report of the ACCF/AHA Task Force on Practice Guidelines. JACC. 2010a;56(25):e50.
18. Greenland P, Alpert JS, Beller GA, Benjamin EJ, Budoff MJ, Fayad ZA, Foster E, Hlatky MA, Hodgson JM, Kushner FG, Lauer MS, Shaw LJ, Smith SC Jr, Taylor AJ, Weintraub WS, Wenger NK. 2010 ACCF/AHA guideline for assessment of cardiovascular risk in asymptomatic adults: a report of the American College of Cardiology Foundation/American Heart Association task force on practice guidelines. J Am Coll Cardiol. 2010b;56:50–103.
19. Greenland P, Blaha MJ, Budoff MJ, Erbel R, Watson KE. Coronary calcium score and cardiovascular risk. J Am Coll Cardiol. 2018;72(4):434–47.
20. Grundy SM, Stone NJ, Bailey AL, et al. ACC/AHA/AACVPR/AAPA/ABC/ACPM/ADA/AGS/APhA/ASPC/NLA/PCNA guideline on the Management of Blood Cholesterol: a report of the American College of Cardiology Foundation/American Heart Association Task Force on Clinical Practice Guidelines. J Am Coll Cardiol. 2018a;139(25):e1082–143.
21. Grundy SM, Stone NJ, Bailey AL, Beam C, Birtcher KK, Blumenthal RS, Braun LT, de Ferranti S, Faiella-Tommasino J, Forman DE, Goldberg R, Heidenreich PA, Hlatky MA, Jones DW, Lloyd-Jones D, Lopez-Pajares N, Ndumele CE, Orringer CE, Peralta CA, Saseen JJ, Smith SC Jr, Sperling L, Virani SS, Yeboah J. AHA/ACC/AACVPR/AAPA/ABC/ACPM/ADA/AGS/APhA/ASPC/NLA/PCNA guideline on the management of blood cholesterol: a report of the American College of Cardiology/American Heart Association Task Force on Clinical Practice Guidelines. Circulation. 2018b;2018:e1082–e1143.
22. Jain T, et al. Dallas heart study. J Am Coll Cardiol. 2004;44:1011–7.
23. Joshi PH, Blaha MJ, Budoff MJ, Miedema MD, McClelland RL, Lima JAC, Agatston AS, Blankstein R, Blumenthal RS, Nasir K. The 10-year prognostic

value of zero and minimal CAC. JACC Cardiovasc Imaging. 2017;10:957–8.

24. Khaleeli E, Peters SR, Bobrowsky K, Oudiz RJ, Ko JY, Budoff MJ. Diabetes and the associated incidence of subclinical atherosclerosis and coronary artery disease: implications for management. Am Heart J. 2001;141:637–44.

25. Malik S, Zhao Y, Budoff M, et al. Coronary artery calcium score for long-term risk classification in individuals with type 2 diabetes and metabolic syndrome from the multi-ethnic study of atherosclerosis. JAMA Cardiol. 2017;2:1332–40.

26. Mao SS, et al. Comparison of coronary artery calcium scores between electron beam computed tomography and 64-multidetector computed tomographic scanner. J Comput Assist Tomogr. 2009;33(2):175–8.

27. Margolis JR, et al. The diagnostic and prognostic significance of coronary artery calcification. A report of 800 cases. Radiology. 1980;137(3):609.

28. Miedema MD, Duprez DA, Folsom AR. The use of coronary calcium testing to guide aspirin utilization for primary prevention: estimates from the multi-ethnic study of atherosclerosis. Circ Cardiovasc Qual Outcomes. 2014;7(3):453–60.

29. Mielke C, Shields J, Broemeling L. Coronary artery calcium, coronary artery disease, and diabetes. Diabetes Res Clin Pract. 2001;53:55–61.

30. Moebus S, Stang A, Möhlenkamp S, Dragano N, Schmermund A, Slomiany U, Hoffmann B, Bauer M, Broecker-Preuss M, Mann K, Siegrist J, Erbel R, Jöckel KH, Heinz Nixdorf Recall Study Group. Association of impaired fasting glucose and coronary artery calcification as a marker of subclinical atherosclerosis in a population-based cohort–results of the Heinz Nixdorf Recall Study. Diabetologia. 2009;52(1):81–9.

31. Nakanishi R, Li D, Blaha MJ, Whelton SP, Darabian S, Flores FR, Dailing C, Blumenthal RS, Nasir K, Berman DS, Budoff MJ. All-cause mortality by age and gender based on coronary artery calcium scores. Eur Heart J Cardiovasc Imaging. 2016;17(11):1305–14.

32. Nasir K, Bittencourt MS, Blaha MJ, Blankstein R, Agatston AS, Rivera JJ, Miemdema MD, Sibley CT, Shaw LJ, Blumenthal RS, Budoff MJ, Krumholz HM. Implications of coronary artery calcium testing among statin candidates according to American College of Cardiology/American Heart Association Cholesterol Management Guidelines: MESA (Multi-Ethnic Study of Atherosclerosis). J Am Coll Cardiol. 2015;66:1657–68.

33. Nasir K, Clouse M. Role of nonenhanced multidetector CT coronary artery calcium testing in asymptomatic and symptomatic individuals. Radiology. 2012;264:637–49.

34. Raggi P, Shaw LJ, Berman DS, Callister TQ. Prognostic value of coronary artery calcium

screening in subjects with and without diabetes. J Am Coll Cardiol. 2004;43:1663–9.

35. Rozanski A, Gransar H, Shaw LJ, Kim J, Miranda-Peats L, Wong ND, Rana JS, Orakzai R, Hayes SW, Friedman JD, Thomson LEJ, Polk D, Min J, Budoff MJ, Berman DS. Impact of coronary artery calcium scanning on coronary risk factors and downstream testing: the EISNER (Early Identification of Subclinical Atherosclerosis by Noninvasive Imaging Research) prospective randomized trial. J Am Coll Cardiol. 2011a;57:1622–32.

36. Rozanski A, et al. Impact of CAC on coronary risk factors and downstream testing: the EISNER prospective randomized trial. J Am Coll Cardiol. 2011b;57:1622–32.

37. Shareghi S, Ahmadi N, Young E, Liu ST, Gopal A, Budoff MJ. The prognostic significance of zero coronary calcium scores on cardiac computed tomography. J Cardiovasc Comput Tomogr. 2007;1:155–9.

38. Tang W, et al. Racial differences in coronary calcium prevalence among high-risk adults. Am J Cardiol. 1995;75:1088–91.

39. Valenti V, Hartaigh BO, Cho I, et al. Absence of coronary artery calcium identifies asymptomatic diabetic individuals at low near-term but not long-term risk of mortality: a 15-year follow-up study of 9715 patients. Circ Cardiovasc Imaging. 2016;9:e003528.

40. Valenti V, Hartaigh BO, Heo R, et al. A 15-year warranty period for asymptomatic individuals without coronary artery calcium: a prospective follow-up of 9,715 individuals. JACC Cardiovasc Imaging. 2015;8:900–9.

41. Waheed S, et al. Collective impact of conventional cardiovascular risk factors and coronary calcium score on clinical outcomes with or without statin therapy: the St. Francis Heart Study. Atherosclerosis. 2016;255:193–9.

42. Wexler L, et al. Coronary artery calcification: pathophysiology, epidemiology, imaging methods, and clinical implications: a statement for health professionals from the American Heart Association. Writing Group. Circulation. 1996;94(5):1175–92.

43. Wolk MJ, et al. ACCf/AHA/ASE/ASNC/HFSA/HRS/SCAI/SCCT/SCMR/STS 2013 multimodality appropriate use criteria for the detection and risk assessment of stable ischemic heart disease. JACC. 2014;63(4):380–406.

44. Yang L, et al. Prevalence of over-weight and obesity in the United States, 2007–2012. JAMA Intern Med. 2015;175(8):1412–3.

45. Yeboah J, McClelland RL, Polonsky TS, et al. Comparison of novel risk markers for improvement in cardiovascular risk assessment in intermediate-risk individuals. JAMA. 2012;308:788–95.

46. Zheng SL, et al. Association of Aspirin use for primary prevention with cardiovascular events and bleeding events: a systematic review and meta-analysis. JAMA. 2019;321(3):277–87.

Epidemiology of Cardiovascular Disease in African Americans

16

Virginia J. Howard

Introduction

In the reporting of United States health statistics, *cardiovascular disease* is usually defined to include all diseases of the circulatory system and is usually referred to as "total cardiovascular diseases" and abbreviated as CVD. It includes ICD-9 codes 390–459 and ICD-10 codes I00-I99. It includes hypertension, coronary heart disease (CHD), stroke, and heart failure. It normally does not include congenital disease. When examining reports in the literature, readers are advised to carefully review methods and definitions on what is included within the categorization of disease. Throughout this chapter, we will specify CVD, CHD, stroke, or other component of CVD.

Mortality, *incidence*, and *prevalence* are indices used to describe differences in the distribution or "risk" of CVD or the specific component of CVD among selected populations. Each index provides particular information that addresses the burden of CVD for the public and for clinical or public health decision-makers. There are marked differences between these indices in the quantity and quality of the data available. The definitions and properties of these indices should be considered related to describing the burden of

cardiovascular disease in African Americans and all populations.

CVD mortality reflects deaths from CVD. In the United States, the source of mortality data that provide estimates of CVD is the national vital statistics system maintained by the National Center for Health Statistics within the Centers for Disease Control (CDC) (https://www.cdc.gov/nchs/nvss/mortality_methods.htm). It is required that all deaths be reported and the vital statistics system reports all death events, with information on the "underlying" (primary) and "contributing" (secondary) causes as well as demographic variables such as age, sex, and race/ethnicity. The causes of death are coded locally, usually by non-physicians, using the codes in the World Health Organization's International Classification of Diseases (ICD) (https://www.cdc.gov/nchs/icd/icd10.htm). The ICD codes have evolved over the years. Starting with 1999 mortality data, revision 10 was employed.

Mortality data are generally summarized based on underlying cause of death. Based on CVD coded as the underlying cause of death, the *CVD mortality rate* is calculated by dividing the number of CVD deaths occurring over a fixed time (usually a year) by the estimated population at risk. Based on census counts conducted each decade, inter-census estimates can be obtained by adjusting the census counts by regional reports of deaths and births (also part of the vital statistics reporting system). The major strength of mortality

V. J. Howard (✉)
Department of Epidemiology, School of Public Health, University of Alabama at Birmingham, Birmingham, AL, USA
e-mail: vjhoward@uab.edu

© Springer Nature Switzerland AG 2021
K. C. Ferdinand et al. (eds.), *Cardiovascular Disease in Racial and Ethnic Minority Populations*, Contemporary Cardiology, https://doi.org/10.1007/978-3-030-81034-4_16

rate as an index of the burden of CVD is the mandatory reporting of deaths. This allows estimates of CVD mortality rates to be made at the national level as well as for specific regions (e.g., state or county level), and for specific age, race/ethnicity, or sex groups, and to be used for monitoring trends over time.

There are, however, shortcomings in the use of mortality rates as an index of the burden of disease, including CVD. While the vital statistics reporting system is highly accurate in determining vital status, the cause of death information has some limitations that need to be considered related to the potential for inaccuracy. The National Death Index (NDI) is the component of the vital statistics system that contains a central computerized index of death information. The information comes from state vital statistics offices based on death certificates (https://www.cdc.gov/nchs/ndi/index.htm). While there is a complex algorithm for coding a single underlying cause of death that gets re-evaluated regularly, the coding is challenging, requires judgment, and has potential for errors with changes over time. These causes of death are converted into the ICD codes through the NDI Plus System. A 1998 report examining the accuracy of this coding system reported a 4% discrepancy rate between the NDI and trained nosologists who examined the death certificates in determining all cause, but not CHD or CVD mortality [1]. Additionally, death certificates that propagate into NDI may be inaccurate. Doctors are rarely trained in how to fill out death certificates; thus, the input data may be suboptimal [2–4]. The reliability of cause of death from death certificates has been shown to be poor, with error rates ranging from 16% to 40% [5, 6]. Reports of CHD cause of death have been investigated with deaths from CHD found to be overreported [2, 7, 8]. There is some evidence that stroke has less priority in the coding algorithm than other causes of death [9]. An additional shortcoming in the use of mortality data as an index of the burden of stroke is the lack of coding of stroke subtype at the level of infarction versus hemorrhage. An investigation of state-level stroke mortality data for 2007–2009 found that for 53% of the stroke deaths, the deaths were classified as unspecified

[10]. While inaccuracy of race information on death certificates is a potential concern in cases where the physician or funeral director completing the certificate has to rely on observation without access to medical records completed by the decedent, validity studies suggest this is of minimal concern for African American and White races but may be of concern for other race/ethnic groups [11].

Most cohort studies do their own adjudication of cause of death, and follow similar protocols, utilizing information from death certificates but supplementing it with various additional information that may be available including hospital, physician office and nursing home records, autopsy reports, and narrative interviews with proxies about events surrounding the death [5, 12–15]. In the REasons for Geographic and Racial Differences in Stroke (REGARDS) national cohort study of African Americans and White Americans, a comparison of NDI-defined deaths with study-adjudicated deaths found that the sensitivity and positive predictive value of the NDI determination compared to the REGARDS determination for CHD mortality were only modest but the specificity and negative predictive value were high [15]. For the broader category of CVD mortality, the sensitivity and positive predictive value of the NDI determination were slightly better. However, the agreement between the NDI and REGARDS adjudicated cause of death varied by age at death, with the NDI cause of death more often coded as a CHD death in the elderly ($\geq$75 years) when the REGARDS cause of death was coded as something else. Overall mortality rates were similar, though. Thus, a recommendation is to consider the potential for misclassification when using only NDI or death certificates to classify cause of death related to cardiovascular disease.

Differences among mortality rates cannot be assumed to be due to differences in actual number of CVD events, that is, incidence. Mortality rates are a product of the incidence and the case-fatality rates, and differences can come from either of these.

Some of the shortcomings of mortality as an index of the distribution of disease are directly addressed by the use of the incidence rate. The *CVD incidence rate* is defined as the number of new CVD events per population occurring over a fixed time (normally a year). Unfortunately, there are also shortcomings in the use of this index. Most important is that there is no national surveillance system or registry of CVD events [16–18]. Information on CVD incidence rates is based on: (1) clinical reports in populations with tightly controlled referral patterns; (2) funded surveillance projects that capture admissions to medical facilities for a fixed geographic region, such as the Jackson Heart Study (JHS) [19], the Greater Cincinnati/Northern Kentucky stroke project (GCNKSS) [20], and the Atherosclerosis Risk in Communities (ARIC) surveillance program [21]; or (3) longitudinal epidemiologic cohort studies, such as the ARIC cohort study [22], the Cardiovascular Health Study [23, 24], the Multiethnic Study of Atherosclerosis [25], the Northern Manhattan Study (NOMAS) [26], and the REGARDS study [27]. The studies cited are ones that include African Americans [28]. In general, these surveillance and cohort studies provide incidence data for the specific geographic regions and race-ethnic groups they represent but because of differences in study design, including enrollment of different races across different field centers within the study (e.g., ARIC and MESA) and JHS only including African Americans, comparisons are limited. There are also shortcomings of incidence data. One is in the assumptions required to generalize results from specific geographic and racial populations to provide either a national picture or a comparison of the disease burden between groups, such as African Americans and White Americans. A second shortcoming is that differences in access to healthcare and use of diagnostic technologies will differentially identify CVD events. In general, racial and ethnic disparities in the delivery of healthcare are well-documented [29], including a 2017 report related to racial disparities in access to and utilization of neurologic healthcare [30]. However, a 2011 American Heart Association/American Stroke Association statement for healthcare professionals concluded there was "limited evidence showing that minorities are less likely to receive evaluation or testing for car-

diovascular disease and stroke than Whites;" however, the statement also reported that minority patients with stroke were less likely to be evaluated by a neurologist [31]. Improvements in access to care over time have been seen with the Affordable Care Act, with African Americans having a greater increase in healthcare coverage than White Americans [32]. Thus, more CVD events will be found, particularly milder events that previously could have been missed [33]. These newly discovered milder strokes would both raise the incidence rates (by adding to the numerator) and decrease the case-fatality rate because patients with mild disease would tend to survive. Access to care is certainly a complicating factor in the interpretation of incidence data, as well as changes in access to care in the interpretation of temporal changes in incidence, especially related to examining differences by race and ethnicity.

The *prevalence of CVD* is defined as the proportion of the population that has survived a CVD event or, in the case of hypertension, is living with a diagnosis. *Prevalence* is a proportion at a fixed point in time, distinguishing it from incidence and mortality that are rates. In comparing changes in prevalence over time, an increase may not necessarily represent poor health outcomes. CVD prevalence can increase not only due to an increase in incidence rate but also because of a declining case-fatality rate, that is, people are living longer following a CVD event. In the case of coronary heart disease, stroke, and heart failure, improvements in emergency treatment and procedures and aggressive acute management would contribute to increasing prevalence. In describing the distribution and burden of cardiovascular disease, with the exception of hypertension, prevalence is not used as often as mortality and incidence are. This is somewhat surprising because the burden of a disease is borne by the person who has the disease and society in general, relative to the care and attention the disease and its severity require. Prevalence estimates can be useful in planning aspects of the healthcare delivery system such as rehabilitation services, the number of specialists and nursing home beds, and efforts in secondary prevention.

Mortality

Most of what we know about CVD epidemiology comes from mortality data because they are data that are mandated to be collected. As described above, the national vital statistics system compiles the data and the CDC provides the most recent data for calculating age-specific mortality rates for specific causes of death for each of the major race/ethnic groups in the United States.

According to the most recent data available, heart disease is the leading cause of death in the United States (https://www.cdc.gov/nchs/fastats/leading-causes-of-death.htm). African Americans have the highest rates of CHD mortality, with rates especially high in middle-aged African American men relative to other race/sex groups. Although mortality rates for major cardiovascular diseases had been declining since the late 1960s across all major demographic groups [34, 35], the decline was diverging for Black and White individuals in the late 1970s with larger declines through 2015 for Whites than Blacks aged ≥35 years old [35]. Overall, the rate of decline of CVD and CHD mortality decelerated between 2011 and 2014, and the mortality increased for 2015 across most race-ethnic groups; for CHD mortality, there was a slight decline for non-Hispanic Blacks [36]. Figure 16.1a, b are maps of the United States showing the CHD mortality rates by county for non-Hispanic Blacks and Whites, respectively,

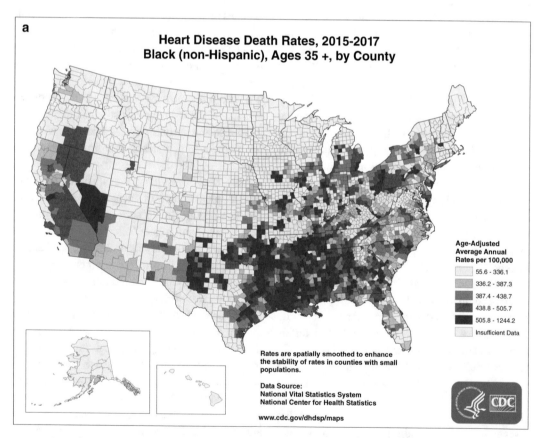

Fig. 16.1 Heart disease mortality rates, the United States, (**a**) black (non-Hispanic) and (**b**) white (non-Hispanic) population ages 35+ years, 2015–2017. Darkest colors represent areas with highest heart disease mortality rates, and lightest colors represent areas with lowest rates. (Retrieved from CDC website https://www.cdc.gov/heart-disease/maps_data.htm (October 18, 2020))

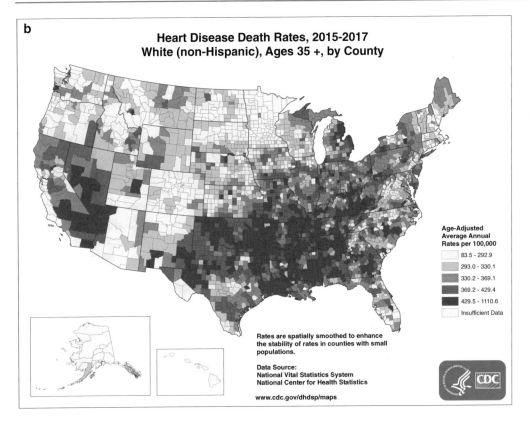

Fig. 16.1 (continued)

for the latest time period available, 2015–2017. Additional maps showing county-level CHD death rates and trends by age group, race, and sex for 1979 through 2017 have been produced by CDC authors [37].

Data from the REGARDS cohort study, based on adjudicated causes of deaths through 2017, also confirmed CVD mortality rates were higher for African Americans than White Americans, and the black-to-white hazard ratio for CVD mortality was larger for participants <65 compared to those who were 65 and older [38]. Data from this study identified that factors such as socioeconomic status and modifiable CVD risk factors explained a substantial amount of the excess CVD mortality in Black compared to White participants [38]. In the ARIC study, also utilizing adjudicated causes of death, Black individuals were found to have

a significantly higher risk of sudden cardiac death compared to White individuals, especially among women [39].

Overall, stroke mortality rates among African Americans are about 40% higher than White Americans with the largest disparity at younger ages [27, 40]. The black–white disparities in the burden of stroke were first recognized in the 1970s based on mortality statistics [41, 42]. While there have been dramatic declines in stroke mortality over the years that have been shared across all race-ethnic groups, the black-to-white mortality ratio has remained significantly higher than 1. It is disproportionately distributed across age groups, with an approximate 2.5 times greater relative risk in Black than White individuals in ages 45–54 and 55–64, and a decreasing black-to-white mortality ratio with increasing age until the oldest age group of 85+ where the ratio is close to 1 [28, 40].

Figure 16.2a, b are maps of the United States showing the stroke mortality rates by county for non-Hispanic Blacks and Whites, respectively, for the latest time period available, 2015–2017.

Incidence

Data on the black–white differences in risk of incident CHD are limited compared to mortality data. In the ARIC study, based on data from 10-year follow-up through 1997, the average age-adjusted incidence rates per 1000 person-years for CHD were 10.6 for Black men, 12.5 for White men, 5.1 for Black women, and 4.0 for White women [43]. Data on total CHD from REGARDS through 2009 with average follow-up of 4.2 years were lower; the age-standardized incidence rates per 1000 person-years were 9.0 for Black men,

8.1 for White men, 5.0 for Black women, and 3.4 for White women [44]. Differences in results between the two studies could be related to time period and that REGARDS did not include coronary revascularizations in the definition of CHD events. REGARDS also found racial and sex differences in fatal versus nonfatal CHD incidence rates; Black men had twice the risk of incident fatal CHD compared to White men but lower nonfatal incident CHD and incident rates for fatal and nonfatal CHD were higher for Black women compared to White women [44]. In an analysis utilizing data from REGARDS (with longer follow-up), ARIC, and CHS, hazard ratios for incident fatal CHD were found to be higher for Black men than White men aged 45–65 years in both ARIC and REGARDS, and nonfatal CHD risk was lower [45]. However, after adjusting for social determinants of health, and CVD risk fac-

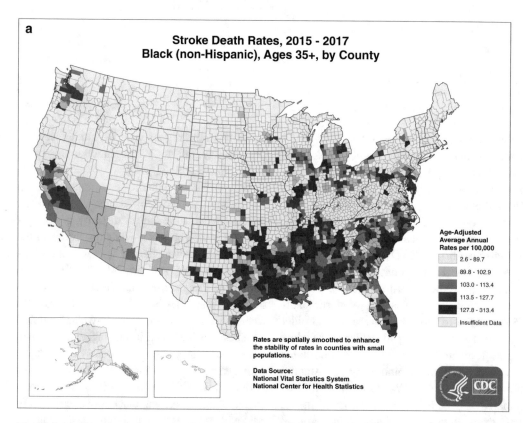

Fig. 16.2 Stroke mortality rates, the United States, (**a**) black (non-Hispanic) and (**b**) white (non-Hispanic) population ages 35+ years, 2015–2017. Darkest colors represent areas with highest stroke mortality rates, and lightest colors represent areas with lowest rates. (Retrieved from CDC website https://www.cdc.gov/heartdisease/maps_ data.htm (October 18, 2020))

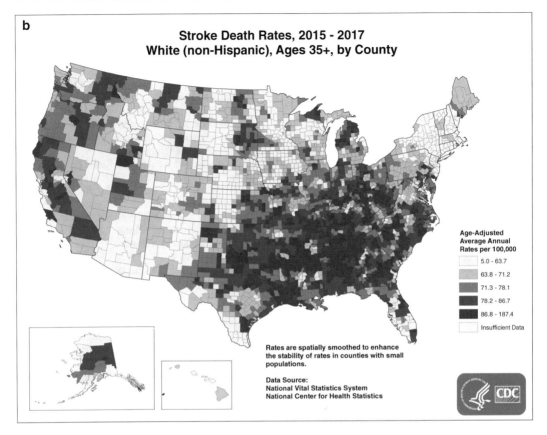

Fig. 16.2 (continued)

tors, Black men and women had similar risk for fatal CHD compared with White men and women. The risk for nonfatal CHD was lower for Black versus White men and women [45]. In the ARIC study, Whites had a significantly higher rate of clinically recognized incident myocardial infarction than Blacks, 5.04 versus 3.24 per 1000 person-years [46]. In examining trends in incidence of CHD, the ARIC study found that the decline among African American men was about half that of White men, about 3.2% per year compared to 6.5%, and for African American women, the decline was 4.0% compared to 5.2% for White women [47].

The increased risk of incident stroke in African Americans compared to Whites has been confirmed across many populations. Data for comparing stroke incidence rates for Black individuals and White individuals from the studies that included physician review of suspected stroke cases has been summarized recently [28, 48, 49]. REGARDS showed a pattern of black–white incidence rate ratios notably similar to the black–white mortality rate ratios, with risk of incident stroke approximately three times greater in Black adults than White adults for ages 45–54 and no difference in stroke risk for those aged 85 years and older [48, 50]. Both NOMAS and the GCNKSS confirmed higher stroke incidence in their African American populations than their White populations, showing black–white incidence rate ratios of 2.0 or greater [51, 52]. Data from the ARIC study showed a black–white incidence rate ratio of 2.77 for ages 45–54 and 2.23 for ages 55–65 [53]. With additional follow-up time through 2011, ARIC found an overall black–white incidence rate ratio of 2.03 [54]. In examining trends in stroke incidence, the GCNKSS found a significant decrease in stroke incidence rates for White but not Black adults over 1993–1994 and 1999 and 2005 [55]. The ARIC study, however, found a significant decrease in stroke incidence rates for both Black and White adults aged 65 and older, over the period of 1987–2011 [54].

Prevalence

For a description of differences in prevalence of CVD across a broad range of ages and by race and sex, it is best to rely on national survey data provided by the National Center for Health Statistics within the CDC. The use of survey data has the strength of a substantial sample size but the weakness of dependence on self-reported conditions. Specifically the National Health Interview Survey (NHIS) (https://www.cdc.gov/nchs/about/factsheets/factsheet_nhis.htm) and the Behavioral Risk Factor Surveillance System (BRFSS) (https://www.cdc.gov/brfss/about/about_brfss.htm) provide prevalence data. With the acknowledgment of the shortcoming of self-report, based on the NHIS, for 2018, the age-adjusted prevalence of all types of heart disease in Blacks was 10.0% and 11.5% in Whites; for CHD, it was 5.4% in Blacks and 5.7% in Whites. The age-adjusted prevalence of stroke in 2018 was 3.9% in Blacks and 2.6% in Whites.

Conclusion

The measures of CVD mortality, incidence, and prevalence provide important insights into the description of the distribution and burden of the disease. Each of these indices has important strengths and limitations. Several recurring patterns are clear. The most critical is the substantially higher risk of heart disease and stroke among African Americans and particularly among younger African Americans for stroke.

References

1. Sathiakumar N, Delzell E, Abdalla O. Using the National Death Index to obtain underlying cause of death codes. J Occup Environ Med. 1998;40(9):808–13.
2. Lakkireddy DR, Gowda MS, Murray CW, Basarakodu KR, Vacek JL. Death certificate completion: how well are physicians trained and are cardiovascular causes overstated? Am J Med. 2004;117(7):492–8.
3. Schuppener LM, Olson K, Brooks EG. Death certification: errors and interventions. Clin Med Res. 2020;18(1):21–6.
4. McGivern L, Shulman L, Carney JK, Shapiro S, Bundock E. Death certification errors and the effect on mortality statistics. Public Health Rep. 2017;132(6):669–75.
5. Ives DG, Samuel P, Psaty BM, Kuller LH. Agreement between nosologist and cardiovascular health study review of deaths: implications of coding differences. J Am Geriatr Soc. 2009;57(1):133–9.
6. Lakkireddy DR, Basarakodu KR, Vacek JL, et al. Improving death certificate completion: a trial of two training interventions. J Gen Intern Med. 2007;22(4):544–8.
7. Lloyd-Jones DM, Martin DO, Larson MG, Levy D. Accuracy of death certificates for coding coronary heart disease as the cause of death. Ann Intern Med. 1998;129(12):1020–6.
8. Agarwal R, Norton JM, Konty K, et al. Overreporting of deaths from coronary heart disease in New York City hospitals, 2003. Prev Chronic Dis. 2010;7(3):A47.
9. Burke JF, Lisabeth LD, Brown DL, Reeves MJ, Morgenstern LB. Determining stroke's rank as a cause of death using multicause mortality data. Stroke. 2012;43(8):2207–11.
10. Cheng TJ, Chang CY, Lin CY, Ke DS, Lu TH, Kawachi I. State differences in the reporting of "unspecified stroke" on death certificates: implications for improvement. Stroke. 2012;43(12):3336–42.
11. Arias E, Heron M, National Center for Health Statistics, Hakes J, Bureau USC. The validity of race and Hispanic-origin reporting on death certificates in the United States: an update. Vital Health Stat. 2016;2(172):1–21.
12. Coady SA, Sorlie PD, Cooper LS, Folsom AR, Rosamond WD, Conwill DE. Validation of death certificate diagnosis for coronary heart disease: the Atherosclerosis Risk in Communities (ARIC) study. J Clin Epidemiol. 2001;54(1):40–50.
13. Curb JD, McTiernan A, Heckbert SR, et al. Outcomes ascertainment and adjudication methods in the Women's Health Initiative. Ann Epidemiol. 2003;13(9 Suppl):S122–8.
14. Halanych JH, Shuaib F, Parmar G, et al. Agreement on cause of death between proxies, death certificates, and clinician adjudicators in the Reasons for Geographic and Racial Differences in Stroke (REGARDS) study. Am J Epidemiol. 2011;173(11):1319–26.
15. Olubowale OT, Safford MM, Brown TM, et al. Comparison of expert adjudicated coronary heart disease and cardiovascular disease mortality with the National Death Index: results from the REasons for Geographic And Racial Differences in Stroke (REGARDS) study. J Am Heart Assoc. 2017;6(5):e004966.

16. Howard VJ, Kissela BM. How do we know if we are making progress in reducing the public health burden of stroke? Stroke. 2012;43(8):2033–4.

17. Sidney S, Rosamond WD, Howard VJ, Luepker RV. The "heart disease and stroke statistics--2013 update" and the need for a national cardiovascular surveillance system. Circulation. 2013;127(1):21–3.

18. Roger VL, Sidney S, Fairchild AL, et al. Recommendations for cardiovascular health and disease surveillance for 2030 and beyond: a policy statement from the American Heart Association. Circulation. 2020;141(9):e104–19.

19. Sempos CT, Bild DE, Manolio TA. Overview of the Jackson Heart Study: a study of cardiovascular diseases in African American men and women. Am J Med Sci. 1999;317(3):142–6.

20. Broderick J, Brott T, Kothari R, et al. The Greater Cincinnati/Northern Kentucky Stroke Study: preliminary first-ever and total incidence rates of stroke among blacks. Stroke. 1998;29(2):415–21.

21. White AD, Folsom AR, Chambless LE, et al. Community surveillance of coronary heart disease in the Atherosclerosis Risk in Communities (ARIC) study: methods and initial two years' experience. J Clin Epidemiol. 1996;49(2):223–33.

22. The Atherosclerosis Risk in Communities (ARIC) study: design and objectives. The ARIC investigators. Am J Epidemiol. 1989;129(4):687–702.

23. Fried LP, Borhani NO, Enright P, et al. The cardiovascular health study: design and rationale. Ann Epidemiol. 1991;1(3):263–76.

24. Gilsanz P, Kubzansky LD, Tchetgen Tchetgen EJ, et al. Changes in depressive symptoms and subsequent risk of stroke in the cardiovascular health study. Stroke. 2017;48(1):43–8.

25. Bild DE, Bluemke DA, Burke GL, et al. Multi-Ethnic Study of Atherosclerosis: objectives and design. Am J Epidemiol. 2002;156(9):871–81.

26. White H, Boden-Albala B, Wang C, et al. Ischemic stroke subtype incidence among whites, blacks, and Hispanics: the Northern Manhattan Study. Circulation. 2005;111(10):1327–31.

27. Howard VJ, Cushman M, Pulley L, et al. The reasons for geographic and racial differences in stroke study: objectives and design. Neuroepidemiology. 2005;25(3):135–43.

28. Elkind M, Lisabeth L, Howard VJ, Kleindorfer D, Howard G. Approaches to studying determinants of racial-ethnic disparities in stroke and its sequelae. Stroke. 2020;51(11):3406–16.

29. Smedley BD, Stith AY, Nelson AR. Unequal treatment: confronting racial and ethnic disparities in health care. Washington, DC: The National Academies Press; 2003.

30. Saadi A, Himmelstein DU, Woolhandler S, Mejia NI. Racial disparities in neurologic health care access and utilization in the United States. Neurology. 2017;88(24):2268–75.

31. Cruz-Flores S, Rabinstein A, Biller J, et al. Racial-ethnic disparities in stroke care: the American experience: a statement for healthcare professionals from the American Heart Association/American Stroke Association. Stroke. 2011;42(7):2091–116.

32. Chen J, Vargas-Bustamante A, Mortensen K, Ortega AN. Racial and ethnic disparities in health care access and utilization under the Affordable Care Act. Med Care. 2016;54(2):140–6.

33. Howard VJ, Lackland DT, Lichtman JH, et al. Care seeking after stroke symptoms. Ann Neurol. 2008;63(4):466–72.

34. Cooper R, Cutler J, Desvigne-Nickens P, et al. Trends and disparities in coronary heart disease, stroke, and other cardiovascular diseases in the United States: findings of the national conference on cardiovascular disease prevention. Circulation. 2000;102(25):3137–47.

35. Van Dyke M, Greer S, Odom E, et al. Heart disease death rates among blacks and whites aged >/=35 years – United States, 1968–2015. MMWR Surveill Summ. 2018;67(5):1–11.

36. Sidney S, Quesenberry CP Jr, Jaffe MG, Sorel M, Go AS, Rana JS. Heterogeneity in national U.S. mortality trends within heart disease subgroups, 2000–2015. BMC Cardiovasc Disord. 2017;17(1):192.

37. Vaughan AS, Schieb L, Casper M. Historic and recent trends in county-level coronary heart disease death rates by race, gender, and age group, United States, 1979–2017. PLoS One. 2020;15(7):e0235839.

38. Tajeu GS, Safford MM, Howard G, et al. Black-white differences in cardiovascular disease mortality: a prospective US study, 2003–2017. Am J Public Health. 2020;110(5):696–703.

39. Zhao D, Post WS, Blasco-Colmenares E, et al. Racial differences in sudden cardiac death. Circulation. 2019;139(14):1688–97.

40. Howard G. Ancel keys lecture: adventures (and misadventures) in understanding (and reducing) disparities in stroke mortality. Stroke. 2013;44(11):3254–9.

41. Wylie CM. Death statistics for cerebrovascular disease: a review of recent findings. Stroke. 1970;1(3):184–93.

42. Oh SJ. Cerebro-vascular diseases in Negroes. J Natl Med Assoc. 1971;63(2):93–8.

43. Jones DW, Chambless LE, Folsom AR, et al. Risk factors for coronary heart disease in African Americans: the atherosclerosis risk in communities study, 1987–1997. Arch Intern Med. 2002;162(22):2565–71.

44. Safford MM, Brown TM, Muntner PM, et al. Association of race and sex with risk of incident acute coronary heart disease events. JAMA. 2012;308(17):1768–74.

45. Colantonio LD, Gamboa CM, Richman JS, et al. Black-white differences in incident fatal, nonfatal, and total coronary heart disease. Circulation. 2017;136(2):152–66.

46. Zhang ZM, Rautaharju PM, Prineas RJ, et al. Race and sex differences in the incidence and prognostic significance of silent myocardial infarction in the Atherosclerosis Risk in Communities (ARIC) study. Circulation. 2016;133(22):2141–8.

47. Rosamond WD, Chambless LE, Heiss G, et al. Twenty-two-year trends in incidence of myocardial

infarction, coronary heart disease mortality, and case fatality in 4 US communities, 1987–2008. Circulation. 2012;125(15):1848–57.

48. Howard VJ, Kleindorfer DO, Judd SE, et al. Disparities in stroke incidence contributing to disparities in stroke mortality. Ann Neurol. 2011;69(4):619–27.

49. Carnethon MR, Pu J, Howard G, et al. Cardiovascular health in African Americans: a scientific statement from the American Heart Association. Circulation. 2017;136(21):e393–423.

50. Howard G, Moy CS, Howard VJ, et al. Where to focus efforts to reduce the Black-White disparity in stroke mortality: incidence versus case fatality? Stroke. 2016;47(7):1893–8.

51. Sacco RL, Boden-Albala B, Gan R, et al. Stroke incidence among white, black, and Hispanic residents of an urban community: the Northern Manhattan Stroke Study. Am J Epidemiol. 1998;147(3):259–68.

52. Kissela B, Schneider A, Kleindorfer D, et al. Stroke in a biracial population: the excess burden of stroke among blacks. Stroke. 2004;35(2):426–31.

53. Rosamond WD, Folsom AR, Chambless LE, et al. Stroke incidence and survival among middle-aged adults: 9-year follow-up of the Atherosclerosis Risk in Communities (ARIC) cohort. Stroke. 1999;30(4):736–43.

54. Koton S, Schneider AL, Rosamond WD, et al. Stroke incidence and mortality trends in US communities, 1987 to 2011. JAMA. 2014;312(3):259–68.

55. Kleindorfer DO, Khoury J, Moomaw CJ, et al. Stroke incidence is decreasing in whites but not in blacks: a population-based estimate of temporal trends in stroke incidence from the Greater Cincinnati/Northern Kentucky Stroke Study. Stroke. 2010;41(7):1326–31.

Cardiac Amyloid Heart Disease in Racial/Ethnic Minorities: Focus on Transthyretin Amyloid Cardiomyopathy

Kevin M. Alexander, Matthew S. Maurer, and Icilma V. Fergus

Overview

Amyloidosis may be systemic or localized and refers to the deposition and infiltration of dysfunctional proteinaceous material in various organs. Systemic amyloidosis includes but is not limited to the heart, kidneys, nerves, liver, and gastrointestinal tract. This is distinct from localized amyloidosis in which infiltration may occur as deposits in the skin, soft tissues, oropharynx, larynx, lung, bladder, or lymph nodes. In both forms, protein with unstable tertiary structures misfold, aggregate, and form fibrils that build up in various organs [1, 2]. Individual amyloid fibrils are insoluble and notably resistant to proteolysis, non-branching, 7–10 nm in width, and are of variable length. Under polarized microscopy, the deposits, when stained with the dye Congo red, display apple-green birefringence. While there are various subtypes of amyloidosis, cardiac amyloidosis is caused predominantly by two precursor proteins, (1) an immunoglobulin light chain, termed light chain (AL) amyloidosis that is a systemic disease resulting in a rapidly fulminant course without treatment [3, 4], or (2) transthyretin (TTR), a liver derived protein that misfolds causing ATTR, with an age-dependent penetrance marked by cardiomyopathy and/or a sensory polyneuropathy [5, 6]. TTR exists as a homotetramer that transports thyroid hormone and retinol; hence, the name *trans* (for transporter), *thy* (for thyroid hormone), and *retin* (for retinol or Vitamin A). In pathologic conditions, mutations in the protein or aging, the tetramer becomes unstable and dissociates into monomers or oligomers, with consequential amyloid fibrils [1, 7]. In this chapter, we focus primarily on variant ATTR (ATTRv) and wild-type ATTR (ATTRwt), as both are underdiagnosed and potentially deadly among Black and Hispanic populations. Of note, approximately 3.4% of Black patients carry a transthyretin variant that confers an increased risk of developing ATTR cardiomyopathy [8]. If not treated, ATTR cardiomyopathy may lead to progressive heart failure and death. Fortunately, effective treatments for ATTR amyloidosis are now available and continue to emerge [4, 9]. Amyloid heart disease in Hispanic individuals has not been well described in the literature, and in this chapter, we will also attempt to shed more light on the manifestations of ATTR in this population.

K. M. Alexander
Stanford University School of Medicine,
Stanford, CA, USA

M. S. Maurer
Columbia University Irving Medical Center,
New York Presbyterian Hospital,
New York, NY, USA

I. V. Fergus (✉)
Icahn School of Medicine at Mount Sinai,
New York, NY, USA
e-mail: icilma.fergus@mountsinai.org

© Springer Nature Switzerland AG 2021
K. C. Ferdinand et al. (eds.), *Cardiovascular Disease in Racial and Ethnic Minority Populations*,
Contemporary Cardiology, https://doi.org/10.1007/978-3-030-81034-4_17

What Is Transthyretin Cardiac Amyloidosis (ATTR)?

Transthyretin (TTR) is a 127-amino acid plasma protein made of four noncovalently associated, β-sheet enriched subunits, which form two thyroxine (T$_4$) binding sites [10]. This protein, originally called prealbumin (because it migrates just slightly albumin in serum protein electrophoresis), is stabilized by retinol binding but can dissociate into individual monomers. TTR amyloidosis (ATTR) is dichotomized into two forms based on the genetic sequence of the TTR protein. There are >130 TTR mutations that have been reported [1, 7, 10]. If there is a mutation in the TTR protein, it is termed ATTRv (previously called ATTRh, where "*h*" stands for hereditary) and manifests as familial amyloid cardiomyopathy or familial amyloid polyneuropathy (FAC or FAP). In the absence of a point mutation, it is called wild-type transthyretin amyloidosis (ATTRwt). TTR point mutations, such as the Val122Ile mutation, result in kinetic instability and dissociation into monomers that misfold forming amyloid fibrils that deposit in the myocardium resulting in ATTRv [7, 10]. Whereas ATTRwt occurs in the seventh or eighth decade of life and thus was previously called senile cardiac amyloidosis [11]. ATTRwt mainly involves the heart but is also associated with bilateral carpal tunnel syndrome, spinal stenosis, and biceps tendon rupture, thus indicating a tissue tropism for ligaments and connective tissues as well. ATTRv results in a progressive, degenerative, multi-systemic disorder with a heterogeneous clinical presentation marked by cardiac and/or peripheral or autonomic nervous system involvement and often mimics other disease entities. Therefore, a careful clinical evaluation and appropriate testing are warranted to make an accurate diagnosis. ATTRv is heritable in an autosomal dominant manner, with first-degree relatives having a 50% chance of inheritance. Particular mutations in the TTR gene affect specific populations; Val122Ile (Afro-Caribbean), Thr60Ala (Irish, so-called Appalachian mutation), Val30Met (Portuguese, Swedish, and Japanese, so-called Portuguese mutation) [12,

13]. Cardiac involvement results in a restrictive cardiomyopathy with an aggressive and progressive form of heart failure that initially occurs in the setting of preserved ejection fraction. Amyloid heart disease should be suspected when a patient does not appear to respond to, or is intolerant of standard treatments for heart failure, including angiotensin converting enzyme inhibitors (ACEi), angiotensin receptor blockers (ARBs), beta-blockers, or angiotensin receptor neprilysin inhibitor (ARNi) therapy [2, 5, 14]. If untreated, patients with ATTRv cardiomyopathy experience accelerating symptoms until death occurs, typically 3–5 years after clinical presentation [5, 9, 12]. Population studies suggest that carriers of the Val122Ile mutation develop symptoms of congestive heart failure in the seventh decade of life, and that the disease may be clinically quiescent prior to this time [15, 16]. ATTRv is typically characterized according to its predominant clinical presentation, in which two post-mitotic organs, the heart, and the peripheral and autonomic nervous system are typically affected. Those with a predominant cardiac phenotype have heart failure, and those with a predominant neurologic phenotype have a peripheral sensory-motor and autonomic neuropathy [17]. A majority of TTR mutations manifest as a mixed clinical phenotype involving both neurologic and cardiac symptoms [13].

Cardiac Manifestations

Amyloidosis is a heterogeneous clinical condition resulting from deposits of amyloid in multiple organs, but cardiac involvement is common and often the cause of death [3, 13, 17]. Cardiac amyloidosis manifests with cardiac arrhythmias or conduction disease as well as heart failure characterized by a restrictive cardiomyopathy. Deposits within the myocardial interstitium may disrupt normal electrical conduction and contractile function; thus, death secondary to cardiac dysrhythmia or pulseless electrical activity can occur in addition to heart failure [13, 17]. Restrictive pathophysiology initially manifests as diastolic dysfunction in the setting of a reduced left ventricular (LV) capacitance. Echocardiography reveals biatrial dilation and thick ventricular walls with small chamber volumes, as well as increased intra-atrial septal thickness, valve thickening, and small pericardial effusions [18, 19]. Apical strain is preserved on echo compared with some other cardiomyopathies and is discussed later. There are now that are currently available to treat ATTRv that will be discussed later in this chapter, but it is important to remember that drugs typically used to treat heart failure are often not helpful and are potential harmful in patients with cardiac amyloidosis [2, 9, 14]. ACE and ARB drugs may result in hypotension especially in ATTRv patients with concomitant autonomic dysfunction. Beta-blockers may worsen cardiac output as patients with cardiac amyloidosis and restrictive cardiomyopathies are dependent on fast heart rates to maintain cardiac output. Agents with alpha blocking properties, such as carvedilol, should be also be minimized due to the propensity for exacerbating hypotension. Non-dihydropyridine calcium channel blockers, such as verapamil, are contraindicated due to the risk of high-degree heart block and significant negative inotropic effect. As the ATTR cardiomyopathy progresses, patients become generally intolerant of medications with a blood pressure lowering effect and may require the addition of midodrine for symptomatic hypotension. Valves may also be affected due to endocardial deposits, although it remains unclear whether infiltration directly leads to valve dysfunction. This question warrants future study. Ischemia is also possible with ATTRv cardiac infiltration. Ischemia may occur due to mechanisms that involve damage to the microvasculature rather than typical epicardial coronary artery disease [20].

Systemic Manifestations

Extra cardiac manifestations of ATTRv may involve several organs, often resulting in loss of autonomic nervous system control. Manifestations may include sensory and motor impairment, autonomic dysfunction (ortho-static hypotension or recurrent urinary tract infections due to bladder dysfunction), gastrointestinal dysfunction (alternating symptoms of diarrhea and constipation, and unintentional weight loss) [2, 5]. There may also be ocular manifestations, such as opacification of the vitreous humor or glaucoma. Renal involvement can occur with some forms of amyloidosis but is not typical of Val122Ile ATTRv that is the predominant focus of this chapter [2, 5, 21].

A progressive sensorimotor neuropathy termed familial amyloidotic polyneuropathy (FAP) may be manifested by with severely limiting symptoms [22, 23]. The patients may present with debilitating paresis, early impaired nociperception, and anhidrosis in the lower limbs [22–24]. The clinical presentation is phenotypically variable and can differ even among those with the same mutation and among family members. Polyneuropathy, when present, is a progressive sensorimotor and autonomic process, which may mimic other neuropathic conditions, potentially resulting in multiple misdiagnoses, such as chronic inflammatory demyelinating polyneuropathy, prior to identification of the causative condition, namely ATTRv [23, 24]. Disease severity and progression depend on the mutation. The mutation that classically causes FAP is Val30Met that is not commonly found in African American populations but is endemic in other individuals particularly Portuguese, Swedish, or Japanese ancestry [23–25]. It is important to emphasize that carpal tunnel syndrome (CTS) is not the result of peripheral polyneuropathy but due to compression of the median nerve and thus does meet clinical indication to prescribe a TTR silencer therapy. However, when present, CTS can be helpful in diagnosing ATTRv.

ATTR in Black Populations

In the United States, the most common allele of ATTRv is Val122Ile, and is seen almost exclusively in Black people of Afro-Caribbean descent [26]. The mutation is a substitution of isoleucine for valine at position 122 (Val122Ile) [8, 26, 27]. The association of the Val122Ile mutation with amyloid heart disease in elderly Black patients has been confirmed in several studies [8, 26, 27]. Review of various study cohorts reveals that the prevalence of non-light chain cardiac amyloidosis in patients over age 60 was higher in Black compared to White individuals (1.6% vs. 0.42%). Notably higher proportions of Black patients were found to have ATTR cardiomyopathy in the seventh and eighth decades of life (with ratios of 8:1 and 13:1, respectively) in retrospective studies [24, 26, 27]. Of the patients with ATTR cardiomyopathy on autopsy, 23% of Black participants (vs. 0% of White participants) were heterozygous for the Val122Ile mutation. This has been confirmed by DNA samples from over 14,000 patients in which 3.4% of Blacks were noted to have the V122Ile mutation [13, 15, 28]. In an analysis of 207 Black participants in the Beta-Blocker Evaluation in Survival Trial (BEST) trial, which studied the effect of bucindolol in a population with symptomatic systolic heart failure (in whom cardiac amyloidosis was an exclusion), the Val122Ile mutation was higher in the group over 60 years of age compared with younger participants (10% vs. 6.3%) [29]. It may be further noted that the presence of the Val122Ile mutation resulted in higher rates of cardiovascular hospitalization (64% vs. 28%) and decreased survival (73% vs. 22%) with a survival of 25.6 versus 43 months [8, 30]. The Val122Ile mutation is 5 times more prevalent in Black patients with heart failure than in a community cohort of comparable age. In a UK study of Black people of Afro-Caribbean descent with heart failure, ATTR cardiomyopathy was the fourth most common cause identified, with 8% of subjects having the Val122Ile mutation. While a recent retrospective analysis of echocardiographic data suggested low penetrance of Val122Ile (7%), the interpretation was confounded by the low sensitivity of the echocardiographic measures selected. Additionally, the low penetrance was discordant with the observation that the Val122Ile mutation was associated with a 47% increased risk of incident heart failure, suggesting that more sensitive detection methodologies might have better identified in ATTRv disease.

ATTR in Hispanic Populations

Compared to Black patients, there are less data available regarding the prevalence of ATTR among Hispanic patients [31]. The largest study to date comes from the Transthyretin Amyloidosis Outcomes Survey (THAOS) registry [23]. This international registry includes >2500 patients with transthyretin amyloidosis. In 2015, 256 patients from Latin American were enrolled with 148 from Brazil, 57 from Mexico, and 51 from Argentina [32]. In Brazil and Argentina, the most common mutation by far was Val30Met, which was found in 91.9% and 96.1% of patients, respectively. Val30Met is the most common TTR mutation worldwide. One of the Val30Met founder mutations arose from the Portuguese lineage, which likely explains its high prevalence in regions of South America. Further study of the Brazilian cohort revealed that Val30Met ATTR is frequently misdiagnosed (up to 26.6% of patients) [33, 34]. Brazilian Val30Met ATTR patients with a later age of disease onset (>50 years old) tend to have more severe neurologic symptoms and are more likely to have cardiac involvement compared to patients with early onset disease [35]. In contrast to South America, in Mexico, Ser50Arg is the most frequently encountered transthyretin mutation [36, 37]. A recent study of a Mexican database revealed that of the 111 patients identified with a TTR mutation, 74% had the Ser50Arg variant, followed by the Gly47Ala (13%) and Ser52Pro (11%) variants [37]. The authors estimated a prevalence of 0.89 per 100,000 for the Ser50Arg variant in Mexico. For both Val30Met and Ser50Arg, most patients have a neuropathic phenotype. Other rare mutations have been reported in the Hispanic population. An Ecuadorian family was found to have a trinucleotide deletion of the valine codon 122 codon. In the addition to the above-mentioned mutations, it is worth noting that given the West African ancestry of many Hispanic individuals from the Caribbean countries, the V122I variant likely is one of the most common TTR variants in these groups.

Making the Diagnosis of ATTR Cardiomyopathy

Time from symptom onset to ATTR diagnosis can be unacceptably long, often several years due to the non-specific symptoms or symptoms mimicking other potential diagnoses [2, 9]. In part, this delay occurs because patients are not being adequately evaluated and in part, symptoms of ATTRv may be variable in the early phases of disease. Thus, a detailed clinical history and appropriate testing are important (Table 17.1).

Diagnostic Testing

The Role of Biomarkers: Various biomarkers have been increasingly utilized to provide prognostic information for patients with ATTR cardio-

Table 17.1 Making the diagnosis of ATTR cardiomyopathy

History/physical examination	Imaging and testing
Heart failure with preserved ejection in the absence of hypertension, particularly in men	Discordance between ECG voltage and left ventricular wall thickness. Low QRS voltage is a late phase finding
Normotension in a person with previous hypertensive readings	Progressive diminution in QRS voltage on serial ECG
Evidence of right-sided heart failure, including loss of appetite, hepatomegaly, ascites, and lower extremity edema	Pseudo-infarction pattern on ECG
Intolerance of commonly used heart failure medications	Low tissue Doppler velocities, strain, or strain rate; Echo indicating apical preservation
Bilateral carpal tunnel syndrome, lumbar spinal stenosis, biceps tendon rupture, or previous hip or knee replacements	Thick interventricular septum and granular myocardial sparkling on standard 2D TTE
Important labs	Subendocardial late gadolinium enhancement on cardiac MRI
	Elevated natriuretic peptides out of proportion to clinical syndrome
	Positive troponins

myopathy. In study of 869 patients with cardiac ATTR (553 with ATTRwt and 316 with ATTRv), Gilmore et al. studied two widely measured cardiac biomarkers, N-terminal pro-B-type natriuretic peptide (NT-proBNP) and estimated glomerular filtration rate (eGFR) for prognostic staging. Stage I was defined as NT-proBNP ≤3000 ng/L and eGFR ≥45 mL/min [51, 38]. Stage III was defined as NT-proBNP > 3000 ng/L and eGFR < 45 mL/min. In a validation cohort of 318 patients, the median survival for stage I patients was 69.2 months, stage II was 46.7 months, and stage III was 24.1 months ($P < 0.0001$). Another prognostic staging has been developed for ATTRwt cardiomyopathy using NT-proBNP and troponin T with cutoff values of 3000 pg/mL and 0.05 ng/mL, respectively [39]. Stage I was defined as having both biomarker values below the cutoff, stage II as having one value above, and stage III as having both values above the cutoff. The 4-overall survivals for stages I–III were 57%, 42%, and 18%, respectively.

In addition to the abovementioned general cardiac biomarkers, the role of more specific biomarkers has been explored. Retinol-binding protein 4 (RBP4) is a natural TTR ligand, and thus its serum concentration has been hypothesized to be affected in the presence of ATTR disease. In a single center, serum RBP4 concentration was significantly lower in Black patients with Val122Ile ATTR cardiomyopathy ($n = 25$) compared with Black patients with non-amyloid heart failure ($n = 50$) [40]. This finding suggests that RBP4 in the future may be a helpful tool for identifying ATTR. Finally, there is evidence that the serum concentration of TTR itself may provide prognostic information. In a study of 116 ATTRwt patients, a lower baseline TTR level was associated with a shorter survival [41]. Moreover, those who were treated with the TTR stabilizer diflunisal had an increased TTR level. Therefore, serum TTR may serve as both a prognostic marker and a marker of treatment response to TTR stabilizers.

Endomyocardial Biopsy: Endomyocardial biopsy is the gold standard diagnostic test for cardiac amyloidosis, being 100% sensitive and specific, assuming that sufficient samples are obtained (i.e., at least four samples) [42]. Although the procedure carries some risk (e.g., bleeding, vascular injury, pericardial tamponade), it is considered to be safe and well tolerated, particularly when performed by a high-volume proceduralist. Tissue samples are initially stained with Congo Red. Under light microscopy, amyloid deposits will appear as light material in extracellular spaces. Under polarized light, amyloid deposits will display characteristic "apple green" birefringence (Fig. 17.1). Additional analysis is needed to determine the specific amyloid precursor protein (e.g., TTR or immunoglobulin free light chain). Immunohistochemistry is a frequently used test to define the amyloid precursor protein. The tissue samples are exposed to various antibodies, and depending on the protein present in the amyloid fibrils, the appropriate antibody will bind. Occasionally, there can be false positives or negatives with immunohistochemistry. Thus, the authors favor obtaining mass spectrometry analysis when possible. For this assay, areas of amyloid deposition are microdissected from the tissues slides using a laser, and then the peptides in the fibrils are digested and sequence by mass spectrometry. The amino acid sequence will definitively identify the amyloid precursor protein.

The ECG: The hallmark finding suggestive of cardiac amyloidosis is discordance between the QRS voltage and the wall thickness on echocardiography (Fig. 17.2). While low voltage is highly specific for an infiltrative process, it is not diagnostic of amyloidosis. Low voltage may be present in a myriad of conditions such as pericardial effusion, chronic obstructive pulmonary disease, or other conditions that increase the distance of the heart from the surface ECG. It is important to note that 15% of patients with ATTRv due to Val122Ile may present with ECG evidence of left ventricular hypertrophy. When low voltage is evident on an ECG due to ATTRv, this represents late-stage disease. A more important clue in the diagnosis may be progressive diminution of voltage over time in a tracing that previously demonstrated left ventricular hypertrophy [30, 43]. Another clue may be ECG changes indicative of a previous MI (Q waves) without corroboration of a segmental wall motion abnormality on echocardiography, the so called "pseudoinfarct pattern" or even poor precordial R wave progression. Both pseudoinfarcts and poor precordial R wave progression are more common in patients with cardiac amyloidosis (~70–80%) than low voltage (<40%). ECG findings while not that sensitive can be highly specific in the right clinical context when there is supporting history to suggest the diagnosis of ATTRv cardiomyopathy. This should prompt further testing to confirm the diagnosis [30, 43].

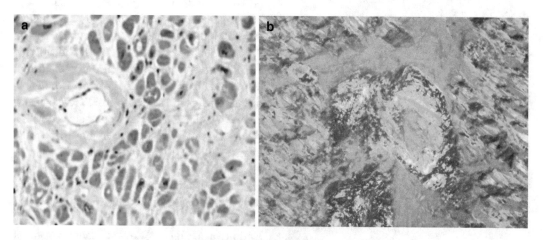

Fig. 17.1 Amyloid deposits reflecting "Apple Green" birefringence (Pink (**a**) and Green (**b**))

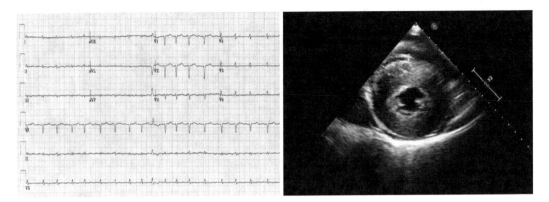

Fig. 17.2 ECG-echo discordance

Echocardiography: Echocardiography is a useful tool in the diagnosis of ATTRv; however, certain advanced evaluations such as strain and strain may require analysis in an advanced laboratory. Early echocardiography manifestations of amyloidosis include "diastolic dysfunction" that evolves to a restrictive filling pattern accompanied by significant infiltration of the myocardium [43–45]. The appearance of a bright or speckled myocardium has been described in cardiac amyloidosis, or the so called "starry night sky" but is non-specific and now with the use of harmonic imaging can be seen even in non-amyloid hearts; hence, this finding is not specific for diagnosing cardiac amyloidosis [44, 45]. A "thick" appearing myocardium on an echocardiogram but a relatively low voltage on ECG or the QRS to wall thickness ratio has a >80% sensitivity and specificity for distinguishing cardiac amyloidosis from hypertensive heart disease or hypertrophic cardiomyopathy [30, 43]. Note that the muscle is not truly hypertrophied as seen in hypertension or aortic valve disease; thus, there is discordance with high voltage on the ECG [30, 43]. A wall thickness of >1.2 cm in the absence of a condition such as hypertension or aortic stenosis is suggestive of cardiac amyloidosis. Thus, this voltage/myocardium mismatch has become a hallmark in making the diagnosis of ATTR cardiomyopathy. Other 2D findings may include a small left ventricular diameter, dilated atrial, and pericardial effusion [43, 44] In advanced echocardiography labs, strain imaging technology has increased the sensitivity and specificity in the diagnosis of cardiac amyloidosis [45]. In patients with diastolic dysfunction, Doppler assessment is made of both the mitral inflow velocities and myocardial tissue velocities, and the ratio assessed (E/e' ratio). However, the typical findings of an early diastolic relaxation pattern, followed by pseudonormalization then restrictive pattern—elevated E/e' ratio, may be manifested with a recurrence of a diminished E/e' ratio may be seen in restrictive or infiltrative cardiomyopathies and may be seen also in cardiac amyloidosis but is not specific for ATTRv [45, 46]. Strain measures myocardial deformation, which is longitudinal, radial, or circumferential, whereas strain rate refers to the temporal intensity in the change of myocardial deformation. If there is myocardial infiltration by amyloid with increased wall thickness of over 12 mm, there may be reduced systolic and diastolic longitudinal strain and strain rate at the mid and basal segments of the ventricle. Apical strain is preserved. This distinct pattern should raise suspicion of cardiac amyloidosis (Fig. 17.3). Tissue Doppler, while used to evaluate diastolic parameters in heart failure, is less accurate in assessing for cardiac amyloidosis compared with strain analysis [45, 47, 48]. Radial and circumferential strain imaging is also helpful in distinguishing hypertrophic cardiomyopathy from cardiac amyloidosis [47–49] with severely reduced measures seen in those with amyloidosis, but most of the shortening occurs in the longitudinal plane. Another useful

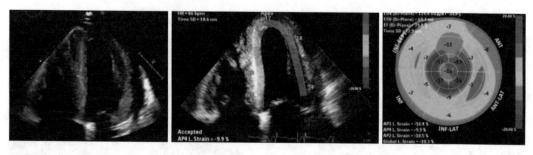

Fig. 17.3 Echo images showing strain imaging. (Reproduced with permission from Ruberg et al. [76])

measure in echocardiography is myocardial contraction fraction (MCF) [29, 50]. This index is related to the longitudinal shortening of the myocardium and is independent of LV size and geometry. It is related to longitudinal strain and is a ratio of stroke volume (SV) from myocardial volume (MV). The MCF has been shown to differentiate between other causes of increased myocardial thickness such as LVH from amyloid infiltration and is prognostic.

Nuclear Imaging: Technetium pyrophosphate (^{99m}Tc-PYP), DPD, and HMDP are radiotracers with predilection for bone enhancement. While other imaging modalities are being used to identify cardiac amyloidosis, these are the only non-invasive techniques to diagnose ATTR [51, 52]. The data supporting the diagnosis of ATTR cardiac involvement are based on a large multicenter study of patients with biopsy-proven amyloidosis who were evaluated with a semi-quantitative visual score of myocardial uptake compared with bone uptake (0 = no cardiac uptake to 3 = high uptake). Further analysis was performed in which a region of interest (ROI) was drawn over the heart and corrected for contralateral counts by calculating a heart-to-contralateral (H/CL) ratio. An H/CL ratio ≥1.5 was consistent with 97% sensitivity and 100% specificity for identifying ATTRv. 99mTc-DPD is 100% sensitive to identify cardiac ATTR and 100% specific to distinguish from AL; however, mild uptake is noted in other subtypes of cardiac amyloidosis. Since normal myocardium does not have affinity for radiolabeled phosphate derivatives, it will not demonstrate significant tracer uptake. However, it

is postulated that the amyloid infiltrated myocardium in ATTRv may contain micro-calcifications that could account for the uptake. It must be emphasized that the presence does not allow for discernment among patients with AL and therefore monoclonal protein must be excluded [52, 53]. Tc99-PYP has been confirmed to have high specificity and sensitivity (92% and 91%, respectively) [52, 53] for ATTRv cardiomyopathy. Furthermore, in patients with clinical findings consistent with cardiac amyloid, a positive 99mTc-PYP scan is 100% specific for TTR when grade 2 or 3 uptake was present without a monoclonal protein by serum and urine testing, solidifying this testing as a gold standard.

Cardiac MRI: Cardiac magnetic resonance imaging (CMRI) has become a useful tool when assessing for cardiomyopathies, particularly those that are infiltrative. MRI is now being more widely use to raise the suspicion of cardiac amyloid [54, 55]. In advanced laboratories, CMRI captures the anatomy of the heart with diagnostic precision. The cardiac structures are clearly delineated including the chambers and the valves and especially the myocardium and can distinguish between the three compartments—interstitium, muscle, and endothelium. Additionally, as the extracellular matrix expands with the infiltration of amyloid fibrils, CMRI detects the change in kinetics between normal and abnormal tissue [54–57]. This results in delayed enhancement of the myocardium and is highly indicative of cardiac amyloid infiltration (Fig. 17.4). However, CMRI cannot be used to discern whether the amyloid infiltration is due to ATTR or AL.

Genetic Testing: Genetic evaluation and assessment is clearly important as the diagnosis of ATTRv cannot be made without TTR gene sequencing. It is important to recognize that even community clinical providers can now acquire test kits so that blood and saliva samples can be

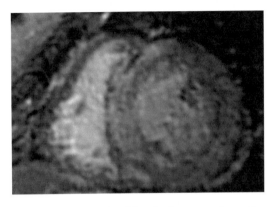

Fig. 17.4 MRI showing delayed enhancement in cardiac amyloid

provided and sent to laboratories which can provide the analysis [58, 59]. Genetic sequencing of the TTR gene will confirm the presence or absence of a mutation [59]. In patients with clinical findings suggestive of ATTR including a positive biopsy or positive scintigraphy, full-gene sequencing of TTR may be performed. In such cases, identifying a pathogenic TTR variant will be diagnostic for ATTRv. Clearly, access to genetic testing has the potential to enhance patient care by shortening the time to accurate diagnosis and identifying relatives at risk for disease. Inheritance in ATTRv is typically autosomal dominant, although homozygous and compound heterozygous cases have been reported [60]. All first-degree relatives of a proband—including children, siblings, and parents—are at 50% risk of carrying the familial TTR variant. Given the expected benefits of early recognition in ATTRv, an important conversation needs to be considered about when genetic testing should be

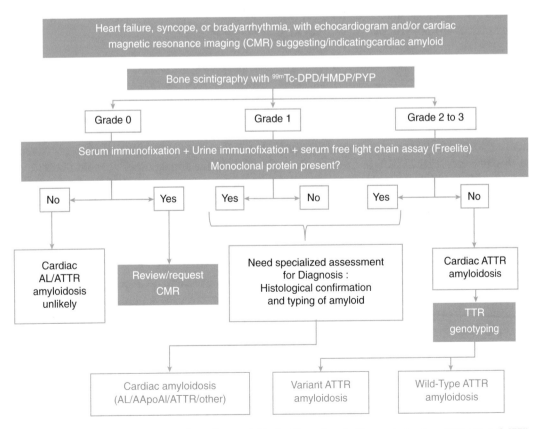

Fig. 17.5 Flowchart for diagnosis ATTR cardiac amyloidosis. (Reproduced with permission from Gillmore et al. [77])

offered to at-risk adult relatives of patients with a pathogenic TTR variant at the time of diagnosis [58–60].

Since ATTRv onset is typically no earlier than the third to fifth decade of life, genetic testing is not recommended for very young family members (Fig. 17.5). Another factor to consider is that true penetrance of ATTRv is unknown and also that disease expression is variable. Therefore, even if a relative of a patient is genetically identified, disease manifestation may vary. Therefore, ATTRv carriers should undergo a comprehensive history and physical examination to assess for any signs of cardiac or extra cardiac amyloidosis.

Therapeutic Options

Typical Heart Failure Medications May Not Work: It is important to recognize that several new therapies are available for ATTRv and that standard pharmacologic treatments for heart failure are of little efficacy [14, 61]. In fact, they may be deleterious to the patient. Bioavailable loop diuretics in conjunction with aldosterone antagonists are aimed at maintaining euvolemia, which is challenging in patients with cardiac amyloidosis often with low blood pressure due to either low cardiac outputs and/or concomitant autonomic dysfunction. The neurohormonal blocking agents such as ACEi and ARBs and beta-blockade are generally not well tolerated [14]. Cardiac glycosides such as digoxin are also of limited utility and may also result in higher toxicity risk due to concomitant renal dysfunction. Sudden cardiac death in patients with cardiac amyloidosis was historically thought to be largely due to electromechanical dissociation. Emerging evidence, however, suggests that these patients are also at a significant risk of developing ventricular arrhythmias [2]. There is a role for pacemakers in those patients with symptomatic bradyarrhythmias and also potentially a role for defibrillators. Given the failure of the typical CHF drugs, targeted therapies are designed to help in correcting or mitigating the underlying protein dysgenesis or dysfunction in patients with ATTRv cardiomy-

opathy thus ameliorating the vicious cycle of progressive heart failure. Treatments are categorized based on the mechanism of action.

TTR Stabilizers: One approach involves the stabilization of the tetramer called TTR stabilizers. The nonsteroidal anti-inflammatory drug (NSAID) diflunisal has been found to be beneficial as it binds to the thyroxine binding sites on TTR, preventing dissociation of the TTR tetramer and amyloid fibril formation [62–65]. However, since NSAIDs can cause numerous adverse outcomes including renal dysfunction, hypertension, volume overload gastrointestinal disorders (GI), and bleeding, the use is limited especially in patients with an advanced disease [37–67]. Diflunisal is, however, more easily available and affordable than some other treatments, so it continues to be of use for the management of ATTRv. The GI side effects may be mitigated with concurrent use of proton pump inhibitors and hence can be used reasonably well in patients.

Tafamidis, another TTR stabilizer, has been shown to slow disease progression in patients with TTR cardiomyopathy and improve survival [68–70]. Tafamidis binds to the thyroxine binding sites of the TTR tetramer and is able to prevent dissociation into the monomers thereby inhibiting the formation of amyloid fibrils. This promotes stability in Pro BNP and echocardiographic markers. Tafamidis is well tolerated and reduces cardiovascular hospitalizations. Tafamidis is now approved in the United States for ATTR cardiomyopathy [68–70].

TTR Suppressors: A second approach to treat ATTRv involves the suppression of TTR expression. Small interfering RNA (siRNA) agents bind to conserved sequences on TTR messenger RNA (mRNA), leading to degradation of the mRNA and reducing TTR gene expression [71] Since the particles are lipid based, the treatment requires intravenous infusion but results in a significant reduction of TTR by more than 50% by day 3 and nadir at day 10. There is continued suppression beyond the 10 days with recovery beyond day 70. Thus, the siRNA patisiran has been shown to significantly reduce serum TTR levels. In the phase 3 APOLLO study, patisiran met primary and all secondary endpoints, and demonstrated an encouraging safety profile [71]. The US Food and Drug Administration (FDA) has approved patisiran, which is the first siRNA to be approved for treating ATTRv amyloidosis. The cost remains prohibitive and limits the availability to those most in need of it.

Other strategies for TTR suppression are also currently being used such as anti-sense oligonucleotides (ASO) for reduction of TTR translation through suppression of gene expression [61]. These ASOs inhibit hepatic expression of misformed TTR but are currently aimed at targeting FAP. Continued research focuses on ATTR cardiac involvement.

Organ Transplantation: Given the advance of numerous effective therapies, organ transplantation is becoming obsolete. However, there are two types of organ transplantation that may be helpful for cardiac amyloidosis—orthotopic liver and heart transplantation. The majority of TTR is produced by the liver, and hence, orthotopic liver transplantation (OLT) has been used for halting production of TTR in patients with early stage ATTR amyloidosis [72, 73]. However, most benefit is derived in patients with Val130Met manifested mostly as familial amyloid polyneuropathy (FAP), and not in patients with cardiac involvement as seen in Val122Ile mutation which is seen more commonly in Black individuals. Furthermore, OLT does not eliminate progression of cardiac amyloid deposition, ATTRwt can form deposits on the preexisting template of mutant TTR deposits [72, 73]. Disease progression and acceleration of amyloid deposition have also been reported with OLT. Patients with significant cardiac involvement can be considered for heart transplantation (OHT), but without OLT, the liver will continue to produce mutant TTR that can deposit in the new graft. Many patients may not be candidates for heart transplantation due to advanced age and comorbidities especially in Black subjects. Other limitations of transplantation include organ availability, surgical morbidity and mortality, need for immunosuppression, as well as high cost [74, 75].

Many limitations could be surmised including the fact that the patients with ATTRv are at more advanced age as mentioned, but may do surprisingly well The ideal patient for OHT would be a younger patient with severe amyloid related cardiomyopathy and no other significant systemic manifestations, although there may still be a tendency for amyloid progression [66, 67].

Considerations

ATTRv cardiomyopathy results in a debilitating condition with a shortened lifespan but need no longer be a death sentence as treatments are available. Many healthcare providers consider this deadly condition to be rare and untreatable and so their patients may succumb to the disease due to lack of knowledge in the general group of healthcare providers. Does this condition contribute to the shortened life expectancy for Black men with heart failure compared with higher expectancies for White men, and women? Congestive heart failure is more devastating for Black individuals due to more frequent hospitalizations, comorbidities, and deaths. Are treatment centers adequately making the diagnosis of ATTRv? There is a disparity in that providers and healthcare centers in underserved communities may be ill equipped in providing the necessary testing for the diagnosis. Healthcare providers in the same communities may also not be aware of the disease and even thus less able to make accurate diagnosis, and may not know when to refer. The disease is frequently misunderstood and complicated, but it is certainly not rare, being more widely prevalent than recognized. In multiple studies and cohorts, the prevalence stands at about 4%, which accounts for over 1 million Black participants. Thus, education about ATTRv is crucial in these communities and more emphasis should be placed on providing education for healthcare providers in these communities as well as potential patients themselves. There are recognizable clinical clues in basic tools such as the ECG and a good history and physical are paramount. Genetic testing kits are now available to be used in offices. Early assessment will lead to appropriate referrals and the time to diagnosis could be shortened.

Treatment presents another potential disparity as the cost for the new and available therapies are prohibitive and may be unattainable for many of these patients. Concerted efforts by governmental agencies, payors, and pharmacies as well as organizations should be spent generating mechanisms to provide access to these treatments.

Finally, we know that ATTRv is autosomal dominant but has variable penetration so many cases will be missed [31]. The available data we have are mostly from studies of those with fully penetrant disease in the seventh and eighth decades. There is an opportunity to recognize early signs, perhaps forestalling deadly cardiac manifestations. Clearly more research and clinical studies should be conducted and on a larger scale. As such, efforts should be augmented such that there is enrollment of study participants in clinical trials for ATTRv. With such a high prevalence in Black populations is a condition that is inherently treatable, it is hoped that more engagement and education will result in mitigation and management of ATTRv cardiomyopathy.

References

1. Sipe JD, Benson MD, Buxbaum JN, et al. Amyloid fibril protein nomenclature: 2012 recommendations from the Nomenclature Committee of the International Society of Amyloidosis. Amyloid. 2012;19:167–70.
2. Siddiqi OK, Ruberg FL. Cardiac amyloidosis: an update on pathophysiology, diagnosis, and treatment. Trends Cardiovasc Med. 2018;28:10–21.
3. Muchtar E, Gertz MA, Kumar SK, Lacy MQ, Dingli D, Buadi FK, et al. Improved outcomes for newly diagnosed AL amyloidosis over the years 2000–2014: cracking the glass ceiling of early death. Blood. 2017;129:2111–9.
4. Dubrey SW, Cha K, Anderson J, et al. The clinical features of immunoglobulin light-chain (AL) amyloidosis with heart involvement. QJM. 1998;91:141–57.
5. Gertz MA. Hereditary ATTR amyloidosis: burden of illness and diagnostic challenges. Am J Manag Care. 2017;23(7 Suppl):S107–12.
6. Rapezzi C, Arbustini E, Caforio ALP, et al. Diagnostic work-up in cardiomyopathies: bridging the gap between clinical phenotypes and final diagnosis. A position statement from the ESC Working Group on Myocardial and Pericardial Diseases. Eur Heart J. 2013;34(19):1448–58.
7. Jiang X, Buxbaum JN, Kelly JW. The V122I cardiomyopathy variant of transthyretin increases the velocity of rate-limiting tetramer dissociation, resulting in accelerated amyloidosis. Proc Natl Acad Sci U S A. 2001;98:14943–8.
8. Quarta CC, Buxbaum JN, Shah AM, et al. The amyloidogenic V122I transthyretin variant in elderly black Americans. N Engl J Med. 2015;372(1):21–9.
9. Shah K, Mankad A, Castano A, Akinboboye O, Duncan P, Fergus I, Maurer M. Transthyretin cardiac amyloidosis in black Americans. Circ Heart Fail. 2016;9(6):e002558.
10. Blake CC, Geisow MJ, Oatley SJ, Rérat B, Rérat C. Structure of prealbumin: secondary, tertiary and quaternary interactions determined by Fourier refinement at 1.8 A. J Mol Biol. 1978;121:339–56.
11. Cornwell GG, Murdoch WL, Kyle RA, Westermark P, Pitkänen P. Frequency and distribution of senile cardiovascular amyloid. A clinicopathologic correlation. Am J Med. 1983;75:618–23.
12. Dungu JN, Papadopoulou SA, Wykes K, Mahmood I, Marshall J, Valencia O, et al. Afro-Caribbean heart failure in the United Kingdom: cause, outcomes, and ATTR V122I cardiac amyloidosis. Circ Heart Fail. 2016;9(9):e003352.
13. Ruberg FL, Maurer MS, Judge DP, Zeldenrust S, Skinner M, Kim AY, et al. Prospective evaluation of the morbidity and mortality of wild-type and V122I mutant transthyretin amyloid cardiomyopathy: the Transthyretin Amyloidosis Cardiac Study (TRACS). Am Heart J. 2012;164:e1.
14. Konstam MA, Rousseau MF, Kronenberg MW, et al. Effects of the angiotensin converting enzyme inhibitor enalapril on the long-term progression of left ventricular dysfunction in patients with heart failure. Circulation. 1992;86:431–8.
15. Buxbaum J, Alexander A, Koziol J, Tagoe C, Fox E, Kitzman D. Significance of the amyloidogenic transthyretin Val 122 Ile allele in African Americans in the Arteriosclerosis Risk in Communities (ARIC) and Cardiovascular Health (CHS) Studies. Am Heart J. 2010;159:864–70.
16. Yamashita T, Hamidi Asl K, Yazaki M, Benson MD. A prospective evaluation of the transthyretin Ile122 allele frequency in an African-American population. Amyloid. 2005;12:127–30.
17. Gonzalez-Lopez E, Gallego-Delgado M, Guzzo-Merello G, de Haro-Del Moral FJ, Cobo-Marcos M, Robles C, et al. Wild-type transthyretin amyloidosis as a cause of heart failure with preserved ejection fraction. Eur Heart J. 2015;36:2585–94.
18. Dorbala S, et al. Writing Group. ASNC/AHA/ASE/EANM/HFSA/ISA/SCMR/SNMMI expert consensus recommendations for multimodality imaging in car-

diac amyloidosis: Part 1 of 2—evidence base and standardized methods of imaging. J Nucl Cardiol. 2019;26(6):2065–123.

19. Falk RH, Quarta CC. Echocardiography in cardiac amyloidosis. Heart Fail Rev. 2015;20:125–31.

20. Dorbala S, Vangala D, Bruyere J, et al. Coronary microvascular dysfunction is related to abnormalities in myocardial structure and function in cardiac amyloidosis. JACC Heart Fail. 2014;2(4):358–67.

21. Said SM, Sethi S, Valeri AM, et al. Renal amyloidosis: origin and clinicopathologic correlations of 474 recent cases. Clin J Am Soc Nephrol. 2013;8(9):1515–23.

22. Plante-Bordeneuve V. Update in the diagnosis and management of transthyretin familial amyloid polyneuropathy. J Neurol. 2014;261(6):1227–33.

23. Maurer MS, Hanna M, Grogan M, et al. Genotype and phenotype of transthyretin cardiac amyloidosis: THAOS (transthyretin amyloid outcome survey). J Am Coll Cardiol. 2016;68(2):161–72.

24. Nagasaka T. Familial amyloidotic polyneuropathy and transthyretin. Subcell Biochem. 2012;65:565–607.

25. Connors LH, Lim A, Prokaeva T, Roskens VA, Costello CE. Tabulation of human transthyretin (TTR) variants, 2003. Amyloid. 2003;10(3):160–84.

26. Jacobson DR, Alexander AA, Tagoe C, Buxbaum JN. Prevalence of the amyloidogenic transthyretin (TTR) V122I allele in 14 333 African-Americans. Amyloid. 2015;22(3):171–4.

27. Arvanitis M, Chan GG, Jacobson DR, Berk JL, Connors LH, Ruberg FL. Prevalence of mutant ATTR cardiac amyloidosis in elderly African Americans with heart failure. Amyloid. 2017;24(4):253–5.

28. Buxbaum J, Jacobson DR, Tagoe C, et al. Transthyretin V122I in African Americans with congestive heart failure. J Am Coll Cardiol. 2006;47:1724–5.

29. Tendler A, Helmke S, Teruya S, Alvarez J, Maurer MS. The myocardial contraction fraction is superior to ejection fraction in predicting survival in patients with AL cardiac amyloidosis. Amyloid. 2015;22:61–6.

30. Dubrey SW, Cha K, Simms RW, Skinner M, Falk RH. Electrocardiography and Doppler echocardiography in secondary (AA) amyloidosis. Am J Cardiol. 1996;77:313–5.

31. Alexander KM, Orav J, Singh A, Jacob SA, Menon A, Padera RF, Kijewski MF, Liao R, Di Carli MF, Laubach JP, Falk RH, Dorbala S. Geographic disparities in reported US amyloidosis mortality from 1979 to 2015: potential underdetection of cardiac amyloidosis. JAMA Cardiol. 2018;3(9):865–70.

32. Cruz MW, Barroso F, González-Duarte A, Mundayat R, Ong ML, On behalf of the THAOS Investigators. The demographic, genetic, and clinical characteristics of Latin American subjects enrolled in the Transthyretin Amyloidosis Outcomes Survey. Amyloid. 2017;24(sup1):107–8.

33. Cruz MW, Pinto MV, Pinto LF, Gervais R, Dias M, Perez C, Mundayat R, Ong ML, Pedrosa RC, Foguel D. Baseline disease characteristics in Brazilian patients enrolled in Transthyretin Amyloidosis

Outcome Survey (THAOS). Arq Neuropsiquiatr. 2019;77(2):96–100.

34. González-Duarte A, Soto KC, Martínez-Baños D, Arteaga-Vazquez J, Barrera F, Berenguer-Sanchez M, Cantu-Brito C, García-Ramos G, Estañol Vidal B. Familial amyloidosis with polyneuropathy associated with TTR Ser50Arg mutation. Amyloid. 2012;19(4):171–6.

35. Pinto MV, Pinto LF, Dias M, Rosa RS, Mundayat R, Pedrosa RC, Waddington-Cruz M. Late-onset hereditary ATTR V30M amyloidosis with polyneuropathy: characterization of Brazilian subjects from the THAOS registry. J Neurol Sci. 2019;403:1–6.

36. González-Duarte A, Lem-Carrillo M, Cárdenas-Soto K. Description of transthyretin S50A, S52P and G47A mutations in familial amyloidosis polyneuropathy. Amyloid. 2013;20(4):221–5.

37. González-Duarte A, Cárdenas-Soto K, Bañuelos CE, Fueyo O, Dominguez C, Torres B, Cantú-Brito C. Amyloidosis due to TTR mutations in Mexico with 4 distincts genotypes in the index cases. Orphanet J Rare Dis. 2018;13(1):107.

38. Klaassen SHC, Tromp J, Nienhuis HLA, et al. Frequency of and prognostic significance of cardiac involvement at presentation in hereditary transthyretin-derived amyloidosis and the value of N-terminal pro-B-type natriuretic peptide. Am J Cardiol. 2018;121(1):107–12.

39. Grogan M, Scott CG, Kyle RA, Zeldenrust SR, Gertz MA, Lin G, Klarich KW, Miller WL, Maleszewski JJ, Dispenzieri A. Natural history of wild-type transthyretin cardiac amyloidosis and risk stratification using a novel staging system. J Am Coll Cardiol. 2016;68(10):1014–20.

40. Arvanitis M, Koch CM, Chan GG, Torres-Arancivia C, LaValley MP, Jacobson DR, Berk JL, Connors LH, Ruberg FL. Identification of transthyretin cardiac amyloidosis using serum retinol-binding protein 4 and a clinical prediction model. JAMA Cardiol. 2017;2(3):305–13.

41. Hanson JLS, Arvanitis M, Koch CM, Berk JL, Ruberg FL, Prokaeva T, Connors LH. Use of serum transthyretin as a prognostic indicator and predictor of outcome in cardiac amyloid disease associated with wild-type transthyretin. Circ Heart Fail. 2018;11(2):e004000.

42. Maurer MS, Hanna M, Grogan M, Dispenzieri A, Witteles R, Drachman B, Judge DP, Lenihan DJ, Gottlieb SS, Shah SJ, Steidley DE, Ventura H, Murali S, Silver MA, Jacoby D, Fedson S, Hummel SL, Kristen AV, Damy T, Planté-Bordeneuve V, Coelho T, Mundayat R, Suhr OB, Waddington Cruz M, Rapezzi C, THAOS Investigators. Genotype and phenotype of transthyretin cardiac amyloidosis: THAOS (transthyretin amyloid outcome survey). J Am Coll Cardiol. 2016;68(2):161–72.

43. Jacobson D, Tagoe C, Schwartzbard A, Shah A, Koziol J, Buxbaum J. Relation of clinical, echocardiographic and electrocardiographic features of cardiac amyloidosis to the presence of the transthyretin V122I

allele in older African-American men. Am J Cardiol. 2011;108:440–4.

44. Cueto-Garcia L, Reeder GS, Kyle RA, et al. Echocardiographic findings in systemic amyloidosis: spectrum of cardiac involvement and relation to survival. J Am Coll Cardiol. 1985;6:737–43.

45. Klein AL, Hatle LK, Burstow DJ, et al. Doppler characterization of left ventricular diastolic function in cardiac amyloidosis. J Am Coll Cardiol. 1989;13:1017–26.

46. Koyama J, Ray-Sequin PA, Falk RH. Prognostic significance of ultrasound myocardial tissue characterization in patients with cardiac amyloidosis. Circulation. 2002;106:556–61.

47. Koyama J, Falk RH. Prognostic significance of strain Doppler imaging in light-chain amyloidosis. JACC Cardiovasc Imaging. 2010;3:333–42.

48. Liu D, Hu K, Herrmann S, Cikes M, Ertl G, Weidemann F, et al. Value of tissue Doppler-derived Tei index and two-dimensional speckle tracking imaging derived longitudinal strain on predicting outcome of patients with light-chain cardiac amyloidosis. Int J Cardiovasc Imaging. 2017;33:837–45.

49. Liu D, Hu K, Stork S, Herrmann S, Kramer B, Cikes M, et al. Predictive value of assessing diastolic strain rate on survival in cardiac amyloidosis patients with preserved ejection fraction. PLoS One. 2014;9:e115910.

50. Arenja N, Fritz T, Andre F, Riffel JH, Aus dem Siepen F, Ochs M, et al. Myocardial contraction fraction derived from cardiovascular magnetic resonance cine images-reference values and performance in patients with heart failure and left ventricular hypertrophy. Eur Heart J Cardiovasc Imaging. 2017;18:1414–22.

51. Gillmore JD, Damy T, Fontana M, et al. A new staging system for cardiac transthyretin amyloidosis. Eur Heart J. 2018;39(30):2799–806.

52. Bokhari S, Castaño A, Pozniakoff T, Deslisle S, Latif F, Maurer MS. (99m)Tc-pyrophosphate scintigraphy for differentiating light-chain cardiac amyloidosis from the transthyretin-related familial and senile cardiac amyloidoses. Circ Cardiovasc Imaging. 2013;6:195–201.

53. Rapezzi C, Quarta CC, Guidalotti PL, et al. Usefulness and limitations of 99mTc-3,3-diphosphono-1,2-propanodicarboxylic acid scintigraphy in the aetiological diagnosis of amyloidotic cardiomyopathy. Eur J Nucl Med Mol Imaging. 2011;38:470–8.

54. Fontana M, Pica S, Reant P, Abdel-Gadir A, Treibel TA, Banypersad SM, et al. Prognostic value of late gadolinium enhancement cardiovascular magnetic resonance in cardiac amyloidosis. Circulation. 2015;132:1570–9.

55. Vogelsberg H, Mahrholdt H, Deluigi CC, Yilmaz A, Kispert EM, Greulich S, et al. Cardiovascular magnetic resonance in clinically suspected cardiac amyloidosis: noninvasive imaging compared to endomyocardial biopsy. J Am Coll Cardiol. 2008;51:1022–30.

56. Syed IS, Glockner JF, Feng D, Araoz PA, Martinez MW, Edwards WD, et al. Role of cardiac magnetic resonance imaging in the detection of cardiac amyloidosis. JACC Cardiovasc Imaging. 2010;3:155–64.

57. Zhao L, Tian Z, Fang Q. Diagnostic accuracy of cardiovascular magnetic resonance for patients with suspected cardiac amyloidosis: a systematic review and meta-analysis. BMC Cardiovasc Disord. 2016;16:129.

58. Kufova Z, Sevcikova T, Januska J, Vojta P, et al. Newly designed 11-gene panel reveals first case of hereditary amyloidosis captured by massive parallel sequencing. BMJ. 2018;71:687–94.

59. McKenna A, Hanna M, Banks E, et al. The genome analysis toolkit: a mapreduce framework for analyzing next-generation DNA sequencing data. Genome Res. 2010;20:1297–303.

60. Kontorovich A, McClellan A, Cullina S, Belbin G, Gorevic P. Genotype-first analysis of *TTR* variant carriers identifies novel traits associated with heritable amyloidosis. Circulation. 2019;140:A13496.

61. Benson MD, Waddington-Cruz M, Berk JL, et al. Inotersen treatment for patients with hereditary transthyretin amyloidosis. N Engl J Med. 2018;379(1):22–31.

62. Diflunisal Sekijima Y, Dendle MA, Kelly JW. Orally administered diflunisal stabilizes transthyretin against dissociation required for amyloidogenesis. Amyloid. 2006;13:236–49.

63. Castaño A, Helmke S, Alvarez J, Delisle S, Maurer MS. Diflunisal for ATTR cardiac amyloidosis. Congest Heart Fail. 2012;18:315–9.

64. Tojo K, Sekijima Y, Kelly JW, Ikeda S. Diflunisal stabilizes familial amyloid polyneuropathy-associated transthyretin variant tetramers in serum against dissociation required for amyloidogenesis. Neurosci Res. 2006;56:441–9.

65. Sultan MB, Gundapaneni B, Schumacher J, et al. Treatment with tafamidis slows disease progression in early-stage transthyretin cardiomyopathy. Clin Med Insights Cardiol. 2017;11:1179546817730322.

66. Davis MK, Lee PH, Witteles RM. Changing outcomes after heart transplantation in patients with amyloid cardiomyopathy. J Heart Lung Transplant. 2015;34(5):658–66.

67. Mehra MR, Canter CE, Hannan MM, Semigran MJ, Uber PA, Baran DA, Danziger-Isakov L, Kirklin JK, Kirk R, Kushwaha SS, Lund LH, Potena L, Ross HJ, Taylor DO, Verschuuren EA, Zuckermann A, International Society for Heart Lung Transplantation (ISHLT) Infectious Diseases Council; International Society for Heart Lung Transplantation (ISHLT) Pediatric Transplantation Council; International Society for Heart Lung Transplantation (ISHLT) Heart Failure and Transplantation Council. The 2016 International Society for Heart Lung Transplantation listing criteria for heart transplantation: a 10-year update. J Heart Lung Transplant. 2016;35(1):1–23.

68. Maurer MS, Elliott P, Merlini G, et al. Design and rationale of the phase 3 ATTR-ACT clinical trial (tafamidis in transthyretin cardiomyopathy clinical trial). Circ Heart Fail. 2017;10(6):e003815.

69. Rosenblum H, Castano A, Alvarez J, et al. Improved survival in patients with transthyretin cardiac amyloidosis treated with TTR stabilizers. J Card Fail. 2017;23(8):S20.

70. Rosenblum H, Castano A, Alvarez J, Goldsmith J, Helmke S, Maurer MS. TTR (transthyretin) stabilizers are associated with improved survival in patients with TTR cardiac amyloidosis. Circ Heart Fail. 2018;11(4):e004769.

71. Adams D, Gonzalez-Duarte A, O'Riordan WD, et al. Patisiran, an RNAi therapeutic, for hereditary transthyretin amyloidosis. N Engl J Med. 2018;379(1):11–21.

72. Suhr OB, Holmgren G, Steen L, et al. Liver transplantation in familial amyloidotic polyneuropathy. Follow-up of the first 20 Swedish patients. Transplantation. 1995;60(9):933–8.

73. Liepnieks JJ, Benson MD. Progression of cardiac amyloid deposition in hereditary transthyretin amyloidosis patients after liver transplantation. Amyloid. 2007;14:277–82.

74. Conner R, Hosenpud JD, Norman DJ, Pantely GA, Cobanoglu A, Starr A. Heart transplantation for cardiac amyloidosis: successful one-year outcome despite recurrence of the disease. J Heart Transplant. 1988;7:165–7.

75. Kpodonu J, Massad MG, Caines A, Geha AS. Outcome of heart transplantation in patients with amyloid cardiomyopathy. J Heart Lung Transplant. 2005;24:1763–5.

76. Ruberg FL, Grogan M, Hanna M, Kelly JW, Maurer MS. Transthyretin amyloid cardiomyopathy: JACC state-of-the-art review. J Am Coll Cardiol. 2019;73(22):2872–91. https://doi.org/10.1016/j.jacc.2019.04.003. PMID: 31171094; PMCID: PMC6724183.

77. Gillmore JD, Maurer MS, Falk RH, Merlini G, Damy T, Dispenzieri A, Wechalekar AD, Berk JL, Quarta CC, Grogan M, Lachmann HJ, Bokhari S, Castano A, Dorbala S, Johnson GB, Glaudemans AW, Rezk T, Fontana M, Palladini G, Milani P, Guidalotti PL, Flatman K, Lane T, Vonberg FW, Whelan CJ, Moon JC, Ruberg FL, Miller EJ, Hutt DF, Hazenberg BP, Rapezzi C, Hawkins PN. Nonbiopsy diagnosis of cardiac transthyretin amyloidosis. Circulation. 2016;133(24):2404–12.

Imaging for the Assessment and Management of Cardiovascular Disease in Women and Minority Populations

18

Carola Maraboto Gonzalez, Vanessa Blumer, and Robert C. Hendel

Introduction

Substantial ethnic and sex differences exist regarding risk, prevalence, clinical presentation, disease severity, response to treatment, and clinical outcomes of cardiovascular disease (CVD) in diverse populations in the United States. Therefore, it is not surprising that the diagnostic and prognostic value of various imaging techniques is often unique for each studied cohort, although there is often a limited amount of data available.

The field of cardiovascular imaging has undergone significant growth in recent years, with the emergence of new imaging modalities and improvement in technology that has allowed a more detailed and accurate evaluation of the cardiovascular system. In this chapter, we review the different available techniques of cardiovascular imaging in this multimodality era, and the implications of their use for diagnosis and risk stratification on patients in diverse populations based on currently available evidence in the literature.

Background

For the past few decades, dramatic declines in heart disease mortality have been observed; nonetheless, CVD still represents one of the leading causes of death for men and women in the United States [1]. Awareness about CVD on ethnic minorities has increased and, over the past years, multiple studies have been performed so as to identify and better define differences among patients from different racial/ethnic backgrounds and different sex in order to ensure appropriate and individualized use of our available resources to diagnose and manage these highly prevalent conditions.

Ethnic minorities are disproportionally affected by multiple cardiovascular risk factors, including but not limited to hypertension, diabetes, obesity, and chronic kidney disease. Furthermore, socioeconomic disparities and differences in access to healthcare also play a major role in the development on CVD in these populations.

A substantial number of large-scale population studies have examined the impact of cardiovascular disorders on minority populations in the United States. The Multi-Ethnic Study of

C. M. Gonzalez · R. C. Hendel (✉)
Tulane University School of Medicine, New Orleans, LA, USA
e-mail: cmarabotogonzalez@tulane.edu; rhendel@tulane.edu

V. Blumer
Division of Cardiology, Duke University Medical Center, Durham, NC, USA
e-mail: vanessa.blumer@duke.edu

© Springer Nature Switzerland AG 2021
K. C. Ferdinand et al. (eds.), *Cardiovascular Disease in Racial and Ethnic Minority Populations*,
Contemporary Cardiology, https://doi.org/10.1007/978-3-030-81034-4_18

Atherosclerosis (MESA) is a 10-year longitudinal study conducted with the aim to evaluate the characteristics of subclinical CVD and the risk factors that predict its progression among a multiethnic population [1]. Another large cohort looking at this was the Atherosclerosis Risk in Communities (ARIC) study, a prospective community-based project that included individuals from a racially diverse population in the United States [2]. Similarly, the Hispanic Communities Health Study—Study of Latinos (HCHS-SOL) study focused on the evaluation of prevalence, risk factors, and development of disease in the Hispanic community [3]. The Dallas Heart Study was a single-centered, population-based study that included 52% African Americans, aimed to improve prevention, diagnosis, and treatment of CVD [4]. Looking particularly at young adults, CARDIA (Coronary Artery Risk Development in Young Adults) included participants aged 18–30 years, with approximately equal proportions of Black and White individuals [5]. Finally, the Hypertension Genetic Epidemiology Network (HyperGEN) study included African American and White individuals with the main objective of characterizing hypertension-promoting genes, as well as elucidating the epidemiology and pathophysiology of hypertension and its complications [6]. These major cohort trials, among other studies, have provided the foundation of our current knowledge on ethnic differences related to CVD, helping elucidate variations in prevalence of risk factors (obesity, diabetes, hypertension), and phenotypic variation on development of left ventricular hypertrophy (LVH), as well as the impact of socioeconomic factors in healthcare access and its effect on long-term outcomes.

Focusing on women, a unique population with particular pathophysiology and clinical manifestations of heart disease, there have been some efforts to incorporate sex-specific evidence and adopt female-specific diagnostic guidelines [7, 8]. Heart disease is the leading cause of death for African American and White women in the United States. Among American Indian and Alaska Native women, heart disease and cancer cause roughly the same number of deaths each year, whereas for Hispanic and Asian or Pacific Islander women, heart disease is second only to cancer as a cause of death [9, 10]. As a matter of fact, it has been known for many years that women tend to present with atypical symptoms, making the diagnostic process challenging [2]. A large observational study found that, from patients with myocardial infarction, women were more likely than men to present without chest pain; additionally, women had higher mortality [11]. Despite the overall decline in CVD, recent data suggest stagnation in the improvements in incidence and mortality of heart disease, specifically among younger women (<55 years) [12]. Noninvasive testing carries inherent differences between women and men, with variation in sensitivity and specificity, which are included in Table 18.1. It is thus pivotal that we understand

Table 18.1 Differences in sensitivity and specificity of noninvasive cardiovascular testing among men and women

Test	Sensitivity (%)		Specificity (%)		Reference
	Men	Women	Men	Women	
Exercise ECG	61 (54, 68)	68 (23–100[a])	70 (64, 75)	77 (17–100[a])	[77, 78]
Stress echocardiography	79 (74, 83)	76 (71, 80)	83 (74, 89)	88 (81, 93)	[79]
SPECT MPI	84 (79, 89)	89 (84, 93)	79 (70, 85)	71 (61, 80)	[80]
PET MPI	81[b]	81[b]	86[b]	89[b]	[81]
Cardiac MRI	89 (75, 95)	86 (80, 90)	84 (77, 88)	83 (77, 87)	[82]
Coronary CT angiography	90 (56, 100)	96 (85, 100)	89 (74, 94)	78 (68, 86)	[62]

Loosely based on https://www.acc.org/latest-in-cardiology/articles/2018/09/14/09/54/imaging-of-heart-disease-in-women. Accessed 22 Dec 2020

Note: Data are presented as mean sensitivity and specificity; numbers in parentheses indicate reported 95% confidence intervals

[a]Indicates range (no confidence interval was reported in this source)

[b]Confidence interval or range was not reported in this source

the mechanisms that contribute to worsening risk factor profiles in young women to reduce cardiovascular-specific morbidity and mortality.

Cardiac Imaging Modalities and Applications in Diverse Populations

Echocardiography

Echocardiography remains one of the most valuable resources in cardiac evaluation, being widely available, easily performed, and allowing a comprehensive assessment of cardiac morphology, function, and hemodynamics. This technique employs the principles of ultrasound imaging, relying on the interaction between high-frequency sound waves emitted from a transducer and diverse body structures, which result in the generation of a digital image. Several modalities are currently available, including M-mode, two-dimensional (2D), three-dimensional (3D), color Doppler, pulsed-wave Doppler, and continuous-wave Doppler, all of them with their own advantages and limitations. Based on large cohorts, reference ranges of normal have been set for various morphologic and functional parameters; in addition, echocardiographic examination can provide substantial information on various pathologies including coronary artery disease, valvular heart disease, cardiomyopathies, pericardial disease, vascular disease, congenital heart disease, as well as systemic conditions such as infiltrative processes, among other entities.

Hypertension, the most prevalent and potent CVD risk factor, is disproportionately uncontrolled in US minorities. Although reasons for these disturbing disparities are unclear, it is probably a multifactorial problem, with genetic predisposition, co-morbidities, and unacceptable socioeconomic, and geographic disparities in CVD and risk factors having a major impact on this. In addition, LVH, an increase in left ventricular mass (LVM) that develops as an adaptive response, has been proven to be a strong marker of CVD morbidity and mortality [13]. In this regard, echocardiography has been widely used for evaluation of LVM, in the past based on M-mode and now with the use of 2D-echo, which has led to lower variability (Fig. 18.1).

A disparity in prevalence of LVH between African Americans and Caucasians has been previously described. A retrospective study analyzed electrocardiographic (ECG) and echocardiographic criteria for LVH among patients with

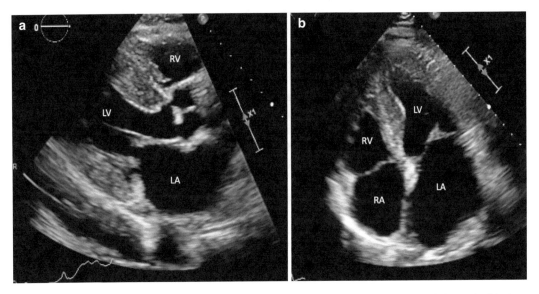

Fig. 18.1 2D-echocardiogram images obtained in the parasternal long axis (**a**) and parasternal short axis (**b**) views demonstrating severe concentric left ventricular hypertrophy (LA: left atrium, LV: left ventricle, RV: right ventricle)

hypertension and found that the prevalence of LVH by echocardiography was higher in African Americans than Whites, although the difference was even more apparent when analyzing ECG data. The reason for such differences was unclear, but the authors hypothesized that these could be due to anthropomorphic racial differences, such as greater LVM in the Black population [14]. Another analysis from the ARIC study aimed to increase our understanding of the observed racial disparities in predisposition to left ventricular remodeling by evaluating differences in arterial elastance as a measure of arterial afterload, and its association with cardiac structure and function. The authors found that Black individuals not only display a higher arterial afterload compared to White individuals, but they also develop more adverse changes in cardiac morphology and function, which suggest greater vulnerability to elevated afterload. This susceptibility may contribute to the higher risk of cardiovascular complications seen in the Black population and establishes a case for more aggressive blood pressure control in these patients [15]. Moreover, Gardin et al. analyzed data from the CARDIA study aiming to assess demographic differences in echocardiography measured LVM; after adjustment for blood pressure and anthropometric measures, LVM was again noted to be higher in Blacks, and in men when compared to women [16]. Similarly, examination of a population-based cohort among hypertensive adults found that both LVM and relative wall thickness were higher in Black adults, and these differences persisted after controlling for clinical and hemodynamic parameters (cardiac index, peripheral resistance index, and pulse pressure/stroke index). Therefore, Black adults had higher prevalence of LVH and concentric remodeling [17]; differences in left ventricular structure were thought to be possibly related to ethnicity-specific genetic predisposition, presence of increased vascular reactivity or maybe intermittent episodes of blood pressure elevation (stress-response, nocturnal hypertension) in the Black population. Furthermore, a study from the Northern Manhattan Study (NOMAS) examined the relationship of socioeconomic status and ethnicity with LVM measured by echocardiogram.

The authors found that socioeconomic status was a predictor of LVM among Black individuals, displaying an inverse and graded relationship, independent of hypertension. Of note, this relationship was not observed among Hispanics or Whites, even those with low socioeconomic status. The mechanism behind these findings remains obscure but the authors hypothesized that increased sympathetic stimulation due to chronic psychosocial stress could have a greater impact in Black patients leading to the structural changes observed [18].

Regarding the Hispanic community, prior studies have shown that Mexican Americans, constituting a substantial part of Hispanics in the United States, have lower coronary heart disease mortality compared with non-Hispanic US populations, despite having increased rates of cardiovascular risk factors [19–21]. This has been referred to as the "Hispanic paradox," which has been a matter of discussion and hypothesis generation, some theories suggesting that genetic [21] or phenotypical differences in subclinical cardiovascular disease could account for this phenomenon [19]. Additionally, socioeconomic and cultural factors have also been proposed as factors influencing this enigma [21, 22]. The Echocardiographic Study of Latinos (ECHO-SOL) intended to define the normal reference values of left ventricle and left atrium measurements in healthy individuals of Hispanic origin, since the current recommendations provided by the American Society of Echocardiography (ASE) are mainly based on studies including White patients with small numbers of ethnic minorities. The authors found gross differences between Hispanics and the established normal reference values for chamber quantification, suggesting that the ASE cutoffs underestimate the measures of left ventricular mass index (LVMI), interventricular septal diameter, and regional wall thickness. Furthermore, normal reference values for Hispanic patients overestimate the left ventricular end-diastolic volume (LVEDV), left ventricular internal diameter in diastole, and left ventricular posterior wall diameter, indicating that this population tends to have thicker and smaller hearts. These differences should be taken into consideration prior to making decisions on diagnosis or treatment of these patients [23].

In order to obtain ethnic-appropriate reference values for chamber quantification, the echoNoR-MAL study compiled data from population-based datasets including Africans, American Blacks, East Asians, Australian Aboriginals, Europeans, Middle Easterns, Pacifics, or South Asians. Noteworthy differences were found in this database, mainly when using nonindexed values. The upper reference values for LVEDV, left ventricular end-systolic volume (LVESV), and left ventricular stroke volume (LVSV) were highest in Europeans and lowest in South Asians; in addition, the upper reference values for left ventricular end-diastolic diameter and left ventricular end-systolic diameter were higher for Europeans than for East Asians, South Asians, and Africans; left atrial diameter and volume were also highest for Europeans (Table 18.2) [24]. Current guidelines present a statement regarding differences in 3D echocardiographic left ventricular volumes among different ethnic groups, reporting that volumes were smaller among Asian Indians than White Europeans. Despite these observations, at this time, specific normal reference ranges for left ventricle volume and size according to ethnic differences have not been delineated [25].

Racial/ethnic and sex differences in valvular heart disease have been well-described. For example, mitral annular calcification (MAC) was associated with CAD to a greater extent among non-Hispanic Whites compared with Hispanics [26]. In the same way, ethnic differences in aortic valve thickness were explored in a large multi-ethnic population-based cohort from the NOMAS study. Echocardiographic evaluation of the aortic valve thickness was performed and then classified according to severity. Hispanics were found to have significantly less moderate/severe aortic valve thickness (OR 0.43%, 95% CI 0.25–0.73) than non-Hispanic Whites. Notably, men had almost twofold increased risk of having moderate/severe aortic valve thickness compared to women (OR 1.96, 95% CI 1.24–3.10). In a multivariate analysis, only age, Hispanic ethnicity, sex, and hypertension were independently linked with severity of aortic valve thickness [27].

As previously pointed out, echocardiography also plays a notable role in the evaluation of infiltrative diseases, including amyloidosis, which is characterized by amyloid fibrils deposit in the extracellular space of various organs. It has been increasingly recognized as a cause of heart failure, primarily with transthyretin amyloid (ATTR), of which two main subtypes exist: wild and mutant. Remarkably, African Americans are more frequently affected by this condition since 3.5% of the Black population carry the most common amyloidogenic mutation [28]. Cardiac involvement in amyloidosis presents with numerous characteristic features on echocardiogram, including increased wall thickness, biatrial enlargement, advanced diastolic dysfunction, and a "sparkling" appearance of the myocardium, although this last finding is common with the use of harmonic imaging in patients without cardiac amyloidosis (Fig. 18.2). In addition, multivalvular regurgitation, pericardial effusion, and the classic "cherry-on-top" pattern on strain imaging can be visualized [29, 30] which is highly suggestive of cardiac amyloidosis.

The use of stress echocardiography for the evaluation of patients with known/suspected ischemic heart disease is a well-accepted approach but one where ethnic/racial and sex differences are of critical importance. Although only few studies have compared the performance of stress echocardiography to detect CAD between sexes, diagnostic accuracy is regarded as comparable in women and men [7]. Echocardiography also offers the advantage of using no ionizing radiation, conferring a potential preference in pregnant and young women. Evidence regarding its prognostic utility among diverse ethnic/racial groups is also limited. In a retrospective study, out of patients with a negative dobutamine stress echocardiogram (DSE), African American patients had higher incidence of nonfatal myocardial infarction and major adverse cardiovascular events (MACE) during 3-year follow-up, compared with Caucasians. The authors noted that, at baseline, African American patients had higher rates of diabetes and hypertension; furthermore, during the test, they were also more likely to have a hypertensive

Table 18.2 Reference values for left ventricular volume and ejection fraction for men and women according to ethnicity

Men	European			East Asian			South Asian	
Number subjects/studies	1107/10			523/6			329/5	
Age, years	30	50	70	30	50	70	50	70
LVEDV, mL	151 (3.8)	138 (1.9)	126 (3.3)	140 (3.0)	127 (1.9)	113 (3.4)	102 (3.1)	84 (4.5)
LVEDV/BSA, mL/m^2	72 (1.9)	66 (0.9)	61 (1.5)	72 (1.9)	71 (1.3)	69 (2.5)	52 (1.5)	46 (2.7)
LVEDV/height, mL/m	83 (2.0)	78 (1.1)	73 (2.0)	80 (2.2)	74 (1.5)	68 (2.8)	58 (2.0)	48 (2.5)
LVESV, cm	65 (2.0)	59 (1.0)	54 (1.7)	56 (1.3)	50 (1.1)	45 (2.2)	42 (1.6)	34 (4.0)
LVESV/BSA, mL/m^2	31 (0.8)	29 (0.4)	27 (0.8)	30 (0.6)	28 (0.7)	26 (1.3)	22 (0.5)	21 (1.6)
LVESV/height, mL/m	36 (0.8)	34 (0.5)	31 (1.0)	32 (0.8)	29 (0.6)	27 (1.1)	24 (0.7)	22 (1.8)
SV, mL	91 (2.8)	83 (1.3)	75 (1.7)	87 (0.9)	82 (1.8)	77 (3.4)	61 (2.1)	50 (1.3)
SV, mL (lower reference value)	39 (1.0)	37 (0.5)	35 (1.0)	43 (1.7)	39 (1.1)	36 (1.9)	26 (1.0)	24 (1.6)
SV/BSA, mL/m^2	44 (1.2)	41 (0.6)	37 (0.8)	46 (1.6)	46 (0.8)	47 (1.2)	32 (1.0)	28 (2.0)
SV/BSA, mL/m^2 (lower reference value)	20 (0.8)	19 (0.4)	18 (0.7)	24 (1.0)	22 (0.7)	20 (1.2)	14 (0.5)	14 (0.7)
SV/height, mL/m	50 (1.8)	46 (0.9)	43 (1.0)	50 (1.1)	48 (0.9)	47 (1.8)	35 (1.3)	30 (0.8)
SV/height, mL/m (lower reference value)	23 (0.8)	21 (0.4)	20 (0.6)	24 (1.0)	23 (0.6)	21 (1.1)	16 (0.5)	15 (0.8)
EF, % (lower reference value)	49 (0.9)	50 (0.6)	50 (1.3)	55 (0.7)	56 (0.5)	56 (0.9)	52 (0.6)	52 (0.9)

Women	European			East Asian			South Asian	
Number subjects/studies	1107/10			418/6			235/4	
Age, years	30	50	70	30	50	70	50	70
LVEDV, mL	116 (3.0)	106 (1.7)	95 (3.0)	109 (3.2)	103 (1.6)	96 (1.7)	80 (2.8)	73 (6.2)
LVEDV/BSA, mL/m^2	62 (0.9)	58 (0.6)	53 (1.3)	68 (1.5)	66 (1.2)	64 (2.3)	47 (1.2)	46 (2.4)
LVEDV/height, mL/m	68 (0.9)	63 (0.7)	59 (1.3)	67 (1.5)	65 (1.1)	62 (2.2)	50 (1.3)	46 (2.6)
LVESV, cm	48 (1.0)	44 (0.7)	41 (1.4)	40 (1.3)	38 (1.2)	36 (2.3)	35 (1.3)	27 (3.5)
LVESV/BSA, mL/m^2	26 (0.5)	24 (0.4)	23 (0.8)	25 (0.9)	24 (0.5)	23 (0.8)	20 (0.7)	17 (2.1)
LVESV/height, mL/m	28 (0.4)	27 (0.3)	25 (0.7)	24 (0.8)	24 (0.8)	23 (1.5)	22 (0.8)	17 (2.1)
SV, mL	72 (1.7)	66 (1.0)	60 (1.8)	72 (3.6)	67 (2.1)	63 (3.8)	48 (1.5)	46 (3.6)
SV, mL (lower reference value)	34 (0.7)	30 (0.5)	27 (1.0)	32 (1.7)	30 (1.2)	28 (2.3)	22 (1.3)	19 (0.9)
SV/BSA, mL/m^2	39 (0.9)	37 (0.5)	35 (0.9)	45 (1.6)	44 (0.9)	44 (1.4)	29 (0.6)	29 (1.3)
SV/BSA, mL/m^2 (lower reference value)	20 (0.4)	17 (0.4)	15 (0.8)	21 (1.2)	20 (0.7)	18 (1.1)	14 (0.6)	12 (0.6)
SV/height, mL/m	42 (1.0)	39 (0.5)	37 (0.9)	45 (2.2)	42 (1.2)	40 (2.0)	30 (1.0)	29 (2.5)
SV/height, mL/m (lower reference value)	21 (0.5)	19 (0.3)	16 (0.7)	20 (1.1)	19 (0.8)	19 (1.5)	15 (0.7)	12 (0.3)
EF, % (lower reference value)	51 (0.5)	51 (0.5)	51 (1.0)	57 (0.8)	57 (0.6)	57 (1.2)	53 (1.0)	53 (3.1)

From Ref. [24]

response and present LVH. Also, in a multivariate analysis, African Americans were two-times more likely to suffer from any cardiac event compared with Caucasians. The authors postulated that their findings could be related to more severe subclinical disease with active atherosclerosis and endothelial dysfunction that could be underappreciated with evaluation of solely wall motion abnormalities [31], since we know that these patients carry a significantly elevated risk of CVD. Moreover, Sutter et al. [32] conducted a study looking at several variables to identify predictors of major cardiac events in African American individuals with normal stress echocardiogram, finding that increased age, smoking history, CAD, LVH, and poor exercise capacity

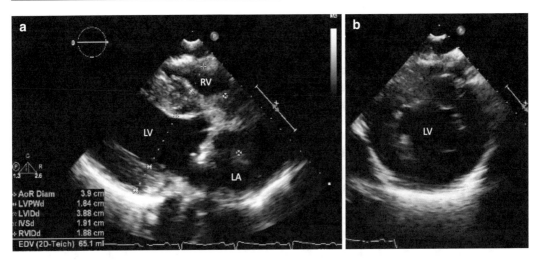

Fig. 18.2 2D-echocardiogram images obtained in the parasternal long axis (**a**) and apical four-chamber (**b**) views showing increased wall thickness seen in classic left ventricular hypertrophy, in this case, also associated with biatrial enlargement in the setting of cardiac amyloidosis (LA: left atrium, RA: right atrium, LV: left ventricle, RV: tight ventricle)

were independent risk factors for cardiovascular events. On the other hand, a British study evaluated the prognostic value of DSE among Indian Asian, European White, and Afro-Caribbean patients, concluding that no significant differences exist in the predictive utility of DSE between these populations [33].

Radionuclide Imaging

CAD represents a major cause of death in adult population in the United States; however, it carries inherent disparities among different ethnic groups and has substantial differences based on sex. Single Photon Emission Computed Tomography (SPECT) myocardial perfusion imaging (MPI) is the most widely used cardiac nuclear imaging technique, obtained by employing either exercise or pharmacologic stress followed by the injection of a pharmaceutical radiotracer and image acquisition with gamma cameras that capture the gamma ray photons and transform the information into a three-dimensional digital image. SPECT has been established as a powerful noninvasive tool for evaluation of patients with suspected CAD, demonstrating a high diagnostic accuracy and providing valuable prognostic and risk-stratifying information. Nevertheless, few studies have addressed its utility among various racial/ethnic populations.

In African Americans, the prognostic value of SPECT MPI was unknown given the lack of studies enrolling a significant sample of this particular population. A study by Alkeylani et al. [34] approached this specific question and compared the prediction of cardiac events of stress technetium-99m sestamibi SPECT in Caucasians and African Americans, finding that this imaging technique provides important prognostic information, with equally predictive value for cardiac outcomes in both racial groups. Interestingly, all-cause mortality for African Americans with normal SPECT MPI was significantly higher compared with Caucasians. Similarly, Akinboboye et al. [35] reported that African American patients with normal stress MPI had a slightly increased rate of major cardiovascular events per year (2%), higher than previously described; in addition, from individuals with normal MPI, those that underwent pharmacologic stress test or had history of myocardial infarction were at increased risk, which is likely due to the inability to exercise and the known CAD; therefore, these patients may require increased surveillance.

In order to provide further evidence regarding the use of MPI among ethnic minorities, Shaw et al. [36] analyzed data from a large registry that included a total of 1993 African American, 464 Hispanic, and 5258 Caucasian non-Hispanic patients undergoing exercise or pharmacologic stress technetium-99m tetrofosmin SPECT myocardial perfusion imaging. The authors found that risk stratification with SPECT was highly effective in predicting cardiac death and myocardial infarction for all ethnic cohorts, including African American and Hispanic patients. Moreover, cardiovascular events were noted to be higher than expected at all levels of scan severity for these ethnic minorities when compared with Caucasian non-Hispanics, suggesting that it would be reasonable to establish a more aggressive approach in these populations to effectively and timely manage their cardiovascular risk.

Some studies have found an increased rate of false positive SPECT results in patients with LVH, which we tend to encounter more frequently among African Americans compared to other racial/ethnic groups, as previously described in this chapter. A retrospective study suggested an overall reduction in the specificity of this test for detection of obstructive CAD during chest pain evaluation in those patients [37]. Potential explanations for the perfusion defects seen in patients with LVH are presence of microvascular disease or angiographically underestimated CAD [38]. Evidence for this is mixed though, since other studies have reported that LVH does not affect the sensitivity or specificity of the study [39, 40], and that the prognostic value of MPI SPECT remains in patients with LVH [41]. Despite this conflicting data, these studies provide useful information to consider in this discussion since, as mentioned before, several ethnic disparities exist in prevalence of LVH. Additionally, current evidence implies that the sensitivity, specificity, and normalcy rates of SPECT for detection of CAD are equivalent in diabetic and nondiabetic patients; nevertheless, the event-free survival is worse for diabetic patients with mildly to moderately abnormal MPI scans, compared to nondiabetic patients [42]. Likewise, one study showed that cardiac event

rate increased after 2 years of a normal MPI in diabetics, but not in nondiabetics [43]. Prevalence of diagnosed and undiagnosed diabetes mellitus is substantially variable among ethnic groups, being more prevalent among Asians, non-Hispanic Blacks, and Hispanics, compared to non-Hispanic Whites [44], which should be taken in consideration during study interpretation in these high-risk populations.

Stress imaging with echocardiography or radionuclide MPI, SPECT or positron emission tomography (PET), is recommended for the initial evaluation of symptomatic women at intermediate to high risk for CAD who have resting ECG ST-segment abnormalities, poor exercise capacity, or abnormal (intermediate to high risk) exercise ECG [7, 8, 45]. However, among women at low or low–intermediate risk for ischemic heart disease, an exercise ECG stress test appears to provide similar prognostic information [46].

In regard to SPECT MPI, this technique has shown to have sex-specific challenges in women, such as reduced LV size and breast attenuation, that may confer reduced accuracy to detect CAD [47]. However, with contemporary gating and attenuation-correction techniques, performance in women is comparable to stress echocardiography and is also comparable to that in men. When compared to SPECT MPI, PET MPI allows higher spatial resolution and reduced artifact. Although studies evaluating the diagnostic performance of PET MPI in women are not as numerous as for SPECT MPI, recent evidence suggests improved accuracy over SPECT MPI to detect CAD in women. Improved performance is partly due to decreased soft tissue attenuation experienced by high-energy PET. PET agents also have a shorter half-life, conferring lower radiation exposure [45].

A number of advances in radionuclide imaging have been developed in recent years, with new applications of these imaging modalities, in this case, for evaluation of infiltrative diseases. In this regard, ^{99m}Tc-Pyrophosphate scintigraphy (^{99m}Tc-PYP) has become an attractive tool for noninvasive identification of ATTR cardiac amyloidosis since it is widely available and it has proven to have high sensitivity and specificity, allowing to differentiate it from light chain (AL) amyloid [48, 49] (Fig. 18.3). Among other infiltrative processes, sarcoidosis is a multisystem granulomatous disease that affects the heart in 20–25% of the cases, conveying major prognostic implications [50]. Thus, noninvasive testing is generally considered in patients with biopsy-proven extracardiac sarcoidosis that presents with symptoms or ECG changes suggestive of cardiac involvement, as well as those with suspected relapse and those receiving chronic immunosuppressive treatment to monitor response to therapy. Fluorodeoxyglucose positron emission tomography (FDG-PET) provides excellent image quality with high temporal and special resolution, allowing detection of both active inflammation and scar. Nevertheless, adequate patient preparation is critical to obtain a reliable study, composed of high-fat and low-carbohydrate diet followed by fasting, with the purpose of suppressing physiologic myocardial glucose uptake [51, 52]. These specific modalities have major implications particularly in the Black population, which is disproportionally affected by these systemic conditions.

Cardiac Computed Tomography

Cardiac computed tomography is a rapidly growing imaging modality that has established itself as a valuable tool for examination of cardiac structure and function, allowing detailed anatomical delineation that makes it key for assessment of congenital heart and vascular disease, as well as evaluation of ischemic heart disease, pericardial disease, and cardiac masses, among other conditions (Fig. 18.4). The major limitations of this modality are the exposure to a small amount of ionizing radiation and the need for iodinated intravenous contrast, which restricts its use particularly in patients with renal dysfunction, iodine allergy, and pregnant women. In addition, in order to obtain adequate images, a slow heart rate is required, necessitating prior planning with oral beta-blocker administration. Nonetheless, with the advent of multi-detector spiral CT, dual-energy CT, and improved gating and decreased radiation dosing techniques, the use of coronary CT angiography (CCTA) scan has become more widely employed.

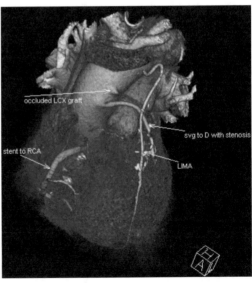

Fig. 18.4 CCTA provides detailed imaging of native coronary arteries and bypasses grafts anatomy. In this case, a reconstruction image was obtained revealing the presence of a stent in the right coronary artery, patent left internal mammary artery graft to the left anterior descending artery, stenosis of the saphenous vein graft to a diagonal branch, and occlusion of the saphenous vein graft to the left circumflex artery

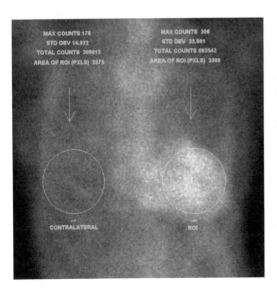

Fig. 18.3 ^{99m}Tc-PYP scan from a patient with a nonischemic cardiomyopathy. The study revealed myocardial uptake greater than rib uptake (semiquantitative grade 3), as well as an elevated heart-to-contralateral lung ratio to 1.7, strongly suggestive of ATTR amyloidosis

In the matter of anatomical parameters, CT has shown analogous findings to other imaging modalities, with outstanding spatial resolution. A retrospective analysis by Takx et al. [53] examined CT-derived cardiac measurements with the aim to compare these between Black patients with acute chest pain and age- and gender-matched White patients. The authors found that Black patients had larger myocardial mass compared with Whites, as noted echocardiography.

The Prospective Multicenter Imaging Study for Evaluation of Chest Pain (PROMISE) was a major community-based population trial looking at the diagnostic value of CCTA in the evaluation of patients with chest pain or dyspnea on exertion. They included 10,003 patients and randomized them to CCTA versus functional testing (exercise ECG, nuclear stress, or stress echocardiography). The strategy of anatomical testing with CCTA did not improve clinical outcomes over 2 years of follow-up [54]. A few years later, the Scottish Computed Tomography of the Heart (SCOT-HEART) investigators conducted a large landmark trial of patients with stable chest pain that were randomized to standard care plus CCTA versus standard care alone, resulting in a notable decline in rate of death from CAD or nonfatal myocardial infarction at 5 years in the CTA group, without a significant increase in coronary angiography or revascularization [55]. These studies suggest that cardiac CT angiography has at least clinical equipoise with functional testing, if not superior to other imaging modalities for diagnosis of ischemic heart disease.

Expanding on CAD evaluation, global plaque burden, a predictor of major cardiac adverse events, has been also successfully measured with CCTA. Naoum et al. analyzed data from patients from the CONFIRM registry (Coronary CT Angiography Evaluation for Clinical Outcomes) and developed age- and sex-specific nomograms of CAD extent with the use of CCTA, providing a comparison point for further patient evaluation [56]. In addition to global burden, plaque characteristics seem to differ between ethnic groups. This was seen in a study of patients from the Coronary CT Angiography Evaluation for

Clinical Outcomes: An International Multicenter (CONFIRM) study [57], which demonstrated that African Americans and East Asians were more likely to have ε1 calcified segments and less likely to have ε1 noncalcified segments compared to Caucasians [55].

Computed tomography-derived fractional flow reserve (CT-FFR), obtained based on computational fluid dynamics, has recently emerged and gained popularity as a noninvasive tool able to provide important information regarding hemodynamic significance of coronary artery lesions. The main trials studying this technique have included mainly Caucasians and Asians, with some including a small number of Hispanic and African American patients [58–60]. Notably, epidemiological data have suggested an increased prevalence of coronary artery disease and mortality in South Asians, and a lower prevalence in East Asians, when compared with Caucasians. A study including 300 patients was done with the aim of determining differences in CT coronary angiography to explain this finding, and showed that South Asians had the lowest coronary luminal volumes, left ventricular mass and LAD FFRct, compared with Caucasians and East Asians [61]. However, due to the lack of inclusion of a significant sample of patients from ethnic minorities in most trials, the diagnostic and prognostic value of this particular tool among ethnic minorities remains to be further explored before conclusions can be made across various ethnic groups. Regarding the impact of sex in diagnostic accuracy of this modality, no definite conclusions can be derived as this particular question has not been specifically addressed, with the majority of patients included in the main trials being men.

Per American Heart Association recommendations, coronary CT angiography "may be reasonable" in symptomatic women at intermediate risk for CAD, including those with equivocal stress test results [7]. While few studies have compared sex differences in the performance of coronary CT angiography, the available evidence suggests that sensitivity and specificity are overall comparable in men and women. In the recent ACCURACY trial, which prospectively enrolled

230 patients undergoing coronary CT angiography and invasive coronary angiography, reported sensitivity and specificity were similar between the sexes (sensitivity and specificity of 90% and 89% in women vs 96% and 78% in men, respectively) [62]. Another study aiming to compare use and prognostic value of anatomic (CT) versus stress testing (exercise ECG, stress echocardiography, or stress nuclear) in stable men and women revealed that women appear to derive more prognostic information from CT; men, on the other hand, seemed to obtain similar prognostic information from both tests [63]. As far as cardiac outcomes, one study showed that women and men had comparable rates of incident mortality and myocardial infarction after adjusting for age, risk factors, anginal symptoms, and nonobstructive CD extent [64].

Use of coronary calcium score and its implications among racial/ethnic minorities are outlined in Chap. 15.

Cardiac Magnetic Resonance

Cardiac magnetic resonance (CMR) stands out as an invaluable resource for cardiovascular evaluation, offering high-resolution images that provide accurate volumetric assessments independent of geometric assumptions, as well as measurements of diverse anatomic and physiology parameters, and quantification of myocardial blood flow without exposure to ionizing radiation [65]. Furthermore, CMR can assess valvular abnormalities and provide information about tissue characterization and metabolism. The contrast agent used in this modality is gadolinium and, while it is usually well tolerated, it has been associated with the development of nephrogenic systemic fibrosis in patients with renal dysfunction; additionally, its restricted availability and cost may limit its use (Fig. 18.5).

Given the advantages of CMR, it is now considered the criterion standard for LVM measurement, a marker of subclinical disease, providing excellent quality and quantification [66–68]. The use of CMR in the MESA study provided, for the first time, normal parameters for LVM and volumes for White Americans, African Americans, Hispanics, and Asian-Americans. The authors showed that African Americans have higher LVM, and Asian Americans have lower LVM and volumes compared with other ethnicities. Similarly, Asian American women had smaller left ventricular volumes and mass compared to other ethnic groups, even after adjusting for body

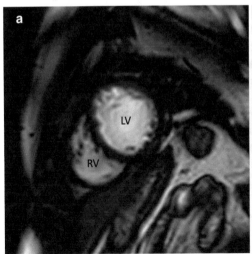
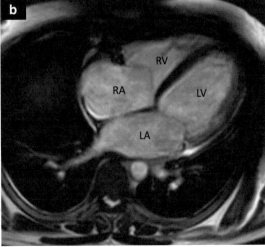

Fig. 18.5 CMR images from a patient with heart failure, consistent with dilated nonischemic cardiomyopathy. A short axis view (**a**) and four-chamber view by axial acquisition (**b**) are shown (LA: left atrium, RA: right atrium, LV: left ventricle, RV: right ventricle)

surface area [69]. Another study from the same cohort demonstrated that right ventricle structure and function differ among races and ethnic groups [70]. In their study, the authors found that Black individuals had lower right ventricular ejection fraction than White individuals. Interestingly, right ventricular mass was lower in Black adults compared with White adults, in contrast to LVM, which has been demonstrated to be greater in Black individuals compared with White individuals in prior studies, as mentioned before [71]. A study from the same database [72] compared the racial differences on LVMI obtained from CMR, as well as the impact of these differences on various cardiovascular outcomes. The authors found that African Americans and Hispanics had, overall, higher LVMI compared with non-Hispanic Whites and Chinese. There was a strong relationship between LVMI and incident CVD in Chinese and Hispanics, but less so for non-Hispanic Whites, and there was no significant racial/ethnic difference between LVMI and heart failure, atrial fibrillation, and all-cause mortality. Furthermore, another analysis from the same cohort looking at Hispanic subgroups found that both Caribbean-origin and Mexican-origin Hispanics had a twofold increased risk of LVH compared with non-Hispanic Whites; in the Caribbean-origin Hispanics this was thought to be explained by higher prevalence of hypertension; however, interestingly enough, the Mexican-origin Hispanics, contrary to Caribbean-origin Hispanics, had lower prevalence of hypertension, so LVH development could not be attributed to this [73]. Correspondingly, one analysis from the Dallas Heart Study revealed that Black, compared to White men and women, have increased LV mass and a two- to threefold higher prevalence of LVH measured by CMR, independent of systolic blood pressure, age, gender, socioeconomic status, and body composition (fat mass and fat-free mass) [71].

With regard to infiltrative diseases, CMR plays a major diagnostic and prognostic role. In cardiac amyloidosis, extracellular volume increases as amyloid is deposited in the tissue, which can be estimated with T1 mapping. Also,

valvular thickening and regurgitation are frequently seen, as well as a unique pattern of late gadolinium enhancement (LGE), which is usually global subendocardial, but can also present as patchy, diffuse or transmural [30]. In the case of sarcoidosis, LGE is often patchy and multifocal, usually with subepicardial involvement along the basal septum; however, it can also be intramural, with no pattern being specific for sarcoid [74]. In addition, detection of edema and inflammation has been achieved with the use of T2 mapping, adding valuable information. Once again, these applications take major relevance in that these conditions present in a disproportionate manner within our community, with higher prevalence among African Americans.

This imaging modality is also being increasingly used for evaluation of the vascular system and its properties. Aortic stiffness has been recognized as a potential risk factor but also a consequence of hypertension and, in a multiethnic study, African Americans and Hispanic Americans had higher proximal aortic stiffness compared to White Americans, independent of traditional cardiovascular risk factors [75].

Evidence regarding the diagnostic accuracy of CMR imaging in women is less extensive than for stress echocardiography and radionuclide MPI. However, recent studies suggest superior performance compared with SPECT MPI [7, 65]. The sensitivity and specificity of CMR imaging for the detection of CAD were found to be comparable between the sexes (89% and 84% for women, 86% and 83% for men, respectively), with CMR imaging having higher sensitivity than SPECT MPI in both women and men. Also notable from this study was the lower sensitivity of SPECT MPI in women compared with men [65, 76]. Although the American Heart Association provides a class I recommendation for stress echocardiography and radionuclide MPI in the workup of symptomatic women at intermediate to high risk for CAD, these guidelines indicate that stress MPI with MR imaging may also be reasonable in this same group (class IIb recommendation) [7]. MR imaging may also be well suited for women who are poor candidates for echocardiography or in young or pregnant women, in whom radiation is of greater concern [76].

Clinical Implications

A comprehensive medical assessment should allow a proper identification of patient's sex, ethnic and cultural background with consideration of the clinical implications regarding risk factors, clinical manifestations and prognosis. At this time, it is unclear whether early and targeted interventions in the most susceptible minority groups would have an impact on long term outcomes; nevertheless, it would be reasonable to pursue a more intense treatment approach and tailor therapy for patients from sex/ethnic/racial minorities known to have increased risk of CVD based on available data to address every patient's individual risk. In addition, current evidence underlines the importance of developing sex/racial/ethnic-specific guidelines that consider the increased cardiovascular risk seen in these minority groups to establish suitable screening measures and management recommendations in these populations to improve their outcomes.

Although differences in diagnostic and prognostic value may exist, most of these imaging modalities serve underrepresented populations. Moreover, as previously indicated, certain imaging techniques are of increased utility in specific communities due to inherent differences among them in prevalence and presentation of cardiovascular disease.

Conclusion

In order to provide patients with valuable medical care, it is crucial for healthcare providers to be aware of the differences in risk factors and clinical presentation of heart disease among individuals from different racial/ethnic groups, as well as the variations appreciated between men and women (Table 18.3). Furthermore, it is important to underscore that the diagnostic accuracy of each cardiovascular imaging modality depends largely on disease prevalence, which

Table 18.3 Key points in use of different modalities of cardiovascular imaging in woman and minority populations

Several variations exist in prevalence of heart disease among different racial/ethnic groups, and between men and women, which dictate the disparities observed in diagnostic accuracy of various imaging modalities

Differences in risk factors and disease presentation between minority groups should be contemplated to select the appropriate diagnostic test

Each patient should be approached in an individualized manner, and clinical practice guidelines should be reviewed to ensure proper patient care

Racial/ethnic minorities and women continue to be substantially underrepresented in major clinical trials

Future research is needed to focus on further delineating these disparities to obtain accurate reference values for these groups and be able to properly evaluate our patients

dictates the disparities noted in these assessments. Understanding these differences will ensure the appropriate use of these techniques and allow more accurate conclusions leading to the establishment of a proper and individualized treatment strategy for patients of diverse populations. Clinical practice guidelines, including those addressing appropriate use criteria for each and every cardiovascular imaging modality, should be reviewed to ensure proper resource utilization and patient care.

References

1. Menet A, et al. Prognostic importance of postoperative QRS widening in patients with heart failure receiving cardiac resynchronization therapy. Heart Rhythm. 2016;13(8):1636–43.
2. Pilote L, et al. A comprehensive view of sex-specific issues related to cardiovascular disease. CMAJ. 2007;176(6):S1–44.
3. Warriner DR, Lawford P, Sheridan PJ. Cardiac resynchronization therapy leads to improvements in handgrip strength. Cardiol Res. 2016;7(3):95–103.
4. Iyengar A, et al. The in-hospital cost of ventricular assist device therapy: implications for patient selection. ASAIO J. 2017;63(6):725–30.
5. Cutter GR, et al. Cardiovascular risk factors in young adults. The CARDIA baseline monograph. Control Clin Trials. 1991;12(1 Suppl):1s–77s.
6. Williams RR, et al. NHLBI family blood pressure program: methodology and recruitment in the

HyperGEN network. Hypertension genetic epidemiology network. Ann Epidemiol. 2000;10(6):389–400.

7. Mieres JH, et al. Role of noninvasive testing in the clinical evaluation of women with suspected ischemic heart disease: a consensus statement from the American Heart Association. Circulation. 2014;130(4):350–79.

8. Shaw LJ. Sex differences in cardiovascular imaging. JACC Cardiovasc Imaging. 2016;9(4):494–7.

9. Bairey Merz CN, et al. Insights from the NHLBI-sponsored Women's Ischemia Syndrome Evaluation (WISE) study: Part II: gender differences in presentation, diagnosis, and outcome with regard to gender-based pathophysiology of atherosclerosis and macrovascular and microvascular coronary disease. J Am Coll Cardiol. 2006;47(3 Suppl):S21–9.

10. Centers for Disease Control and Prevention. Women and heart disease fact sheet. May 14, 2019 [June 6, 2019]. Available from: https://www.cdc.gov/heartdisease/women.htm?CDC_AA_refVal=https%3A%2F%2Fwww.cdc.gov%2Fdhdsp%2Fdata_statistics%2Ffact_sheets%2Ffs_women_heart.htm.

11. Canto JG, et al. Association of age and sex with myocardial infarction symptom presentation and in-hospital mortality. JAMA. 2012;307(8):813–22.

12. Wilmot KA, et al. Coronary heart disease mortality declines in the United States from 1979 through 2011: evidence for stagnation in young adults, especially women. Circulation. 2015;132(11):997–1002.

13. Whelton PK, et al. 2017 ACC/AHA/AAPA/ABC/ACPM/AGS/APhA/ASH/ASPC/NMA/PCNA guideline for the prevention, detection, evaluation, and management of high blood pressure in adults: a report of the American College of Cardiology/American Heart Association Task Force on Clinical Practice Guidelines. Hypertension. 2018;71(6):e13–e115.

14. Chapman JN, et al. Ethnic differences in the identification of left ventricular hypertrophy in the hypertensive patient. Am J Hypertens. 1999;12(5):437–42.

15. Fernandes-Silva MM, et al. Race-related differences in left ventricular structural and functional remodeling in response to increased afterload: the ARIC study. JACC Heart Fail. 2017;5(3):157–65.

16. Gardin JM, et al. Relationship of cardiovascular risk factors to echocardiographic left ventricular mass in healthy young black and white adult men and women. The CARDIA study. Coronary Artery Risk Development in Young Adults. Circulation. 1995;92(3):380–7.

17. Kizer JR, et al. Differences in left ventricular structure between black and white hypertensive adults: the Hypertension Genetic Epidemiology Network study. Hypertension. 2004;43(6):1182–8.

18. Rodriguez CJ, et al. Relation between socioeconomic status, race-ethnicity, and left ventricular mass: the Northern Manhattan study. Hypertension. 2004;43(4):775–9.

19. Gardin JM, et al. Do differences in subclinical cardiovascular disease in mexican americans versus European americans help explain the Hispanic paradox? Am J Cardiol. 2010;105(2):205–9.

20. Friis R, et al. Coronary heart disease mortality and risk among Hispanics and non-Hispanics in Orange County, California. Public Health Rep. 1981;96(5):418–22.

21. Mitchell BD, et al. Myocardial infarction in Mexican-Americans and non-Hispanic whites. The San Antonio Heart Study. Circulation. 1991;83(1):45–51.

22. Supariwala A, et al. Impact of ethnic variation and residential segregation on long-term survival following myocardial perfusion SPECT. J Nucl Cardiol. 2012;19(5):987–96.

23. Qureshi WT, et al. Comparison of echocardiographic measures in a Hispanic/Latino population with the 2005 and 2015 American Society of Echocardiography reference limits (the echocardiographic study of Latinos). Circ Cardiovasc Imaging. 2016;9(1):e003597.

24. Poppe KK, et al. Ethnic-specific normative reference values for echocardiographic LA and LV size, LV mass, and systolic function: the EchoNoRMAL study. JACC Cardiovasc Imaging. 2015;8(6):656–65.

25. Lang RM, et al. Recommendations for cardiac chamber quantification by echocardiography in adults: an update from the American Society of Echocardiography and the European Association of Cardiovascular Imaging. J Am Soc Echocardiogr. 2015;28(1):1–39.e14.

26. Willens HJ, Chirinos JA, Hennekens CH. Prevalence and clinical correlates of mitral annulus calcification in Hispanics and non-Hispanic whites. J Am Soc Echocardiogr. 2007;20(2):191–6.

27. Sashida Y, et al. Ethnic differences in aortic valve thickness and related clinical factors. Am Heart J. 2010;159(4):698–704.

28. Buxbaum JN, Ruberg FL. Transthyretin V122I (pV142I)* cardiac amyloidosis: an age-dependent autosomal dominant cardiomyopathy too common to be overlooked as a cause of significant heart disease in elderly African Americans. Genet Med. 2017;19(7):733–42.

29. Ruberg FL, et al. Transthyretin amyloid cardiomyopathy: JACC state-of-the-art review. J Am Coll Cardiol. 2019;73(22):2872–91.

30. Agha AM, et al. Role of cardiovascular imaging for the diagnosis and prognosis of cardiac amyloidosis. Open Heart. 2018;5(2):e000881.

31. Srivastava AV, et al. Prognostic implications of negative dobutamine stress echocardiography in African Americans compared to Caucasians. Cardiovasc Ultrasound. 2008;6:20.

32. Sutter DA, et al. Improving prediction of outcomes in African Americans with normal stress echocardiograms using a risk scoring system. Am J Cardiol. 2013;111(11):1593–7.

33. O'Driscoll JM, et al. The prognostic value of dobutamine stress echocardiography amongst British Indian Asian and Afro-Caribbean patients: a comparison with European white patients. Cardiovasc Ultrasound. 2015;13:36.

34. Alkeylani A, et al. Influence of race on the prediction of cardiac events with stress technetium-99m sesta-

mibi tomographic imaging in patients with stable angina pectoris. Am J Cardiol. 1998;81(3):293–7.

35. Akinboboye OO, et al. Incidence of major cardiovascular events in black patients with normal myocardial stress perfusion study results. J Nucl Cardiol. 2001;8(5):541–7.

36. Shaw LJ, et al. Ethnic differences in the prognostic value of stress technetium-99m tetrofosmin gated single-photon emission computed tomography myocardial perfusion imaging. J Am Coll Cardiol. 2005;45(9):1494–504.

37. Bartram P, et al. False-positive defects in technetium-99m sestamibi myocardial single-photon emission tomography in healthy athletes with left ventricular hypertrophy. Eur J Nucl Med. 1998;25(9):1308–12.

38. Ammann P, et al. Characteristics of patients with abnormal stress technetium Tc 99m sestamibi SPECT studies without significant coronary artery diameter stenoses. Clin Cardiol. 2003;26(11):521–4.

39. Elhendy A, et al. Impact of hypertension on the accuracy of exercise stress myocardial perfusion imaging for the diagnosis of coronary artery disease. Heart. 2001;85(6):655–61.

40. Vaduganathan P, et al. Diagnostic accuracy of stress thallium-201 tomography in patients with left ventricular hypertrophy. Am J Cardiol. 1998;81(10):1205–7.

41. Amanullah AM, et al. Enhanced prognostic stratification of patients with left ventricular hypertrophy with the use of single-photon emission computed tomography. Am Heart J. 2000;140(3):456–62.

42. Kang X, et al. Incremental prognostic value of myocardial perfusion single photon emission computed tomography in patients with diabetes mellitus. Am Heart J. 1999;138(6 Pt 1):1025–32.

43. Giri S, et al. Impact of diabetes on the risk stratification using stress single-photon emission computed tomography myocardial perfusion imaging in patients with symptoms suggestive of coronary artery disease. Circulation. 2002;105(1):32–40.

44. Centers for Disease Control and Prevention. National diabetes statistics report, 2017. Atlanta: Centers for Disease Control and Prevention, US Department of Health and Human Services; 2017.

45. American College of Cardiology. Imaging of heart disease in women: an updated review. 2018 [June 23, 2019]. Available from: https://www.acc.org/latest-in-cardiology/articles/2018/09/14/09/54/imaging-of-heart-disease-in-women.

46. Shaw LJ, et al. Comparative effectiveness of exercise electrocardiography with or without myocardial perfusion single photon emission computed tomography in women with suspected coronary artery disease: results from the What Is the Optimal Method for Ischemia Evaluation in Women (WOMEN) trial. Circulation. 2011;124(11):1239–49.

47. Nevsky G, et al. Sex-specific normalized reference values of heart and great vessel dimensions in cardiac CT angiography. AJR Am J Roentgenol. 2011;196(4):788–94.

48. Bokhari S, et al. (99m)Tc-pyrophosphate scintigraphy for differentiating light-chain cardiac amyloidosis from the transthyretin-related familial and senile cardiac amyloidoses. Circ Cardiovasc Imaging. 2013;6(2):195–201.

49. Castano A, et al. Multicenter study of planar technetium 99m pyrophosphate cardiac imaging: predicting survival for patients with ATTR cardiac amyloidosis. JAMA Cardiol. 2016;1(8):880–9.

50. Sharma OP, Maheshwari A, Thaker K. Myocardial sarcoidosis. Chest. 1993;103(1):253–8.

51. Piekarski E, Benali K, Rouzet F. Nuclear imaging in sarcoidosis. Semin Nucl Med. 2018;48(3):246–60.

52. Bois JP, Muser D, Chareonthaitawee P. PET/CT evaluation of cardiac sarcoidosis. PET Clin. 2019;14(2):223–32.

53. Takx RA, et al. Computed tomography-derived parameters of myocardial morphology and function in black and white patients with acute chest pain. Am J Cardiol. 2016;117(3):333–9.

54. Douglas PS, et al. Outcomes of anatomical versus functional testing for coronary artery disease. N Engl J Med. 2015;372:1291–300.

55. Newby DE, et al. Coronary CT angiography and 5-year risk of myocardial infarction. N Engl J Med. 2018;379(10):924–33.

56. Naoum C, et al. Predictive value of age- and sex-specific nomograms of global plaque burden on coronary computed tomography angiography for major cardiac events. Circ Cardiovasc Imaging. 2017;10(3):e004896.

57. Sanders D. Ethnic differences of coronary atherosclerosis in computed tomography angiography and subsequent risk of major adverse cardiovascular events: The CONFIRM registry. J Am Coll Cardiol. 2017;69(11):1596.

58. Min JK, et al. Diagnostic accuracy of fractional flow reserve from anatomic CT angiography. JAMA. 2012;308(12):1237–45.

59. Norgaard BL, et al. Diagnostic performance of noninvasive fractional flow reserve derived from coronary computed tomography angiography in suspected coronary artery disease: the NXT trial (Analysis of Coronary Blood Flow Using CT Angiography: Next Steps). J Am Coll Cardiol. 2014;63(12):1145–55.

60. Thompson AG, et al. Diagnostic accuracy and discrimination of ischemia by fractional flow reserve CT using a clinical use rule: results from the Determination of Fractional Flow Reserve by Anatomic Computed Tomographic Angiography study. J Cardiovasc Comput Tomogr. 2015;9(2):120–8.

61. Ihdayhid A. Ethnic differences in coronary luminal volume, left ventricular mass and CT-derived fractional flow reserve. J Am Coll Cardiol. 2018;72:B156.

62. Tsang JC, et al. Sex comparison of diagnostic accuracy of 64-multidetector row coronary computed tomographic angiography: results from the multicenter ACCURACY trial. J Cardiovasc Comput Tomogr. 2012;6(4):246–51.

63. Pagidipati NJ, et al. Sex differences in functional and CT angiography testing in patients with suspected coronary artery disease. J Am Coll Cardiol. 2016;67(22):2607–16.

64. Leipsic J, et al. Sex-based prognostic implications of nonobstructive coronary artery disease: results from the international multicenter CONFIRM study. Radiology. 2014;273(2):393–400.

65. Greenwood JP, et al. Comparison of cardiovascular magnetic resonance and single-photon emission computed tomography in women with suspected coronary artery disease from the Clinical Evaluation of Magnetic Resonance Imaging in Coronary Heart Disease (CE-MARC) trial. Circulation. 2014;129(10):1129–38.

66. Jain A, et al. Cardiovascular imaging for assessing cardiovascular risk in asymptomatic men versus women: the multi-ethnic study of atherosclerosis (MESA). Circ Cardiovasc Imaging. 2011;4(1):8–15.

67. de Simone G, et al. Left ventricular mass predicts heart failure not related to previous myocardial infarction: the Cardiovascular Health Study. Eur Heart J. 2008;29(6):741–7.

68. Bluemke DA, et al. The relationship of left ventricular mass and geometry to incident cardiovascular events: the MESA (multi-ethnic study of atherosclerosis) study. J Am Coll Cardiol. 2008;52(25):2148–55.

69. Natori S, et al. Cardiovascular function in multi-ethnic study of atherosclerosis: normal values by age, sex, and ethnicity. AJR Am J Roentgenol. 2006;186(6 Suppl 2):S357–65.

70. Kawut SM, et al. Sex and race differences in right ventricular structure and function: the multi-ethnic study of atherosclerosis-right ventricle study. Circulation. 2011;123(22):2542–51.

71. Drazner MH, et al. Left ventricular hypertrophy is more prevalent in blacks than whites in the general population: the Dallas Heart Study. Hypertension. 2005;46(1):124–9.

72. Akintoye E, et al. Racial/ethnic differences in the prognostic utility of left ventricular mass index for incident cardiovascular disease. Clin Cardiol. 2018;41(4):502–9.

73. Rodriguez CJ, et al. Left ventricular mass and ventricular remodeling among Hispanic subgroups compared with non-Hispanic blacks and whites: MESA (multi-ethnic study of atherosclerosis). J Am Coll Cardiol. 2010;55(3):234–42.

74. Komada T, Suzuki K, Ishiguchi H, Kawai H, Okumura T, Hirashiki A, Naganawa S. Magnetic resonance imaging of cardiac sarcoidosis: an evaluation of the cardiac segments and layers that exhibit late gadolinium enhancement. Nagoya J Med Sci. 2016;78:437–46.

75. Goel A, et al. Ethnic difference in proximal aortic stiffness: an observation from the Dallas Heart Study. JACC Cardiovasc Imaging. 2017;10(1):54–61.

76. Tailor TD, et al. Imaging of heart disease in women. Radiology. 2017;282(1):34–53.

77. Kwok Y, et al. Meta-analysis of exercise testing to detect coronary artery disease in women. Am J Cardiol. 1999;83(5):660–6.

78. Gianrossi R, et al. Exercise-induced ST depression in the diagnosis of coronary artery disease. A meta-analysis. Circulation. 1989;80(1):87–98.

79. Kim C, et al. Pharmacologic stress testing for coronary disease diagnosis: a meta-analysis. Am Heart J. 2001;142(6):934–44.

80. Iskandar A, et al. Gender differences in the diagnostic accuracy of SPECT myocardial perfusion imaging: a bivariate meta-analysis. J Nucl Cardiol. 2013;20(1):53–63.

81. Bateman TM, et al. Diagnostic accuracy of rest/stress ECG-gated Rb-82 myocardial perfusion PET: comparison with ECG-gated Tc-99m sestamibi SPECT. J Nucl Cardiol. 2006;13(1):24–33.

82. Greenwood John P, et al. Comparison of cardiovascular magnetic resonance and single-photon emission computed tomography in women with suspected coronary artery disease from the Clinical Evaluation of Magnetic Resonance Imaging in Coronary Heart Disease (CE-MARC) trial. Circulation. 2014;129(10):1129–38.

Index